Peripheral Nerve Injuries in the Athlete

Peripheral Nerve Injuries in the Athlete

Joseph H. Feinberg, MD, MS
Hospital for Special Surgery
New York City

Neil I. Spielholz, PT, PhD
Professor Emeritus
University of Miami, Florida

Editors

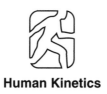

Human Kinetics

BS

Library of Congress Cataloging-in-Publication Data

Peripheral nerve injuries in the athlete / Joseph H. Feinberg, Neil I.
Spielholz, editors.
    p. ; cm.
  Includes bibliographical references and index.
  ISBN 0-7360-4490-6 (hard cover)
  1. Nerves, Peripheral--Wounds and injuries. 2. Sports injuries.
  [DNLM: 1. Peripheral Nerves--injuries. 2. Athletic
Injuries--diagnosis. 3. Athletic Injuries--rehabilitation. 4. Athletic
Injuries--therapy. WL 500 P44456 2003] I. Feinberg, Joseph H., 1955-
II. Speilholz, Neil Irwin.
  RD595 .P465 2003
  617 .4'83044-dc21   2002007975

ISBN: 0-7360-4490-6

Acquisitions Editor: Loarn D. Robertson, PhD; **Developmental Editor:** Elaine H. Mustain;
Assistant Editor: Maggie Schwarzentraub; **Copyeditor:** Brian C. Mustain; **Proofreader:**
Julie A. Marx; **Indexer:** Nancy Ball; **Permission Manager:** Dalene Reeder; **Graphic
Designer:** Fred Starbird; **Graphic Artist:** Yvonne Griffith; **Photo Manager:** Leslie A.
Woodrum; **Cover Designer:** Keith Blomberg; **Photographer (interior):** Photographs
provided by lead authors of their respective chapters unless otherwise noted; **Art Manager:**
Kelly Hendren; **Medical Illustrator:** Jason McAlexander of Interactive Composition
Corporation; **Mac Artist:** Brian McElwain; **Printer:** Sheridan

Printed in the United States of America   10 9 8 7 6 5 4 3 2 1

Human Kinetics
Web site: www.HumanKinetics.com

United States: Human Kinetics, P.O. Box 5076, Champaign, IL 61825-5076
800-747-4457
e-mail: humank@hkusa.com

Canada: Human Kinetics, 475 Devonshire Road Unit 100, Windsor, ON N8Y 2L5
800-465-7301 (in Canada only)
e-mail: orders@hkcanada.com

Europe: Human Kinetics, 107 Bradford Road, Stanningley
Leeds LS28 6AT, United Kingdom
+44 (0) 113 255 5665
e-mail: hk@hkeurope.com

Australia: Human Kinetics, 57A Price Avenue, Lower Mitcham, South Australia 5062
08 8277 1555
e-mail: liahka@senet.com.au

New Zealand: Human Kinetics, P.O. Box 105-231, Auckland Central
09-523-3462
e-mail: hkp@ihug.co.nz

4/14/03

This book is dedicated to my parents, Len and Rozanne; my brother, Matt; my sisters, Melanie and Dawne; and to those teachers and mentors of mine—Dr. Helen Birecka, Dr. Werner Straus, Dr. Neil Spielholz, Dr. Peter Bullough, Dr. Adele Boskey, Dr. Oheneba Boachie-Adjei, and Dr. Richard Brand—who guided and inspired me.

Joseph H. Feinberg

To my mentor, Dr. Joseph Goodgold, and to my wife, Harriet.

Nerve injuries have been of interest to me ever since I first encountered them as a student physical therapist in 1955. I was on a clinical affiliation at the Brooklyn VA Hospital, and many of the patients were veterans of the Korean War with various service-connected peripheral nerve problems. The identification and treatment of these injuries fascinated me. Later, as a staff therapist at the Manhattan VA Hospital, I had the good fortune to meet Dr. Joseph Goodgold, who was the electrodiagnostic consultant. He saw something in me and took me under his wing. A few years later, Dr. Goodgold offered me a position with him as research associate in the electrodiagnostic laboratory in what was then the Institute of Physical Medicine and Rehabilitation (now the Rusk Institute of Rehabilitation Medicine) at New York University Medical Center. The offer, however, came with a stipulation: that I would also work for a PhD in the medical school's department of physiology and biophysics. The rest is history. Dr. Goodgold gave me an opportunity on which to build my career. But, of course, none of that would have been possible had not my wife, Harriet, put up with all that I had to do. And, although I am now "retired," she still allows me time to stay involved.

Neil I. Spielholz

Contents

Chapter 8   Rehabilitation of Upper-Extremity Nerve Injuries

Gerard A. Malanga, MD, Robert Savarese, DO

Chapter 9   Rehabilitation in Radiculopathies and Lower-Extremity Peripheral Nerve Injuries

Brian A. Davis, MD, FACSM, FABPMR

Contributors

Jay E. Bowen, DO

Attending Physician, Kessler Institute for Rehabilitation
Sports Medicine Fellowship Coordinator
Assistant Professor, Physical Medicine and Rehabilitation at the
University of Medicine and Dentistry
Newark, NJ

Brian A. Davis, MD, FACSM, FABPMR

Co-Director of Sports Medicine
Director of Spine Care
Co-Director of Adaptive Sports Clinic
Assistant Professor, Department of Physical Medicine
and Rehabilitation
Assistant Professor, Department of Anesthesiology
and Pain Management
University of California, Davis Medical Center
Physician for USA Boxing, USA Swimming/National Disability Sports
Alliance, and USA Track and Field

Joseph H. Feinberg, MD

Director of Electrodiagnostic Lab
Department of Physiatry
Hospital for Special Surgery
New York, NY

Stephen G. Geiger, MD

Assistant Attending Physiatrist
Hospital for Special Surgery
New York, NY
Clinical Instructor, Department of Physical Medicine
and Rehabilitation
Weill Cornel Medical College
New York, NY

Lisa S. Krivickas, MD

Director of Electrodiagnostic Services, Spaulding Rehabilitation
Hospital
Assistant Professor, Department of Physical Medicine
and Rehabilitation
Harvard Medical School
Boston, MA

Gregory E. Lutz, MD

Chief of Physiatry
Hospital for Special Surgery
New York, NY

Gerard A. Malanga, MD

Director of Sports, Spine and Orthopedic Rehabilitation, Kessler
Institute for Rehabilitation
Associate Professor, Physical Medicine and Rehabilitation
UMDNJ-New Jersey Medical School
Newark, NJ

Scott F. Nadler, DO

Director of Sports Medicine
Associate Professor, Physical Medicine and Rehabilitation
UMDNJ-New Jersey Medical School
Newark, NJ

Robert Savarese, DO

Resident UMDNJ/Kessler Institute for Rehabilitation
UMDNJ-New Jersey Medical School
Newark, NJ

Neil I. Spielholz, PhD

Professor Emeritus
University of Miami
Florida

Preface

My first experience with neurologic injuries in the athlete was as team physician with a local high school. To a coach or trainer, a "burner" was one of those common injuries that rarely was serious and usually didn't merit medical attention. I was surprised at how a neurologic injury that caused loss of sensation and temporary paralysis could be treated so casually. Even the medical literature on the etiology, biomechanics, and management of a "burner" or "stinger" was vague. This experience accentuated my desire to learn more about the etiology, management, and means of prevention of these injuries.

Since the majority of sports-related injuries that clinicians regularly treat are musculoskeletal, the focus of most sports medicine texts is on orthopedic problems. Often little attention is given to the less common, but potentially more serious, neurologic injuries. However, a thorough understanding of these injuries is necessary for anyone who manages the medical care of athletes and decides when an athlete may resume competition.

Peripheral nerve injuries are often insidious in their development and may be difficult to identify. This is particularly true in dealing with a motivated athlete who may disregard subtle changes in strength and sensation. The early presentation of a peripheral nerve injury can be misleading. Neurological injuries that primarily involve motor function may cause weakness that might clinically appear to be simple muscle overuse. Both cervical and lumbar radiculopathies may present with referred pain only, making early recognition difficult. The long-term danger is that by the time the problem is identified as a neurologic injury, the neurologic deficits may be irreversible.

The injured athlete represents a challenging situation for the sports medicine clinician. There is usually great urgency for a quick recovery and return to participation—yet the great demands of competition may put an incompletely rehabilitated athlete at great risk for reinjury or for a new injury. Medical clearance for an athlete depends not only on a clinician's assessment of recovery but on the inherent dangers of the sport and the relative consequences of a reinjury. This makes the management of peripheral nerve injuries that much more challenging.

Given these challenges, successful diagnosis and treatment of peripheral nerve injuries require a firm grasp of the following:

- Basic neuroanatomy and neurophysiology of both neurologic injury and recovery

- Which peripheral nerve injuries are associated with what sport
- The biomechanical risk factors presented by various sports
- Available diagnostic procedures, their limitations, and when they should be ordered
- Modern and aggressive rehabilitation strategies
- When surgery should be considered

Peripheral Nerve Injuries in the Athlete should serve as a guide for the sports medicine clinician in the early recognition, diagnosis, and management of these conditions. Although it includes a number of "quick reference" elements, the text is not meant to be just a cookbook reference. Rather, we hope it will provoke more thought and greater respect for these injuries and at the same time broaden the skills of the clinician—thus creating a greater comfort zone in diagnosis and management. As the pathomechanics become better understood, an emphasis can be placed on prevention.

This book has been divided into two parts. Part I focuses on anatomy, etiology, and diagnosis. Part II focuses on prevention and rehabilitation. Part I includes six chapters. Chapter 1 is a review on some of the basic neurophysiology and the pathophysiology relevant to peripheral nerve injuries and their recovery. Chapter 1 also includes a discussion on electrodiagnostic testing, also known as the EMG. Chapters 2 through 6 summarize the peripheral nerve injuries (including nerve root and plexus injuries) reported in the sports medicine/neurology literature, as well as the neuroanatomy, biomechanics, and physical findings associated with these injuries. Although rehabilitation is primarily discussed in part II of this text, we have included some of the rehabilitation strategies in chapters 2 and 5. This has been done because of the complexity in managing nerve root injuries in the cervical and lumbar spines. The role of electrodiagnostic testing and imaging studies (i.e., plain radiographs, CT scans, MRIs) is also discussed.

Because the prevention and rehabilitation of these injuries are the basis for management and optimum recovery, three chapters have been dedicated to this material in part II. Chapter 7 is a comprehensive review of general rehabilitation techniques. This includes a discussion on the appropriate exercises, proprioceptive factors, functional training, and guidelines for returning to participation. The role of various modalities including electrical stimulation and modern strategies in rehabilitation are also outlined. Chapter 8 focuses on rehabilitation techniques for upper-extremity nerve injuries. Chapter 9 discusses rehabilitation techniques for lower-extremity nerve injuries and reviews the role of taping and bracing. Chapters 1 through 6 include case reports. While the chapter on the pathophysiology of nerve injuries establishes a foundation that subsequent chapters further build on, a sports medicine clinician can use this text as a reference for individual nerve injuries as they are encountered.

Several educational tools have been included in this text to help the reader who is less familiar with some of the terminology, anatomy, physical exam skills, mechanics of the sports, and rehabilitation techniques. A running glossary serves as a dictionary on important terminology throughout the text. A glossary at the end of the text includes the running glossary terms as well as other terms that will be helpful to the reader. Diagrams and charts on neuromuscular anatomy should help the reader visualize these structures. The appendix includes nine tables on the innervation of muscles and joints, including nerve roots, groups of muscles, individual muscles, major nerves, and nerve branches. Figures of the mechanisms of injury and rehabilitation techniques serve as instructive aids as well.

Because this is a text on peripheral nerve injuries in athletes, we have targeted the entire medical community that works with athletes. We recommend this book for team physicians, general practitioners, internists, orthopedists, neurologists, physiatrists, physical therapists, occupational therapists, athletic and personal trainers, exercise physiologists, and the nurses who work with athletes.

Acknowledgments

We would like to acknowledge Dr. Richard Herzog, Dr. Hollis Potter, and Dr. Douglas Minz from the department of radiology at the Hospital for Special Surgery for providing MRI studies that appear in this textbook. We would like to acknowledge the staff at Human Kinetics, specifically Dr. Loarn Robertson, Elaine Mustain, and Maggie Schwarzentraub, for their continued support and guidance. We would also like to thank the authors who have contributed to this text for their hard work, diligence, and expertise.

PART

I

Anatomy, Etiology, and Diagnosis

1

Pathophysiology of Nerve Injury and Electrodiagnostics

Scott F. Nadler, DO
Joseph H. Feinberg, MD

Peripheral nerves constitute a complex circuitry. They communicate sensory perceptions from the skin and joints to the spinal cord, and motor commands from the spinal cord to the muscles. Unlike the central nervous system, which is rarely capable of regenerating, injured peripheral nerves frequently do. The success of reinnervation, however, depends in part on the type of nerve injury sustained; and the type of nerve injury sustained depends on the mechanism of injury.

Understanding the biomechanics of sports—as well as musculoskeletal *kinesiology* and some basic neuroanatomy—can help to detect peripheral nerve injuries in a timely manner, to prevent more permanent deficits, and to manage these deficits when they occur. Management may include stretching and range-of-motion exercises when there is a lack of mobility. Strengthening programs are important when weakness leaves an athlete more vulnerable to injury. For example, a cervical radiculopathy resulting from a burner can weaken the deltoid and rotator cuff muscles, increasing the chances of shoulder injury. In this case, protection would stem from correcting biomechanical flaws that lead to tissue overload and from using orthotic devices to unload tissue and improve biomechanical function.

> **kinesiology**—The science or the study of movement and the active and passive structures involved.

3

MECHANISMS OF NERVE INJURY

Nerves can be injured by

- compression, as in carpal tunnel syndrome;
- traction, as with "burners";
- ischemia, due to vascular compromise; or
- laceration, secondary to bone fracture or penetrating injury.

Other causes to consider in an injured athlete include familial (genetic) factors, underlying metabolic diseases such as diabetes, and environmental factors. By helping determine the mechanism of injury, a careful history can improve the prognosis and dictate the appropriate course of treatment.

By appreciating the complexity of nerve structure and physiology, one can better understand nerve injury and recovery. A connective tissue sheath, the epineurium, surrounds peripheral nerves (figure 1.1). Within the interior of the nerve (i.e., beneath the epineurium) are fascicles, which are bundles of individual nerve axons. A second connective tissue sheath, the perineurium, separates these fascicles from one another. The perineurium provides tensile strength and elasticity to the nerve, contains blood vessels, and serves as a diffusion barrier to regulate intrafascicular pres-

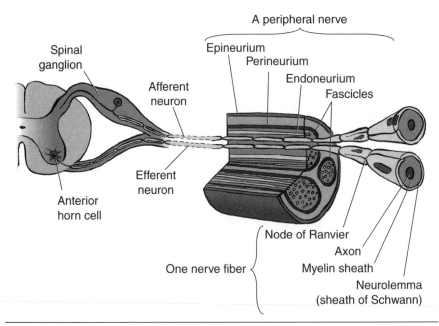

Figure 1.1 Microscopic structure of peripheral nerves.

Adapted, by permission, from A.W. Ham, 1965, *Histology*, 5th ed. (Philadelphia, PA: Lippincott, Williams, and Wilkins), 561.

sure. Within the fascicles are the individual axons, themselves enveloped by a third connective tissue sheath, the endoneurium (figure 1.2). Each axon, therefore, lies within its own connective tissue sheath, which can serve as a guide path for subsequent regeneration if needed.

These various connective tissue sheaths are composed of collagen and elastic fibers, which protect the axons from compressive forces (within limits, of course) and impart some stretchability to the nerves. However, once slack is removed, continued elongation beyond about 12% can cause conduction defects, and elongation beyond 30% can lead to mechanical failure (i.e., rupture) (Sunderland and Bradley 1961, Wall et al. 1992).

The vascular supply to the peripheral nerve is a longitudinal network of nutrient vessels anastomosing on the surface of the nerve and penetrating to the perineurium. Capillaries lie within the fascicles themselves. The blood supply within the peripheral nerve is vital to the survival and functional integrity of the axons (Sunderland 1968). The unique collateral network of vessels makes peripheral nerves somewhat resistant to local ischemic changes.

CLASSIFICATION OF NERVE INJURIES

Two systems are commonly used to classify nerve injuries (table 1.1). A third less commonly used system by Lundborg merely breaks down Seddon's neurapraxia stage, the physiologic conduction block, into type a and type b. Seddon (1943) devised a three-stage scheme to describe microanatomic changes in the nerve after injury. A type 1 injury, or neurapraxia, is a focal conduction block along a length of axon secondary to either acute local demyelination or some other temporary loss of

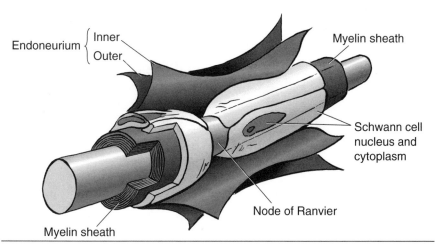

Figure 1.2 Myelinated peripheral nerve fiber.

Adapted from Sir Sydney Sunderland, 1968, *Nerves and nerve injuries* (Philadelphia, PA: Churchill Livingstone), 2.

Table 1.1   Classification of Nerve Injuries

Type	Function	Pathological basis	Prognosis
Lundborg			
Physiologic conduction block: type a	Focal conduction block	Intraneural ischemia Metabolic (ionic) block No nerve fiber pathology	Excellent; immediately reversible
Phsysiologic conduction block: type b	Focal conduction block	Intraneural edema Increased endoneurial fluid pressure Metabolic block; little or no fiber pathology	Recovery in days or weeks
Seddon			
Neurapraxia (*Sunderland* type 1)	Focal conduction block Primarily motor function and proprioception affected Some sensation and sympathetic function can be present	Local myelin injury, primarily larger fibers Axonal continuity No wallerian degeneration	Recovery in weeks to months
Axonotmesis (*Sunderland* type 2)	Loss of nerve conduction at injury site and distally	Disruption of axonal continuity with wallerian degeneration Endoneurial tubes, perineurium, and epineurium intact	Axonal regeneration required for recovery Good prognosis since original end organs reached

(Sunderland type 3)	Loss of nerve conduction at injury site and distally	Loss of axonal continuity and endoneurial tubes Perineurium and epineurium preserved	Disruption of endoneurial tubes, hemorrhage, and edema produce scarring Axonal misdirection Poor prognosis Surgery may be required
(Sunderland type 4)	Loss of nerve conduction at injury site and distally	Loss of axonal continuity, endoneurial tubes, and perineurium Epineurium remains intact	Total disorganization of guiding elements Intraneural scarring and axonal misdirection Poor prognosis Surgery necessary
Neurotmesis *(Sunderland type 5)*	Loss of nerve conduction at injury site and distally	Severance of entire nerve	Surgical modification of nerve ends required Prognosis guarded and dependent upon nature of injury and local factors

Classification systems in italics.

conductivity, and carries the best prognosis for recovery. Neurapraxia is the most common type of nerve injury in athletes. Type 2 injury, or axonotmesis, consists of axonal degeneration, but without disruption of any of the connective tissue sheaths. Axons degenerate within their endoneurial tubes but also retain a guidance pathway for regeneration. This is a lesion in continuity. Regeneration is possible, though many factors affect the rate at which regeneration occurs. Prognosis for recovery is not as good as for the type 1 lesion, but is better than for the type 3 lesion, or neurotmesis. In this situation, all connective tissue sheaths have been disrupted, for example by laceration. The nerve now consists of proximal and distal "stumps." Microsurgical anastomosis may be required to reconnect the stumps; or if a large segment of nerve has been lost, a graft may be needed to bridge the gap.

Sunderland (1951) added two other types of injuries to Seddon's three by theorizing that some injuries might disrupt the endoneurial tubes (leaving perineurium and epineurium intact), while others might disrupt endoneurium and perineurium (leaving just the epineurium intact). In other words, Sunderland retained Seddon's type 1 and type 2 classifications, but moved Seddon's type 3 to a type 5. Sunderland's type 3 includes disruption of the endoneurial tube; his type 4 refers to disruption of both endoneurium and perineurium.

A third way to classify nerve injuries is simply to divide them into demyelinating conditions (producing either conduction block or pronounced slowing of conduction velocity, but without denervation) and degenerating (axonal) conditions (producing denervation of muscle or skin).

REGENERATION AND RECOVERY OF NERVE FUNCTION

Recovery of nerve function depends in great measure on the mode of injury and the type of nerve damage sustained. The lesion with the best prognosis is neurapraxia. In sports-related neurapraxia the conduction block can last from seconds to weeks and on occasion even months. Such injuries usually occur with sudden compressive forces or traction injuries. The extent of injury depends on the degree to which and length of time the nerve is subjected to these forces. Early recognition and action to counteract the forces involved will therefore aid in recovery. Close to full neurologic recovery can be expected when the compressive or traction forces have been alleviated.

On the other hand, lesions associated with axonal degeneration (types 2 and 3 of Seddon) require more time for recovery, since regeneration is a relatively slow process—a common rule of thumb is 1-2 mm/day, or about 1 inch per month. However, this rate is only an approximation, as different investigators have reported different values (see Sunderland 1968 for review of various clinical studies). The bottom line in determining the feasibility of successful axon regeneration is the viability of the anterior horn cell, an intact conduit for it to regenerate through, a receptive neuromuscular junction, and functional contractile muscle tissue.

If all is going well, motor recovery proceeds in a proximal-to-distal fashion. For example, a regenerating axillary nerve would be expected to first reinnervate the posterior deltoid, followed later by the middle deltoid, and last by the anterior deltoid. Physicians caring for such patients should be familiar with the innervation sequence of peripheral nerves. Careful clinical and electromyographic examinations can help detect early return of voluntary control—information that is quite heartening to the patient.

Since nerve regeneration is a metabolically active process, part of the overall goal in caring for these patients is to maximize the body's ability to repair itself. It is therefore logical to advise the injured person to avoid tobacco, alcohol, and illicit drugs and to follow good nutrition practices.

ELECTRODIAGNOSTIC TESTING

Electrodiagnostic tests can help diagnose, localize, and objectively quantify peripheral nerve injuries. They can also help physicians predict recovery and outcome. There are no absolute contraindications to performing electrodiagnostic tests; but when patients are on anticoagulation therapy, have pacemakers, or are at risk for developing *lymphedema*, physicians should be familiar with the necessary precautions.

lymphedema—Swelling in subcutaneous tissues as a result of obstruction of lymphatic vessels or lymph nodes.

Electrodiagnostic procedures should be planned in view of each patient's history (including the mechanism of injury) and associated deficits determined by physical examination. In addition, the physician should know the amount of time since the injury occurred, any preexisting conditions (injuries or diseases), medications taken, and family history.

Generally, one should wait two to three weeks postinjury before performing the tests, but there are occasions where valuable information can be obtained soon after the injury. Follow-up exams can often provide valuable information on recovery and may be helpful for management and further intervention.

Types of Electrodiagnostic Testing

The two basic components of an electrodiagnostic examination are nerve conduction studies and needle electromyography (EMG). The two components are complementary and both should be a part of the complete electrodiagnostic evaluation of peripheral nerve injury. Both can cause a little pain but should have no lasting effects.

Nerve Conduction Studies

Conventional nerve conduction studies test sensory and motor nerves that are relatively accessible to electrical stimulation at certain sites. The sensory nerves are those that convey cutaneous sensation, while the motor fibers are those that innervate specific muscles. Nerves to deep muscles (e.g., supraspinatus muscle) can also be studied, but this requires an intramuscular (needle or fine wire) electrode and is technically more difficult to perform and interpret.

Distal nerves of the upper extremity—such as the ulnar, median, and radial nerves, and most muscles they innervate—are relatively superficial. As a result, they are easy to stimulate and the responses can be recorded with electrodes placed appropriately on the surface of the skin. Nerves can be stimulated either orthodromically, in the normal direction of nerve propagation, or antidromically, in the reverse direction of normal nerve propagation. Proximal nerves of the upper extremity, however (e.g., suprascapular, axillary, and musculocutaneous), are deeply situated and less accessible to stimulation. These nerves can be excited by stimulating the brachial plexus (proximal to their point of departure) at Erb's point in the supraclavicular fossa (figure 1.3), or by stimulating with a needle electrode one of the nerve roots that contribute to the proximal nerves.

Motor nerves are studied by stimulating them proximally and recording the compound muscle action potential (CMAP) over a muscle belly. The CMAP represents the *depolarization* of muscle fibers innervated by

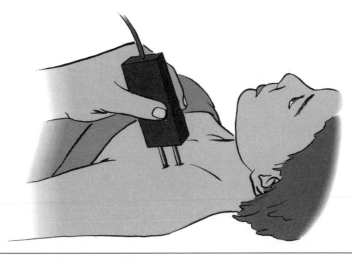

Figure 1.3 Stimulation at Erb's point.

that nerve. If a muscle is relatively superficial, CMAPs can be recorded from it using either surface or intramuscular electrodes. The former are painless. However, if a muscle is deeply situated (e.g., the supraspinatus when one needs to stimulate the suprascapular nerve), then an intramuscular electrode must be placed through the overlying structures (like the upper or middle trapezius in this example) to enter the target muscle.

> **depolarization**—Decrease and ultimate reversal of the transmembrane potential of a muscle (or nerve) fiber. An initial step leading to muscle contraction.

Sensory nerves can usually be studied by placing surface electrodes over a region of skin that is supplied by the nerve or over the nerve trunk itself (e.g., the sural nerve where it passes behind the lateral malleolus to enter the lateral side of the foot). The response recorded from a sensory nerve is called the sensory nerve action potential (SNAP).

Normal values have been determined for conduction velocity, latencies, amplitudes, temporal dispersion, side-to-side differences, etc. Depending on the abnormality detected, conduction studies are useful for distinguishing focal versus diffuse involvement and axonal degeneration versus demyelination (including conduction block); with special techniques, they can even help investigate the possibility of neuromuscular junction defects.

Electromyography

Interpretation of an EMG, or needle examination of muscle, is based on identification of electrical signals coming from that muscle. There are three major components to the examination:

1. With the muscle at rest (the subject is not attempting to contract the muscle), the examiner determines the presence or absence of electrical activity. If activity is present, the next step is to determine if it is "normal" or "abnormal" (figure 1.4, a-b). For example, a denervated muscle generates abnormal spontaneous activity known as fibrillation potentials and positive sharp waves. There are other types of abnormal spontaneous activity, as well, but those are beyond the scope of this presentation. Conversely, other types of spontaneous activity can be found in certain areas of "normal" muscles, so it is imperative to be able to distinguish between the two.

2. With the subject attempting to produce a weak voluntary contraction, the examiner determines if the motor unit potentials fulfill the criteria for "normal." These criteria include the potentials' shape, amplitude, duration, and firing frequency. Experienced examiners rely not only on what these potentials look like on the monitor but also on the sounds that accompany the potentials.

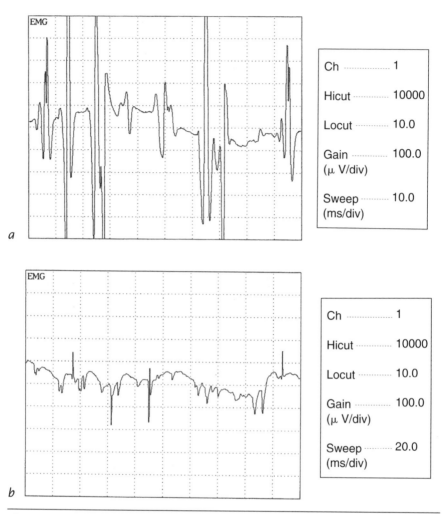

Figure 1.4 *(a)* Normal voluntary motor unit activity. *(b)* Abnormal spontaneous activity. The short-duration spikes are fibrillation potentials; the other wave forms are positive sharp waves.

3. With the subject attempting to produce stronger and stronger contractions, the examiner then determines whether the *recruitment* and firing frequencies of motor units fulfill criteria for being normal. For example, a severely denervated muscle (such as one that has lost almost all of its motor units) has only a few motor units remaining under voluntary control; so even on an attempted strong effort, not many motor unit potentials will appear on the screen. By contrast, a normally innervated muscle will generate so many motor unit potentials on a strong contraction that the screen is filled with activity. The terms "discrete recruitment pattern,"

"reduced recruitment pattern," and "full recruitment pattern" are used to describe the examiner's judgment of this volitional activity.

> **recruitment**—The successive activation of the same and additional motor units with increasing strength of voluntary muscle contraction.

Electrodiagnostic Testing for Regeneration and Reinnervation

If a nerve is injured, axonal degeneration can be followed by regeneration and subsequent reinnervation of denervated motor units. Regeneration is more likely to occur following a type 2 lesion (axonotmesis) than after a type 3 lesion (neurotmesis). Axonotmesis occurs in sports more commonly than does neurotmesis. Recall that in axonotmesis, all connective tissue sheaths of the nerve remain intact, and the axons degenerate within their individual endoneurial tubes. As a result, there is a guidance pathway within which regeneration can occur back to the appropriate target organ. On the other hand, in neurotmesis, the nerve is severed, secondary to either a penetrating wound that cuts the nerve or a fracture that tears a nearby nerve. Surgical repair is frequently required in these cases.

In axonotmesis (i.e., injuries that do not interrupt the continuity of the nerve), two mechanisms can lead to reinnervation of a muscle. Which of these mechanisms predominates depends on the severity and site of the lesion. For example, if an entire nerve trunk is injured, with subsequent degeneration of all the motor axons, reinnervation requires regeneration of axons elongating from the site of the lesion down into the muscle. Regeneration of this type occurs at the rate of (approximately) 1 mm/day, or 1 inch/month. If the lesion affected only some of the motor axons, the muscle is only partially denervated; remaining intramuscular nerve fibers can sprout and reinnervate nearby denervated muscle fibers in a kind of adoption process. This is the phenomenon of collateral sprouting first described by Edds (1950). Since these new terminal nerve fibers do not have to grow over long distances, this type of reinnervation can occur over a shorter time period than if the axons had to regenerate from far away.

Serial EMG studies can help detect evidence of reinnervation even before it is evident on clinical examination. The appearance of motor unit potentials in a muscle previously devoid of them is clear evidence of reinnervation. The potentials produced by these newborn motor units, however, are usually distinctly different from normal motor unit potentials. The potentials produced early in reinnervation frequently exhibit shorter duration and lower amplitude than normal and contain many phases (figure 1.5a). This means that instead of consisting of the usual two or three phases, these units are polyphasic. As reinnervation progresses, the potentials produced by nascent units become longer in duration and frequently larger in amplitude. They are known as long-duration polyphasic motor unit potentials; when heard on the audio system, they have a characteristic "chugging" sound reminiscent of an outboard motor (or Model T Ford, to those of us old enough to remember that) (figure 1.5b). As reinnervation progresses further, polyphasic motor unit potentials may be replaced by normal motor unit potentials—usually associated with return of clinical strength and function.

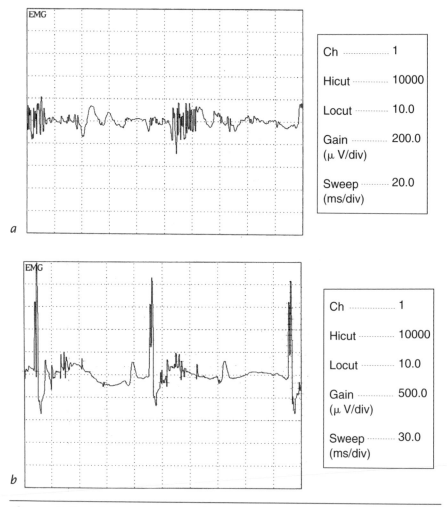

Figure 1.5 *(a)* A nascent or reinnervation potential. *(b)* Long-duration polyphasic potentials, demonstrating terminal collateral sprouting.

> ### Case Report
>
> A 22-year-old college basketball player presented with right wrist drop after an opposing player landed on his forearm during a game.
>
> *Medical history:* He reported that after the injury, he felt a numbness in his hand; he awoke the next morning unable to lift his wrist. He presented for evaluation the following afternoon. He denied any neck pain or other symptoms.
>
> *Surgical history:* None.
>
> *Social history:* Denied smoking and alcohol usage.
>
> *Family history:* Noncontributory.
>
> *Physical examination:* Neck motion was full in all planes. Shoulder, elbow, and wrist motions were full. Strength was 5/5 in bilateral upper extremities. Sensation was normal. Reflexes were normal. Patient was able to extend his wrist in radial deviation with 4/5 strength; finger extensors and extensor carpi ulnaris were 0/5.
>
> *Electrodiagnostic studies:* Consistent with absence of conduction across the forearm with no evidence for spontaneous activity on needle electromyography.
>
> *Diagnosis:* Neuropraxic injury to the posterior interosseous nerve.
>
> *Management and outcome:* The patient was placed in an outrigger splint to allow for more normal use of his digits. Weakness resolved over six weeks, with complete return of motor function by nine weeks.

CONCLUSION

From this brief description of the electrodiagnostic evaluation of peripheral nerve injuries, it should be apparent that the person performing these studies requires not only technical expertise for performing them correctly but the scientific/academic background for properly interpreting them.

REFERENCES

Edds MV: Collateral regeneration of residual motor axons in partially denervated muscles. J Exp Zool 1950; 113:517-552.

Lundborg G: *Nerve injury and repair.* Edinburgh: Churchill Livingstone, 1998.

Seddon HJ: Three types of nerve injury. Brain 1943; 66:237-288.

Sunderland S: A classification of peripheral nerve injuries producing loss of function. Brain 1951; 74:491-516.

Sunderland S: Intraneural topography. In *Nerves and nerve injury.* Edinburgh: E&S Livingstone, 1968; 758-1046.

Sunderland S, Bradley KC: Stress-strain phenomena in human peripheral nerve trunks. Brain 1961; 84:102-127.

Wall EJ, Massie JB, Kwan MK, Rydevik BL, Myers RR, Garfin SR: Experimental stretch neuropathy. Changes in nerve conduction under tension. J Bone Joint Surg Br 1992; 74(1):126-129.

2

Cervical Radiculopathies, Brachial Plexopathies, and the Burner Syndrome

Joseph H. Feinberg, MD
Neil I. Spielholz, PhD

The *burner* or stinger syndrome is the most common neurological injury in sports. Controversy exists as to whether it is primarily a cervical root injury, brachial plexus injury, or both. The athlete's symptoms and physical exam findings may appear similar for both—yet the mechanism of injury, diagnostic studies indicated, management, prognosis, and prevention depend on distinguishing between the two. This chapter reviews the anatomy of the cervical nerve root and brachial plexus, the mechanisms of injury, the clinical symptoms, the physical exam, and physical exam findings. It discusses why the authors believe burners are primarily a cervical root injury. It covers the work-up and presents guidelines on prevention, rehabilitation, and return to participation.

CERVICAL RADICULOPATHIES

The most proximal component of the peripheral nerve, and the most commonly injured in sports, is the cervical nerve root. The confluence of segmental dorsal and ventral roots exiting the spinal cord form each cervical nerve root. The cell bodies of the motor axons forming the ventral root lie in the ventral gray horn of the spinal cord, while the cell bodies of the sensory fibers form the dorsal root ganglia and lie close to the *vertebral foramen*. Just distal to the foramen, the cervical root divides into a posterior primary and an anterior primary ramus. The posterior primary ramus innervates the skin and muscles (paraspinals) of the neck and the posterior elements of the spine. The anterior primary ramus of cervical nerve roots C5-C8, the first thoracic nerve root, and sometimes the C4 and T2 nerve roots, form the brachial plexus and supply sensation and motor function to the upper extremities.

> **vertebral foramen**—A bony canal through which the nerve roots exit the spinal canal. A common site for nerve root compression. There are several anatomic causes for nerve root compression, including uncovertebral bone spurs, disc protrusions, and facet joint hypertrophy. Also known as the **neuroforamen.**

Cervical roots exit the neuroforamen, a bony canal bordered anteromedially by the uncovertebral joint; bordered posterolaterally by the facet or zygoapophyseal joint; bordered superiorly by the pedicle of the vertebra above; and bordered inferiorly by the pedicle of the vertebra below. Medially the foramina are formed by the edge of the vertebral endplates and the intervertebral discs (Ahlgren 1996, Chestnut et al. 1992) (figure 2.1). The nerve exits above its corresponding numbered vertebral body. Therefore the C6 nerve root exits above the C6 vertebral segment through the C5-C6 neuroforamen (figure 2.2). Because the T1 vertebrae lies below C7 with no C8 vertebrae, the C8 nerve root exits between C7 and T1. Thereafter beginning with the T1 nerve root, the nerve exits below its corresponding numbered vertebral body.

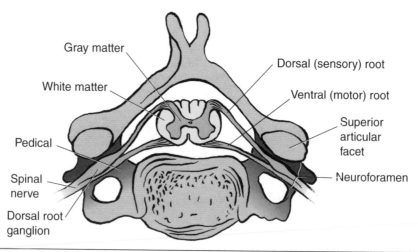

Figure 2.1 Superior view of cervical vertebra.

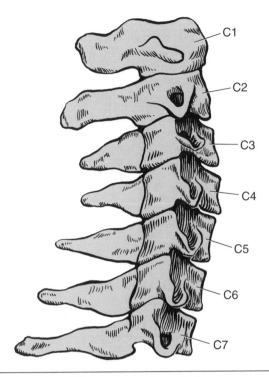

Figure 2.2   Anterior oblique view of cervical spine.

For Further Reading on . . .

Cervical Radiculopathies

Bullough, PG, Boachie-Adjei, O. *Atlas of spinal diseases.* Philadelphia: Lippincott, New York: Gower Medical, 1988.

Brachial Plexopathies

Netter, F.*The CIBA collection of medical illustrations,* volume 8, part 1. p. 28.

The Burner/Stinger Syndrome

Jordan, BD, Tsairis, P, Warren, RF. *Sports neurology,* 2nd edition. Philadelphia: Lippincott-Raven, 1998.

The Cervical Root Versus Brachial Plexus Controversy

Fu, FH, Stone, DA. *Sports injuries.* Baltimore: Williams & Wilkins, 1994

Indications and Applications of Electrodiagnostic Testing

Dumitru, D, Amato, A, Zwarts, M. *Electrodiagnostic medicine,* 2nd edition. Philadelphia: Hanley and Belfus, 2001.

Although about 50% of all cervical rotation occurs at C1-C2, this is rarely the site of pathology in athletes (White and Panjabi 1990). Normally the greatest amount of cervical spine flexion and extension occurs at the C4-C5 and C5-C6 levels (Lind et al. 1989). Degenerative changes most commonly involve levels C5-C6 and C6-C7 (Freidenberg and Miller 1963, Gore et al. 1986). In a 1992 study, Yoo et al. found that

- the C4-C5 neuroforamen is the narrowest in cadaveric cervical spines when compared to the C5-C6 and C6-C7 levels;
- the C4-C5, C5-C6, and C6-C7 neuroforamina further narrow with extension and *ipsilateral rotation;*
- combining extension with ipsilateral rotation had an additive effect on narrowing of all three neuroforamina; and
- the neuroforaminal canals were enlarged with neck flexion and contralateral rotation.

Farmer and Wisneski (1994) studied pressures in the C5, C6, and C7 neuroforamina and found that cervical spine extension increased intraforaminal pressures at all three levels; but with simultaneous arm abduction, the pressures were significantly reduced.

ipsilateral rotation—Rotation to the same side as that on which the patient experiences symptoms.

The cervical roots are among the most commonly injured nerves in athletes (Sallis et al. 1997). The C5 and C6 roots are the most susceptible because they are shorter than the lower cervical roots and are taut when the shoulder is in the dependent position—that is, adducted and hanging down secondary to the forces of gravity. The C5 root is the shortest rootlet of the brachial plexus and emerges from the spinal canal at a more obtuse angle than any other root.

The cervical roots can be injured by direct compression, by traction, or from a combination of the two. A force driving the head and shoulder into opposite directions can lead to excessive nerve root traction. Cervical root compression from a posterolateral disc herniation or endplate spurring can occur before the root enters the neuroforamen. Within the neuroforamen, compression is possible from a foraminal disc extrusion, disc degeneration, uncovertebral joint arthritis, facet joint arthritis/capsulitis (Epstein et al. 1965, Holt and Yates 1966), or neural fibrosis (Hoyland et al. 1989). Neck ipsilateral rotation and oblique hyperextension can lead to a functional narrowing of the neural foramen (Yoo et al. 1992). Rockett (1982) identified scarring primarily involving the C5 nerve root in cases he explored surgically. Scarring occurred at the point where the root emerged from the vertebrae between the anterior and posterior lamellae of the transverse processes. As the root passed between the anterior and medial scalene muscles, it was scarred and fixed to the muscles.

Cervical *disc herniations* account for a very small percentage of cervical radiculopathies in athletes (Albright et al. 1984). Levitz et al. (1997) evaluated 55 athletes referred with chronic recurrent burners. Twenty-two percent had disc herniations and 37% had *disc protrusions*. Levitz et al. (1997) did not specify what percent of the disc protrusions or herniations were central or foraminal. Since herniations must be lateral for cervical root compression to occur (figure 2.3, a-b), the clinical significance of the protrusions and herniations is unclear. Levitz et al. (1997) reported an 85% incidence of degenerative disc disease in athletes with chronic cervical radicular symptoms. They used disc bulges, protrusions, and herniations as criteria for degenerative disc disease. The primary levels involved on MRI were C4-C5, C5-C6, and C6-C7.

> **disc herniation**—The nucleus pulposis (inner portion) of the intervertebral disc has ruptured through the annulus (outer portion) and posterior longitudinal ligament.

> **disc protrusion**—Bulging of the nucleus pulposis through a weakened annulus fibrosis.

BRACHIAL PLEXOPATHIES

The brachial plexus passes through the scalene muscles of the neck, runs between the clavicle and first thoracic rib, courses under the pectoralis

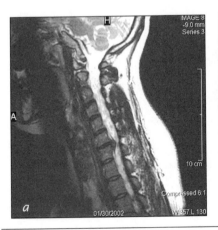 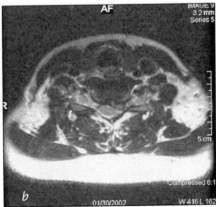

Figure 2.3 Disc herniation laterally compressing nerve root on MRI: *(a)* sagittal slice, *(b)* axial slice.

minor tendon before passing anterior to the glenohumeral joint, and then forms the radial, ulnar, and median nerves. Most proximal are the upper, middle, and lower trunks and most distal are the lateral, posterior, and medial cords (figure 2.4).

Although relatively well protected, the plexus is susceptible to injury at Erb's point, in the supraclavicular fossa posterior to the clavicle and posterolateral to the sternocleidomastoid muscle, where it is somewhat superficial (see figure 1.3, page 10). The upper trunk of the brachial plexus can be injured from a direct blow to Erb's point or when a downward force to the shoulder stretches the plexus. Both mechanisms have been described as causes of a plexopathy (DiBenedetto and Markey 1984, Hoyt 1967, Markey et al. 1993) and are reviewed in the discussion on burners.

Thoracic outlet syndrome (TOS) occurs in athletes from compression within the scalene muscles, between the clavicle and first thoracic rib, or under the insertion of the pectoralis minor tendon into the coracoid process (Johnson 1986). Anatomic variants such as a cervical rib or fibrous band

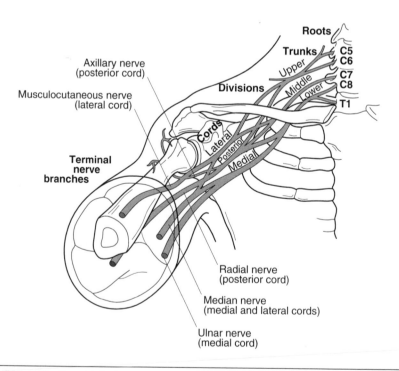

Figure 2.4 Brachial plexus nerve roots as they exit the cervical spine into the upper extremity.

Reprinted, by permission, from S. Shultz, 2000, *Assessment of athletic injuries* (Champaign, IL: Human Kinetics), 59.

can constrict the plexus proximally in the interscalene triangle. Athletes who perform repetitive overhead shoulder motions are at greatest risk for developing TOS (Karas 1990, Leffert 1983, Strukel and Garrick 1978). Poor posture and alignment abnormalities can also contribute to the syndrome. Neurologic symptoms include numbness, tingling, and pain down the medial aspect of the upper extremity and weakness/atrophy in muscles innervated through the C8/T1 or lower trunk distribution. Because arterial or venous compression can also occur, clinicians should look for signs of edema, cyanosis, coolness, and exertional fatigue (Bennett and Mehloff 1994).

> **thoracic outlet syndrome**—Compression of the neurovascular bundle (subclavian artery, subclavian vein, brachial plexus) from either a cervical rib, hypertrophic scalenes, constriction from the pectoralis minor, a narrowed costoclavicular space, or prominent first thoracic rib. Symptoms include numbness, tingling, and weakness corresponding usually to the lower trunk of the brachial plexus. Patients may also complain of pain in the neck or shoulder girdle region.

We have seen scapulothoracic dysfunction and hypermobility syndrome and believe it is a cause of thoracic outlet-type symptoms. These athletes, usually women, complain of numbness, tingling, and pain with certain activities. Their neurologic exam is normal and all thoracic outlet maneuvers are negative. The shoulder complex usually appears to be hypermobile, but closer inspection may find the glenohumeral joint to have normal to limited range. It is the scapulothoracic joint that is hypermobile, and the athlete has difficulty controlling the scapula with active shoulder motion. We suggest that the poorly controlled scapula creates compression/traction where the neurovascular structures pass under the pectoralis minor insertion at the coracoid process.

Brachial neuritis, also known as neuralgic amyotrophy of Parsonage and Turner (Flaggman and Kelly 1980, Tsairis et al. 1972), is an idiopathic brachial plexopathy that can affect athletes (Bergfield et al. 1988). Symptoms often follow a viral illness, immunization, or recent shoulder trauma, or they may develop spontaneously and can be bilateral. Patients usually present with acute shoulder pain, followed several days to weeks later by weakness or frank paralysis. One study showed 37% of patients with a brachial neuritis had complete recovery within one year and 80% within two (Tsairis et al. 1972). The muscle involvement is most often in the distribution of a single proximal peripheral nerve such as the suprascapular, axillary, long thoracic, or the upper trunk of the brachial plexus. Occasionally, two nerves are involved simultaneously, the most common pair being the suprascapular and axillary (Flaggman and Kelly 1980). A case of brachial plexitis has also been reported, presented as an anterior interosseous nerve syndrome (Rennels and Ochoa 1980). Electrodiagnostic studies can help localize the level. Symptoms usually improve gradually over the course of several weeks or months, but not in all patients. Physical therapy can be used to prevent mal-substitution patterns when recovery is expected, develop compensatory substitution patterns when neurological recovery is doubtful, and provide biofeedback techniques to reestablish proper muscle firing patterns during early recovery.

THE BURNER/STINGER SYNDROME

The burner or stinger is a clinical syndrome that produces immediate but usually transitory numbness, tingling, and burning in one upper extremity, usually lasting less than one minute (Rockett 1982). The injured player is often seen shaking the involved extremity as he returns to the huddle or comes to the sideline.

Burners are primarily a football injury (Andrish et al. 1977), and the relative risk is influenced by the position played and by anatomic factors. One study (Castro et al. 1997) found that defensive backs and tight ends had the highest relative risk, while running backs and defensive linemen had the next highest risk.

Burners have been reported by 18% to 70% of college football players (Castro et al. 1997, Clancy et al. 1977, DiBenedetto and Markey 1984, Sallis et al. 1997). They are often recurrent and many can lead to permanent neurologic deficits (Archambault 1983; Speer and Bassett 1990). The natural history and long-term consequences of recurrent burners have not been investigated.

Burners may increase the risk for quadriplegia. Following a burner, athletes often lose some degree of neck extension. More severe or chronic injuries may cause an athlete to keep the head and neck in a slightly flexed position. This posture—along with relative spinal stenosis as indicated by an abnormal Pavlov ratio, additional radiological abnormalities of the cervical spine, and improper tackling techniques—may predispose the athlete to a more catastrophic spinal cord injury (Torg et al. 1993).

The Pavlov ratio is determined on a lateral X ray by dividing the sagittal diameter of the spinal canal by the sagittal diameter of the corresponding vertebral body (Pavlov et al. 1987). Although its role in estimating relative spinal stenosis and the risk of quadriplegia is controversial, some researchers have found that a positive Pavlov ratio (a ratio < 0.8) is associated with burners. Meyer and colleagues (1994) found that players with a Pavlov ratio less than 0.8 had a threefold increased risk of burners. Castro et al. (1997) showed that those with narrower spinal canal diameters and smaller Pavlov ratios (0.75) had a higher risk of recurrent stingers but did not have increased risk of having an initial (first-time) stinger. There was no attempt to correlate the level of stenosis with the level of burner symptoms—in fact, the most common level of stenosis (defined by the Pavlov ratio) was C7.

The Pavlov ratio can help in investigating *relative stenosis*, which is different from true stenosis. The key here is that when it is positive and less than 0.8 it is predictive for recurrent stingers.

Athletes with recurrent burners not only exhibit functional narrowing of the neuroforamen with oblique extension of the neck (Yoo et al. 1992); the foramen is often further compromised from bony hypertrophy (figure 2.5, a-c). Levitz et al. (1997) performed MRIs on 54 athletes with recurrent burners. Only seven athletes did not have degenerative disc disease, and three of those seven had narrowing of the neural foramen secondary to bony hypertrophy.

Burners have been observed in several other sports—in basketball (Chrisman et al. 1965), after a "take down" maneuver or a "fireman's carry" in wrestling (Kelly et al. 1993, Wroble and Albright 1986), and after a collision into the boards in ice hockey. One of our athletes had burner-like symptoms after weightlifting, and a C5 radiculopathy was identified by electrodiagnostic studies.

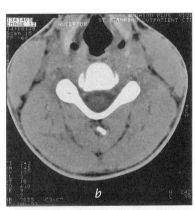

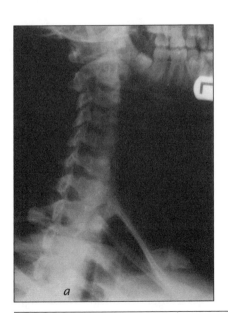

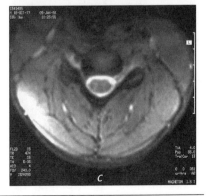

Figure 2.5 *(a)* Cervical spine radiograph demonstrating neuroforaminal narrowing secondary to uncovertebral joint hypertrophy. *(b)* CT scan axial image demonstrating neuroforaminal stenosis. *(c)* MRI axial image demonstrating neuroforaminal stenosis.

Mechanisms of Injury

Several mechanisms of injury have been described. Chrisman and colleagues (1965) demonstrated that a combination of shoulder depression and head/neck contralateral bending led to a traction injury of the C5 or C6 roots (figure 2.6). This happens when a defensive football player lowers his shoulder as he attempts to block or tackle: At the point of contact, the shoulder is forced downward and the head deviates to the opposite side. Watkins (1986) reported that burners resulted from cervical root compression within the neuroforamen during neck oblique extension (figure 2.7). Levitz et al. (1997) felt that nerve root compression could also occur in the intervertebral foramina from a combination of (1) neck oblique extension and (2) the presence of cervical disk disease or of degenerative changes. It appears also that a tackle or collision that forces the head and neck in opposite directions can stretch the upper trunk of the brachial plexus (Barnes 1949, Bateman 1967, Hoyt 1967, Robertson et al. 1979). DiBennedetto and Markey (1984) suggested that another cause is injury to the plexus from a direct blow (figure 2.8). Shoulder dislocations and subluxations can cause burner-like symptoms when a peripheral nerve or the brachial plexus has been injured. The axillary nerve is the most com-

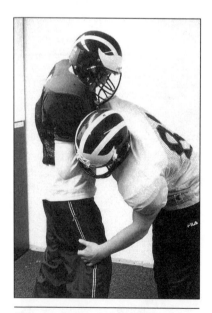

Figure 2.6 A football player using his head and shoulder to tackle an opposing player, resulting in a traction injury that stretches C5-6 roots.

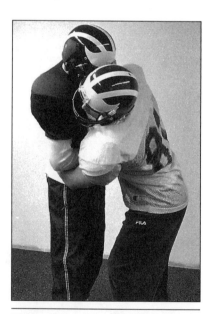

Figure 2.7 A football player striking an opposing player with his head, resulting in oblique extension of his neck and subsequent compression of the upper cervical nerve roots.

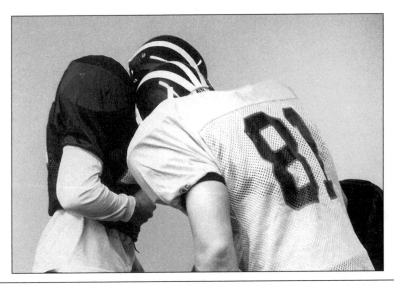

Figure 2.8 A football player driving his head into the region of Erb's point, injuring the opposing player's plexus.

monly injured, followed by the posterior cord, the musculocutaneous nerve, and the suprascapular nerve (Brown 1972, Hoyt 1967, Liveson 1984, Pasila et al. 1978, Travlos et al. 1990).

The Cervical Root Versus Brachial Plexus Controversy

Differentiating a cervical root from a brachial plexus injury can often be very difficult. Moreover, it remains controversial whether root injuries (Levitz et al. 1997, Meyer et al. 1994) or plexus injuries (Hershman et al. 1989, Markey et al. 1993, Sallis et al. 1997) are more common. One study found an equal incidence of both (Wilbourn et al. 1986). Poindexter et al. (1984) found a greater incidence of cervical root injuries, while Clancy et al. (1977) observed a higher incidence of brachial plexopathies.

Contributing to the confusion is an inconsistent nomenclature used to describe cervical root and brachial plexus injuries. Anatomically, the cervical roots become the brachial plexus when the upper, middle, and lower trunks have been formed (see figure 2.4, page 22). Bonney (1959), however, classified both pre- and postdorsal ganglionic nerve root injuries as brachial plexus injuries. Bonney's preganglionic nerve root injuries are equivalent to a cervical radiculopathy. It appears that the nerve between the neuroforamen and trunks of the plexus falls into a gray area for classification.

Although one might expect cervical root injuries to cause neck pain, this is frequently not the case. Moreover, since the clinical presentation for both plexus and root injuries can be very similar, on-the-field diagnoses can be difficult and sometimes unreliable. A careful and thorough neck evaluation, including the *Spurling maneuver* (figure 2.9), is essential and will help determine if the injury is at the root or plexus level. Note: This should be done only after more serious cervical spine injury has been ruled out. If a clinician cannot exclude a cervical spine injury on the playing field, the athlete should be immobilized on a spine board and a neck exam should be delayed until neck radiographs and any other appropriate studies have been done.

> **Spurling maneuver**—Physical exam provocative maneuver to help diagnose a cervical radiculopathy by reproducing radicular symptoms. The patient's head and neck are obliquely extended to the side of symptoms and then axially loaded.

Though injuries to either cervical nerve roots or brachial plexus can lead to burner symptoms, there are several reasons why the cervical roots may be more susceptible to injury than the brachial plexus:

- Because the brachial plexus is plexiform, it can accommodate a significant amount of stretch; the cervical nerve roots, however, are attached to the *dentate ligaments*.
- The cervical roots lack the protective perineural sheath found in the plexus.

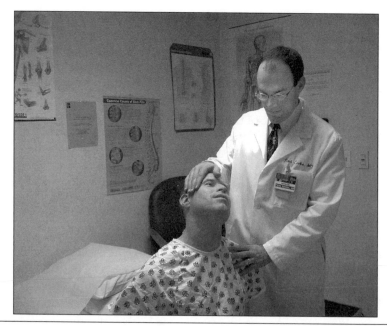

Figure 2.9 Spurling maneuver.

- The cervical roots are pressed against the *vertebral transverse process* by the *adventitia* of the vertebral artery. Additional compression against the transverse process can occur when the scalene muscles tighten.
- Hypertrophy of the scalenes in the muscularly well-developed neck can lead to scarring of the cervical roots.
- The bony neuroforamen becomes the path of greatest resistance when there is traction to both the brachial plexus and cervical nerve roots. It is further compromised with disc and endplate degeneration or when there is uncovertebral spurring.

dentate ligaments—A band of fibrous pia mater extending along the spinal cord on each side between the dorsal and ventral roots; these tissues suspend the spinal cord from the dura mater and help maintain the central position of the cord.

vertebral transverse process—A process that projects on the dorsilateral aspect of each side of a vertebra's neural arch.

adventitia—The outer layer that makes up a tubular organ or structure, is composed of collagenous and elastic fibers, and is not covered with peritoneum.

On- and Off-the-Field Evaluation

On-the-field evaluations of athletes who may have sustained a burner must be thoughtful and thorough. Athletes who have experienced symptoms in two or more extremities should be considered as having had transient quadriparesis until proven otherwise: They should be immobilized on a spine board and sent for an immediate spine evaluation with cervical spine radiographs and the appropriate follow-up imaging (MRI, CT scan, etc.).

All athletes who have experienced burner symptoms should have a thorough neurologic, neck, and upper-extremity exam, in that order. Radicular pain can be so intense that the athlete may deny or fail to describe neck pain. A neck screening evaluation should seek for evidence of a neck injury. Athletes should immediately be immobilized and given radiographic evaluation if they exhibit any significant neurologic deficits, neurologic symptoms, or deficits involving at least two limbs, or if they exhibit obvious swelling or deformity in the spine region or gross limitations in motion. If immobilization is not necessary, the examiner should thoroughly inspect and palpate the neck, then check active and then passive neck motion.

If there are subtle neurologic changes or minor restrictions in neck motion, the athlete should be given tests specific for nerve roots. Vikari-Juntura and colleagues (1989) found the Spurling maneuver (see figure 2.9) and the *shoulder abduction relief sign* to be very specific for radicular pain. We have found the Spurling maneuver to be positive in most athletes with burners, and Torg's group found a positive Spurling maneuver in 71% of their patients with recurrent burners (Levitz et al. 1997). If the neck exam is completely normal, the exam should then focus on the brachial plexus, shoulder, and other potential peripheral nerves.

> **shoulder abduction relief sign**—Physical exam technique designed to help diagnose a cervical radiculopathy at the C5 or C6 level by reducing neural tension. The maneuver is performed by passively abducting the shoulder of the symptomatic side overhead and thus reducing the radicular symptoms.

Injuries to the C5 nerve root lead to weakness in the deltoid, biceps, brachialis, brachioradialis, rotator cuff, and rhomboid muscles. Injuries to the C6 nerve root involve all C5 muscles listed except the rhomboids, and also include the pronator teres, flexor carpi radialis, and extensor carpi radialis. Injuries to the upper trunk of the brachial plexus involve both the C5- and C6-innervated muscles.

Because most athletes make every effort to compensate for any weaknesses they have, it is often difficult to identify such deficits. Athletes also tend to have great baseline strength. To identify weaknesses caused by subtle neurologic damage, clinicians therefore must be familiar with neuroanatomy and possible substitution patterns, and they must be skilled in detecting subtle neurologic deficiencies. They must know how to use mechanical advantage when testing muscle strength—for example, they should test the deltoid by applying downward resistance at the most terminal point in the upper limb (i.e., wrist or hand) as the athlete attempts to forcefully abduct the arm. This gives the examiner the greatest lever arm. We have learned to detect subtle weakness in the biceps and triceps by testing with the elbow maximally flexed.

Imaging Studies

The common burner, which completely resolves within a few minutes and does not recur, can be managed without X rays. When neck motion remains restricted or significant neurologic deficits persist, the clinician should obtain radiographs—including anterior-posterior (AP), lateral, right and left obliques, open-mouth view, and flexion/extension. Additional imaging is unnecessary with a classic burner syndrome when neck motion returns to normal and when neurologic deficits recover. MRIs should be considered when neck motion remains restricted, significant neurologic deficits persist, or clinically the athlete has symptoms at the C7 or C8 root level. This is because these lower root levels are not as susceptible to injury when the shoulder is depressed and the neck is contralaterally flexed. Unlike C5 or C6 radiculopathies, C7 or C8 radiculopathies are more likely to be the result of a disc herniation.

Indications and Applications of Electrodiagnostic Testing

Reports on the role and value of electrodiagnostic studies are limited (Clancy et al. 1977, DiBennedetto and Markey 1984, Markey et al. 1993, Poindexter et al. 1984, Robertson et al. 1979, Speer and Bassett 1990). The results of these studies vary widely, further contributing to the confusion as to whether burner syndromes are primarily root or plexus injuries. EMG can help determine the site and degree of neurologic injury and should be performed when neurologic deficits are significant or symptoms persist (Leffert 1983, Wilbourn 1990). Clinicians should always keep in mind that certain electrodiagnostic abnormalities require time before they become manifest. Even after three to four weeks, an EMG study may not reflect the full degree of neurologic damage. A limited follow-up EMG exam may help further elucidate the situation in another three or four weeks.

In the absence of more significant neurologic damage (e.g., *neurapraxic* injury), electrodiagnostic tests may be normal. Under these circumstances one should rely on clinical findings to localize the level of injury and make an accurate diagnosis.

> **neurapraxic**—An injury to the myelin that results in a temporary conduction block to the axons involved. There is no axonal degeneration. Only the myelin sheath, and not the axon, is damaged.

Differentiating between root and plexus injuries with an electrodiagnostic study can sometimes be difficult. Although abnormal spontaneous activity or polyphasic potentials in the cervical paraspinals indicate a cervical root injury, the absence of abnormal findings in the paraspinals does not completely rule out a cervical radiculopathy. Since the brachial plexus is an extension of the anterior primary rami, it is possible to injure the nerve root and spare the division of the nerve root (posterior ramus) that innervates the paraspinals. This confusion is even more likely with a traction injury, where a stretch to the plexus may create greater tension in the anterior rami divisions of the cervical roots. It may then be difficult to distinguish between a brachial plexopathy from a cervical radiculopathy on EMG studies when the cervical paraspinal muscles are spared. Furthermore, the dorsal scapular nerve—which innervates the rhomboids and branches off the C5 nerve root before the plexus is formed—is also typically involved in C5 radiculopathies but might be spared in a root traction injury. This may account for the higher incidence of brachial plexopathies (as compared to that of radiculopathies) that has been reported in some studies based on electrodiagnostic testing.

Nerve conduction studies are usually normal with cervical nerve root injuries. Significant axonal degeneration can lead to reduced motor amplitudes, but because the great majority of cervical root injuries are proximal to the dorsal root ganglia (preganglionic), sensory amplitudes are usually normal. Plexus injuries are always postganglionic, and when there is axonotmesis both sensory and motor amplitudes may be reduced. Stimulation of Erb's point can help identify distal plexus injuries at the cord level or isolated peripheral nerve injuries to the suprascapular or axillary nerve, which can mimic root or plexus symptoms. Erb's point stimulation may be too distal to pick up an injury to the proximal brachial plexus.

Education and Preventive Rehabilitation

Training in proper techniques of tackling and comprehensive conditioning programs both play important roles in preventing burners and decreasing spine injuries.

Education

Education on proper tackling techniques not only may help prevent burners; it also may decrease the likelihood of more serious cervical spine injuries. It is common during tackling or blocking to lead with the shoulder and make contact by driving the upper shoulder into the opposing athlete (see figure 2.6, page 26). At contact the head and shoulder are driven in opposite directions, creating traction on the upper cervical roots (primarily C5 and C6) or upper trunk of the brachial plexus. Simultaneously, the neck is forcefully extended or laterally flexed. This causes neuroforaminal narrowing and can lead to compression to the upper cervical roots (C5 and C6) on the contralateral side. We recommend instructing athletes to maintain a more upright position and to lead with the upper chest and arms simultaneously.

Another dangerous technique that potentially can lead to catastrophic cervical spine injury is "spear tackling." Athletes who spear tackle lead with the head and use it as a battering ram. This technique, which is no longer permitted in football, can result in quadriplegia (Torg et al. 1993).

Preventive Rehabilitation

Because of the potential seriousness of burner injuries and their high rate of recurrence, one can make a very strong case for comprehensive prevention programs. Rehabilitation should incorporate a comprehensive strengthening program, proprioceptive exercises, and restoration of motion. Strong head and neck muscles (trapezius, paraspinals, scalenes, and sternocleidomastoid) help prevent the violent distraction of the head and shoulder. Just as important as absolute strength is the muscle reaction time and the ability of these muscles to adequately decelerate the head with a strong eccentric contraction after hitting another player or the ground. Excellent isometric strength of the neck stabilizers does not guarantee adequate muscle control in response to a sudden blow to the head and neck. Strengthening of the neck muscles should include exercises that simulate the type of contraction they undergo during a tackle. Proprioceptive exercises improve the athlete's awareness of body position and alignment, so that the tackle is performed in a safe manner while maximizing the efficiency of muscle power. Soft-tissue mobilization techniques, stretching, traction, and judicious use of modalities such as ultrasound or electrical stimulation help athletes to restore motion and to regain proper muscle length, which maximizes a muscles ability to generate power.

Cervical posture can also play an important role. When the head and neck are protracted, additional cervical spine extension is necessary for the athlete to look straight ahead, leading to a functional decrease in diameter of the neuroforamen. A knowledgeable trainer or therapist should instruct athletes in postural exercises—including head, neck, and shoulder retractions, and also stretching of the anterior neck and chest wall muscles.

Orthoses for Prevention

Properly fitted shoulder pads are the first step in preventing burners among football players. When improperly fitted, shoulder pads or cervical rolls may offer little to no protection and only provide a false sense of security. Cervical collars or rolls should be used to help limit end-range neck oblique extension: They should allow some neck extension and bending and should never keep the neck in a flexed or rigid position. A comparison of collars found no significant difference between a cervical roll and a custom orthotic (Hovis and Limbird 1994). Shoulder pad lifters have been used to provide additional protection by elevating the pads and thus further limiting neck motion. Interval pads have also been found to provide a protective cushion to the plexus by shielding it from a direct blow (DiBennedetto and Markey 1984).

CONCLUSION

The burner syndrome, although common, is usually benign and self-limiting. Yet it can remove an athlete from competition for an extended time, limit the athlete's effectiveness during participation, and potentially lead to permanent neurologic injury. Though the controversy continues as to whether it is a brachial plexus or cervical root injury, similar biomechanical principles apply to prevention and management of both. Diagnosis is based primarily on clinical evaluation: While diagnostic tools such as radiographs, MRIs, and EMGs may be helpful, they are necessary in a very small percentage of cases. The key to management is proper education—especially concerning tackling techniques, proper fit and modifications of equipment, and early detection.

Case Report 1

A 15-year-old football player/wrestler presented with right-sided shoulder pain and weakness 10 days after he was injured while wrestling.

Medical history: The patient was injured playing football three months earlier, at which time he complained of right shoulder pain and weakness. Symptoms resolved but returned when he was again injured while wrestling. His pediatrician told him he had a rotator cuff injury. Patient denied any neck pain.

Social history: High-school student athlete, playing football and wrestling.

Family history: Negative.

Physical exam: Clinical assessment demonstrated weakness in the biceps, deltoid, and rotator cuff muscles in the 3/5 range. The biceps reflex was depressed. Sensation was decreased to pin prick along the proximal and lateral aspect of the right shoulder. Neck motion was restricted from end range right lateral bending and right oblique extension. Spurling maneuver on the right was positive, referring pain into the shoulder.

Radiographs: Demonstrated spurring of the uncovertebral joint at C5 (see figure 2.5a, page 25). This led to narrowing of the right C4-C5 neuroforamen. MRI demonstrated no evidence of any disc herniations or degenerative disc disease (see figure 2.5c).

Electrodiagnostic studies: Fibrillation potentials and positive sharp waves in the biceps, deltoid, infraspinatus, and upper cervical paraspinals were in the 2+ and 3+ range. Recruitment was reduced in the biceps and deltoid. There were no polyphasic potentials. Findings were consistent with a C5 radiculopathy with evidence of axonal degeneration to the biceps, infraspinatus, deltoid, and upper cervical paraspinals.

Diagnosis: Right C5 radiculopathy with axonal degeneration.

Management and outcome: The patient was started on a program of physical therapy. This included strengthening of the deltoid, biceps, and rotator cuff muscles, postural reeducation of the head and neck muscles, and proprioceptive muscle training. After regaining full strength and achieving pain-free range of motion with his neck, he was cleared to participate in all sports six months later. The patient decided to return only to wrestling and had no recurrence of the injury.

Case Report 2

Chief complaint: A 19-year-old college defensive back complained of pain in the neck and weakness in the right shoulder.

Medical history: In attempting to tackle an opposing player, the athlete lowered his right shoulder; while making contact, he felt his head deviate to the left. He experienced burning, numbness, and tingling radiating into the right hand. The burning and tingling resolved but the numbness persisted. He was removed from competition and further evaluated.

Social history: College student playing football.

Family history: Negative.

Physical exam: Neck motion was extremely restricted, and the head was kept in a mildly flexed position. There were no palpable masses or areas of tenderness in the neck, but with any attempt to extend or laterally rotate the neck the patient had immediate burning radiating down the extremity. Strength was initially 4/5 in the right deltoid, biceps, and rotator cuff muscles. Sensation was decreased to pinprick in the lateral aspect of the shoulder. All reflexes were 2+.

Radiographs: Cervical spine films (including flexion/extension and oblique views) were normal.

Electrodiagnostic testing: Not performed because of complete return of strength when reexamined two days later.

Diagnosis: Transient right C5 radiculopathy secondary to root traction injury.

Management and outcome: Manual traction with C-spine postural exercises was begun. Strengthening exercises for the right upper extremity were also performed. Exercises were prescribed for the head and neck stabilizers (trapezius, scalenes, sternocleidomastoid, and paraspinals), with a focus on enhancing muscle reaction time and improving head/neck position sense. When full pain-free neck ROM was restored, the athlete was fitted with a cervical collar; he returned to play football two weeks following injury. There were no recurrences.

REFERENCES

Ahlgren, BD. Cervical radiculopathy. Orthop Clin North Am 27:253-262, 1996.

Albright, JP, El-Khoury, G, VanGilder, J, Crowley, E, Foster, D. Head and neck injuries in sports. In Scott, WN, Nisonson, B, Nicholas, JA (eds): *Principles of sports medicine.* Baltimore: Williams & Wilkins, 40-86, 1984.

Andrish, JT, Bergfield, J, Romo, L. A method for the management of cervical injuries in football: a preliminary report. Am J Sports Med 5(2):89-92, 1977.

Archambault, JL. Brachial plexus stretch injury. J Am Coll Health 31:256-260, 1983.

Barnes, R. Traction injuries of the brachial plexus in adults. J Bone Joint Surg 31B(1):10, 1949.

Bateman, JE. Nerve injuries about the shoulder in sports. J Bone Joint Surg 49A:785-792, 1967.

Bennett, JB, Mehloff, TL. Thoracic outlet syndrome. In DeLee, JL, Drez, D. (eds): *Orthopedic sports medicine: principles and practices,* volume 1. Philadelphia: Saunders, 794, 1994.

Bergfield, JA, Hershman, EB, Wilbourn, A. Brachial plexus injury in sports: a five year follow-up. Orthop Trans 12:743-744, 1988.

Brown, JT. Nerve injuries complicating dislocations of the shoulder. J Bone Joint Surg 34B:526, 1972.

Bonney, G. Prognosis in traction injuries of the brachial plexus. J Bone Joint Surg 41B:4-35, 1959.

Castro, FP Jr, Ricciardi, J, Brunet, ME, Busch, MT, Whitecloud III, TS. Stingers, the Torg ratio, and the cervical spine. Am J Sports Med 25(5):603-608, 1997.

Chestnut, RM, Abitro, JJ, Garhn, SR. Surgical management of cervical radiculopathy. Orthop Clin North Am 23:462, 1992.

Chrisman, OD, Snook, GA, Stanitis, JM, Keedy, VA. Lateral flexion injuries in sports. JAMA 192:117-119, 1965.

Clancy, WG Jr, Brand, RL, Bergfield, JA. Upper trunk plexus injuries in contact sports. Am J Sports Med 5:209-216, 1977.

DiBenedetto, M, Markey, K. Electrodiagnostic localization of traumatic upper trunk brachial plexopathy. Arch Phys Med Rehabil 65:15, 1984.

Epstein, J, Lavine, L, Aronson, H, Epstein, B. Cervical spondylotic radiculopathy. Clin Orthop 40:113-122, 1965.

Farmer, JC, Wisneski, RJ. Cervical spine nerve root compression. Spine 19(16):1850-1855, 1994.

Flaggman, PD, Kelly, JJ. Brachial plexus neuropathy. Arch Neurol 37:160-164, 1980.

Freidenberg, ZB, Miller, WT. Degenerative disk disease of the cervical spine. J Bone Joint Surg 45(6):1171-1178, 1963.

Gore, DR, Sepic, SB, Gardner, GM. Roentgenographic findings of the cervical spine in asymptomatic people. Spine 11(6):521-524, 1986.

Hershman, EB, Wilbourn, AJ, Bergfeld, JA. Acute brachial neuropathy in athletes. Am J Sports Med 17:655-659, 1989.

Hirasawa, Y, Sakakida, K. Sports and peripheral nerve injury. Am J Sports Med 11:420-426, 1983.

Holt, S, Yates, PO. Cervical spondylosis and nerve root lesions. J Bone Joint Surg 48B(3):408-423, 1966.

Hovis, WD, Limbird, TJ. An evaluation of cervical orthosis in limiting hyperextension and lateral flexion in football. Med Sci Sports Exerc 26:872-876, 1994.

Hoyland, JA, Freemont, AJ, Jayson, MIV. Intervertebral foramen venous obstruction. Spine 14(6):558-568, 1989.

Hoyt, W. Etiology of shoulder injuries in athletes. J Bone Joint Surg 49A:755-766, 1967.

Johnson, DC. The upper extremity in swimming. In Pettrone, FA (ed): *Symposium in upper extremity injuries in athletes.* St. Louis: Mosby, 36-46, 1986.

Karas, S. Thoracic outlet syndrome. Clin Sports Med 9:297-310, 1990.

Kelly, JD, Marchetto, PA, Odgers, CA, Mayer, RA. The relationship of transient upper extremity paresthesias and cervical stenosis. Orthop Trans 16:732, 1993.

Leffert, RD. Thoracic outlet syndrome and the shoulder. Clin Sports Med 2:439, 1983.

Levitz, CL, Reilly, PJ, Torg, JS. The pathomechanics of chronic, recurrent cervical nerve root neuropraxia. Am J Sports Med 25(1):73-76, 1997.

Lind, B, Sihlbom, H, Nordwall, A, Malchau, H. Normal range of motion of the cervical spine. Arch Phys Med Rehabil 70:692-695, 1989.

Liveson, J. Nerve lesions associated with shoulder dislocations: an electrodiagnostic study of 11 cases. J Neurol Neurosurg Psychiatry 47:742-744, 1984.

Markey, KL, DiBenedetto, M, Curl, WW. Upper trunk brachial plexopathy. The stinger syndrome. Am J Sports Med 21:650-655, 1993.

Meyer, SA, Schulte, KR, Callaghan, JJ, Albright, JP, Powell, JW, El-Khoury, GY. Cervical spinal stenosis and stingers in collegiate football players. Am J Sports Med 22:158-166, 1994.

Pasila, M, Jaroma, H, Kiviluoto, O. Early complications of primary shoulder dislocations. Acta Orthop Scand 49(3):260-263, 1978.

Pavlov, H, Torg, JS, Robie, B, Jahre, C. Cervical spinal stenosis: determination with vertebral body ratio method. Radiology 164:771-775, 1987.

Poindexter, DP, Johnson, EW. Football shoulder and neck injury: a study of the "stinger." Arch Phys Med Rehabil 65:601-602, 1984.

Rennels, GD, Ochoa, J. Neuralgic amyotrophy manifesting as anterior interosseous nerve palsy. Muscle Nerve 3:160-164, 1980.

Robertson, WC Jr, Eichman, PL, Clancy, WG. Upper trunk plexopathy in football players. JAMA 241:1480-1482, 1979.

Rockett, FX. Observations on the burner: traumatic cervical radiculopathy. Clin Orthop 164:18-19, 1982.

Sallis, RE, Jones, K, Knopp, W. Burners: offensive strategy for an under-reported injury. Physician Sportsmed 20(11):47-55, 1997.

Speer, KP, Bassett, FJ III. The prolonged burner syndrome. Am J Sports Med 18:591-594, 1990.

Strukel, R, Garrick, J. Thoracic outlet compression in athletes. Am J Sports Med 6(2):35, 1978.

Torg, JS, Sennett, B, Pavlov, H, Leventhal, MR, Glasgow, SG. Spear tackler's spine. Am J Sports Med 21(5):640-649, 1993.

Travlos, J, Goldberg, I, Boome, R. Brachial plexus lesions associated with dislocated shoulders. J Bone Joint Surg 72B:68-71, 1990.

Tsairis, P, Dyck, P, Mulder, D. Natural history of brachial plexus neuropathy. Arch Neurol 27:109-117, 1972.

Vikari-Juntura, E, Porras, M, Laasonen, EM. Validity of clinical tests in the diagnosis of root compression in cervical disc disease. Spine 14(3):253-257, 1989.

Watkins, RG. Neck injuries in football players. Clin Sports Med 5:215-246, 1986.

White, AA, Panjabi, MM. *Clinical biomechanics of the spine,* 2nd edition. Philadelphia: Lippincott, 102, 1990.

Wilbourn, AJ. Electrodiagnostic testing of neurologic injuries in athletes. Clin Sports Med 9(2):229-245, 1990.

Wilbourn, AJ, Hershman, EB, Bergfield, J. Brachial plexopathies in athletes, the EMG findings. Muscle Nerve 9:254, 1986.

Wroble, RR, Albright, JP. Neck and low back injuries in wrestling. Clin Sports Med 5(2):295-325, 1986.

Yoo, JU, Zou, D, Edwards, WT, Edwards, T, Bayley, J, Yuan, HA. Effect of cervical spine motion on the neuroforaminal dimensions of human cervical spine. Spine 17:1131-1136, 1992.

3
Proximal Upper-Extremity Nerve Injuries

Joseph H. Feinberg, MD
Jay E. Bowen, DO

Proximal upper-extremity nerve injuries in athletes are often related to biomechanical factors and the entire kinetic chain with the more common sites of injury that include the cervical roots, brachial plexus, and the nerves of the shoulder girdle: long thoracic, suprascapular, and axillary. The spinal accessory, dorsal scapular, and musculocutaneous nerves are less commonly involved.

Brachial plexopathies in athletes, whether traumatic or from other causes, can result in significant impairments and limit the athletes' level of achievement or participation in sport. By determining the muscles involved and the sensory abnormalities, one can identify the region affected.

BRACHIAL PLEXOPATHIES

The brachial plexus, which supplies sensation and motor function to the upper extremities, is formed from the anterior rami of nerve roots C5, C6, C7, C8, and T1. C4 and T2 may provide small contributions. The plexus passes between the anterior and middle scalene muscles of the neck, between the clavicle and first rib, under the pectoralis minor tendon, and then passes anterior to the glenohumeral joint to form the radial, ulnar, and median nerves. The upper, middle, and lower trunks of the plexus are supraclavicular; the lateral, posterior, and medial cords are infraclavicular.

Although relatively well protected proximally by overlying soft tissue, the plexus becomes superficial in the supraclavicular fossa after it has exited from between the anterior and middle scalene muscles. This region, known as Erb's point, lies behind the clavicular head of the sternocleido-mastoid muscle and just above the clavicle (see figure 1.3, page 10).

Diagnosis

The most common symptoms of brachial plexopathy are numbness, tingling, weakness, and/or referred pain corresponding to the distribution of a trunk or cord of the plexus. Findings are similar whether or not the etiology of the plexopathy is traumatic.

Because the terminal nerve's fibers traverse different portions of the plexus, examination findings of a partial brachial plexus injury can be mixed and do not necessarily refer to any one root or peripheral nerve distribution (Ferrante and Wilbourn 1995). If a pan-plexus lesion exists, all aspects of the limb demonstrate abnormalities.

Etiology

Severe plexus injuries that result in permanent neurologic sequelae are uncommon. These injuries are associated with compression or traction, or are idiopathic. Traction injuries are usually more devastating and involve the upper trunk with greater frequency.

Brachial Plexus Compression Injuries

Compression or traction can cause severe brachial plexopathies. Hirasawa and Sakakida (1983) observed that Japanese mountain climbers' back-packs caused upper-trunk plexopathies by directly compressing the Erb's point region. Compression of the brachial plexus as it passes through hypertrophied, tight, or scarred muscle can result in thoracic outlet syndrome (TOS) and may produce neurologic symptoms in athletes. Theoretically, compression of the brachial plexus can occur within the interscalene triangle, between the clavicle and first rib, or under the pectoralis minor where the tendon inserts on the coracoid process (Johnson 1986). Anatomic variants such as a cervical rib or fibrous bands can constrict the plexus as it passes between the anterior and middle scalene muscles. A fracture malunion of the clavicle or a healed fracture with excessive callous formation can lead to compression in the costoclavicular space (England and Tiel 1999).

Athletes such as football quarterbacks, tennis players, and baseball players can experience shoulder girdle depression during repetitive overhead shoulder motion (Karas 1990). This depression can compress the brachial plexus as it passes under the pectoralis minor tendon. Kyphotic posture with protracted shoulders produces similar anatomic changes, usually resulting in only sensory complaints of numbness, tingling, or burning in the medial forearm and fourth and fifth digits.

True neurogenic TOS, manifested by thenar muscle wasting and ulnar sensory loss, is extremely rare (Wilbourn 1990). Arterial or venous compression can cause vascular TOS, with symptoms that include edema, cyanosis, coolness, and exertional fatigue (Bennett and Mehloff 1994).

Brachial Plexus Stretch Injuries

The plexus is susceptible to several mechanisms of stretch injury. Common mechanisms include falling on an outstretched abducted arm resulting in anterior glenohumeral dislocation (Liveson 1984, Travlos et al. 1990) and the driving of the head and shoulder in opposite directions during a tackle or collision (Barnes 1949, Bateman 1967, Hoyt 1967) resulting in stretch of the upper trunk of the plexus. The posterior cord is the segment of the plexus most commonly injured with anterior glenohumeral dislocations (Liveson 1984, Travlos et al. 1990). The axillary nerve is the most frequently injured peripheral nerve seen with anterior glenohumeral dislocations (Brown 1972, Hoyt 1967, Liveson 1984, Pasila et al. 1978). One study found that 5 of 11 nerve injuries caused by shoulder dislocations involved the posterior cord—the axillary nerve was involved in 10 of the 11 injuries, the musculocutaneous nerve in 4, and the suprascapular nerve in 1 (Liveson 1984).

Brachial Neuritis

Brachial neuritis, also known as neuralgic amyotrophy of Parsonage and Turner, is an idiopathic cause of brachial plexopathy that can affect athletes (Flaggman and Kelly 1980, Parsonage and Turner 1948). The onset of symptoms often follows a viral illness, an immunization, or recent shoulder trauma, but symptoms may develop spontaneously and can be bilateral (Tsairis et al. 1972). Patients present with acute shoulder pain, followed by weakness several days or weeks later. Gradual improvement occurs over the course of several weeks or months, but permanent paralysis can occur. One study showed 37% of patients with a brachial neuritis had complete recovery in one year and 80% by two years (Tsairis et al. 1972). The neurologic distribution does not always correspond to a particular trunk or cord level. Individual nerves commonly involved are the suprascapular, axillary, and the long thoracic.

Electrodiagnostic studies can help localize the lesions and objectively quantify neurologic injury. Electromyography can identify which muscles are involved when spontaneous activity is seen, denoting acute denervation. The number and type (serrated, polyphasic, or giant) of motor unit potentials seen on recruitment can gauge reinnervation. Motor nerve conduction amplitudes and area can be used to quantify motor axonal involvement. Sensory nerve amplitudes can assist in localizing the site of the lesion (Ferrante and Wilbourn 1995). The lateral antebrachial cutaneous nerve is the most commonly involved in nerve conduction studies and can be used to help distinguish this condition from a cervical radiculopathy. The superficial radial and median sensory response to the thumb can also be involved but less frequently effected.

SPINAL ACCESSORY NEUROPATHY

The spinal accessory nerve (cranial nerve XI) is a pure motor nerve that may have components from nerve roots C3 and C4. It innervates the upper, middle, and lower trapezius and sternocleidomastoid muscles. The spinal accessory nerve becomes superficial in the posterior cervical triangle just posterior to the scalenes, where it is susceptible to injury by a direct blow to the neck or by a lymph node biopsy. The nerve is usually injured at the upper border of the trapezius about one inch above the clavicle (Bateman 1967). Isolated stretch injuries occur as well (Logigian et al. 1988, Wright 1975).

Diagnosis

Athletes with spinal accessory nerve injuries experience weakness when they attempt to elevate or shrug the shoulder. This phenomenon is particularly important in contact sports, where shrugging the shoulder protects the brachial plexus from being stretched during a collision. Injury to the nerve leads to trapezius atrophy (figure 3.1), which is one of the causes of scapular winging—seen on exam by the inferior angle of the scapula pointing midline. The scapula migrates superiorly during shoulder motion.

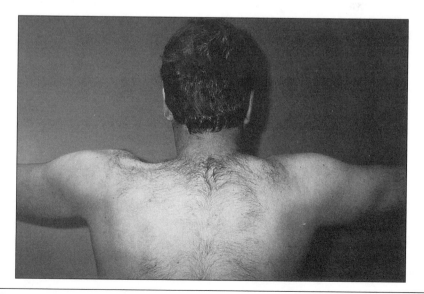

Figure 3.1 Trapezius atrophy in a patient with a spinal accessory neuropathy.

There is also weakness of shoulder abduction because of the lack of scapular stabilization, which in turn is felt to be secondary to muscle imbalances and compensatory overwork of the intact muscles. Even though the spinal accessory nerve is a pure motor nerve, athletes may complain of a dull aching sensation radiating down the arm. The altered motion from muscular imbalance can also cause other problems such as rotator cuff impingement, adhesive capsulitis, or even secondary plexus irritation (Osterman and Babhulkar 1996).

Etiology

Injuries to the spinal accessory nerve have been reported to occur from the use of sticks in such sports as hockey, field hockey, and lacrosse (Bateman 1967, Tsairis 1989). The spinal accessory nerve may also be susceptible to a direct blow to the neck from an opposing football player's helmet.

DORSAL SCAPULAR NEUROPATHY

The dorsal scapular nerve branches off the C5 nerve root immediately after it exits the neural foramen. It innervates the rhomboids and has motor function only. When this nerve is injured, lateral winging of the scapula can be observed at rest and exaggerated by movement, but it is not as prominent as the lateral winging seen with a spinal accessory nerve injury.

Isolated injuries to the dorsal scapular nerve are uncommon. One study reported a combined injury to the dorsal scapular nerve and long thoracic nerve from a shoulder dislocation in judo (Jerosch et al. 1990). Another report described compression of the dorsal scapular nerve, which had a common trunk with the long thoracic nerve through the scalenus medius as an atypical presentation of thoracic outlet syndrome (Chen et al. 1995).

LONG THORACIC NEUROPATHY

The long thoracic nerve is formed from three branches that come off the C5, C6, and C7 nerve roots just distal to the intervertebral foramen and proximal to the trunks of the brachial plexus. The C5 and C6 branches pass between anterior and middle scalenes and unite with the C7 branch just distal to it. The nerve descends deep to the brachial plexus and down the anterolateral aspect of the chest wall to innervate the serratus anterior (figure 3.2). It is a pure motor nerve with no sensory function.

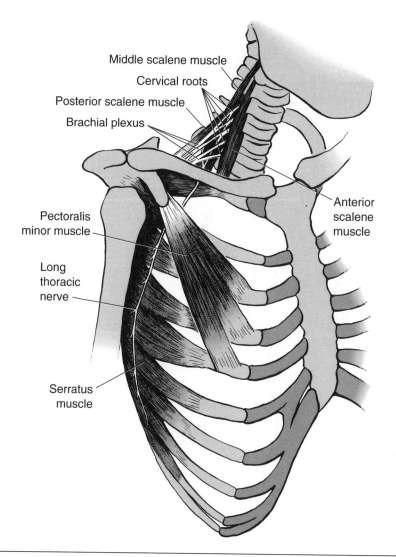

Figure 3.2 The long thoracic nerve.

Diagnosis and Prognosis

Patients with long thoracic neuropathy present with acute pain down the arm or around the scapular region (Johnson and Kendall 1955) followed by weakness, difficulty maintaining shoulder stability, and difficulty elevating the arm. The lack of full scapular lateral rotation and adequate elevation with attempts to abduct the shoulder can lead to supraspinatus

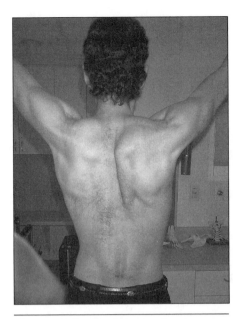

Figure 3.3 Medial winging in a patient with a long thoracic neuropathy.

impingement. Medial scapula winging (figure 3.3) may not be present for up to two weeks following an injury.

Goodman and colleagues (1975) observed that injuries caused by trauma carried a poorer prognosis and greater functional impairment than did neuralgia amyotrophy. This study also showed later institution of therapy (modalities, range of motion, strengthening, and scapular stabilization exercises) after symptom onset led to poorer prognosis as compared with an earlier start to therapy. Individuals who had no recovery of serratus function substituted use of their trapezius and rhomboids.

Etiology

The major causes of a long thoracic neuropathy are trauma, overuse leading to muscular fatigue (which leads to scapulothoracic dysrhythmia resulting in traction of the nerve), and neuralgic amyotrophy. Injuries occur with a shoulder dislocation, a direct blow to the thorax, or faulty biomechanics that repetitively stretch the nerve. Abduction of the shoulder beyond 90 degrees (Prescott and Zollinger 1944) has been reported as a mechanism of injury in basketball and football players (Kaplan 1980). In tennis (Foo and Swann 1983, Goodman 1983, Gregg et al. 1979, Schultz and Leonard 1992) and in baseball (Schultz and Leonard 1992), arm extension or shoulder protraction at end ranges of motion are the mechanical factors believed to be responsible for injury. The follow-through of a golf swing (Overpeck 1940, Schultz and Leonard 1992) and a boxer's missing a punching bag (Overpeck 1940) also put the scapula in a maximally protracted position and are proposed mechanisms of injury. A definite mechanism is often difficult to identify, and one cannot exclude neuralgic amyotrophy.

Long thoracic neuropathy has been reported in many athletic endeavors. Examples include

- a marksman lying in a prone position with prolonged shoulder abduction (Woodhead 1985),
- a ballet dancer performing a cartwheel (Gregg et al. 1979),

- a dancer stretching during warm-up (White and Witten 1993),
- an athlete performing a stretching exercise that included shoulder depression and contralateral neck bending (White and Witten 1993),
- a judo fighter with an anterior shoulder dislocation (Jerosch et al. 1990),
- a hiker who sustained compression from a knapsack strap (Ilfeld and Holder 1942),
- a weightlifter engaging in unusually heavy lifting (Goodman et al. 1975, Hauser and Martin 1943, Schultz and Leonard 1992),
- an individual who was kicked by a horse (Overpeck 1940), and
- an individual who fell on the shoulder (Fardin et al. 1978).

Long thoracic neuropathy also has been reported in an archer (Foo and Swann 1983) and a wrestler, but with no identification of a specific mechanism of injury (Goodman et al. 1975). Gregg and colleagues (1979) described the injury in a hockey player who slid across the ice on an outstretched hand, a gymnast doing exercises on the rings, and a bowler.

SUPRASCAPULAR NEUROPATHY

The suprascapular nerve is a branch of the upper trunk of the brachial plexus. In about half of all people it receives fibers from the C4 nerve root (Sunderland 1990). It rarely arises solely from the distal end of the C5 root (Goss 1973). The nerve passes laterally, deep to the trapezius and omohyoid muscles, and then through the suprascapular notch, which can vary anatomically (Rengachary et al. 1979), and then innervates the supraspinatus. It then courses around the spinoglenoid notch to innervate the infraspinatus. Although it carries no cutaneous sensation, it contains sensory fibers from the scapula, acromioclavicular joint, and glenohumeral joint (figure 3.4).

Diagnosis

Compression of the suprascapular nerve proximally produces shoulder pain in the scapular region and in the acromioclavicular and glenohumeral joints, in addition to weakness of the supraspinatus and infraspinatus muscles. Atrophy is more readily observed in the infraspinatus than in the supraspinatus, which lies beneath the trapezius (figure 3.5, a-b). Entrapment or injury at or proximal to the suprascapular notch includes both supraspinatus and infraspinatus and leads to weakness in abduction and external rotation (Callahan et al. 1991, Hirayama and Takemitsu 1981), while entrapment or injury at the spinoglenoid notch affects only external rotation (Takagishi et al. 1991, Ganzhorn et al. 1981).

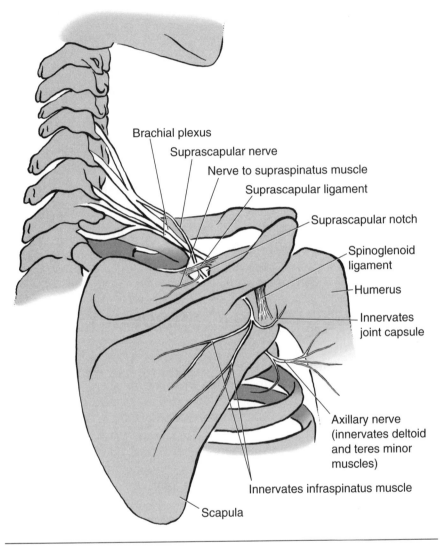

Brachial plexus
Suprascapular nerve
Nerve to supraspinatus muscle
Suprascapular ligament
Suprascapular notch
Spinoglenoid ligament
Humerus
Innervates joint capsule
Axillary nerve (innervates deltoid and teres minor muscles)
Innervates infraspinatus muscle
Scapula

Figure 3.4 The suprascapular nerve.

Nerve conduction studies may help localize the lesion. Erb's point is stimulated, and recordings are taken with needle electrodes superior (supraspinatus) and inferior (infraspinatus) to the spine of the scapula. Two compound motor action potentials (CMAPs) and their latencies are obtained. Side-to-side comparisons should be performed. Needle electromyography of the supraspinatus and infraspinatus should always be performed for a complete study and to obtain the maximum information. Spontaneous activity of either muscle, revealed by positive sharp waves or fibrillations, would demonstrate muscle denervation.

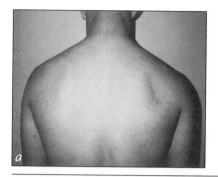
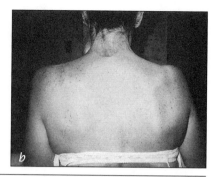

Figure 3.5 *(a)* Atrophy of only the infraspinatus in a patient with a suprascapular neuropathy involving only the branch to the infraspinatus. *(b)* Atrophy of the supraspinatus and infraspinatus in a patient with a suprascapular neuropathy.

If the latency to only the infraspinatus is prolonged, if the distal amplitude is dispersed or significantly reduced, or if spontaneous activity is found in the infraspinatus with no spontaneous activity in the supraspinatus—then the lesion is at the spinoglenoid notch. If both muscles are involved, the lesion will be more proximal, but cannot be definitively localized to the suprascapular notch without further MRI anatomic correlation. We recommend MR imaging in all suprascapular neuropathies (proximal and distal) to look for a source of anatomic compression.

Etiology

The suprascapular notch (Callahan et al. 1991, Fritz et al. 1992, Garcia and McQueen 1981, Post and Mayer 1987, Rengachary et al. 1979) and the spinoglenoid notch (Aiello et al. 1982, Ferretti et al. 1987, Glennon 1992, Henlin et al. 1992, Jackson et al. 1995, Kiss and Komar 1990, Steinman 1988, Takagishi et al. 1991) are the two reported sites of entrapment. The most commonly reported site is the suprascapular notch as the suprascapular nerve courses beneath the superior transverse scapular ligament. Demirhan and colleagues (1998) demonstrated with cadavers that the spinoglenoid ligament is present only about 61% of the time and that it is wider superiorly and fanned and twisted inferiorly, inserting into the posterior shoulder capsule. The researchers observed maximal movement and stretch on the suprascapular nerve with cross-body shoulder adduction and internal rotation of the glenohumeral joint. The suprascapular nerve is also susceptible to a direct blow at its most superficial location, which is Erb's point (Mestdagh et al. 1981).

A ganglion is the most common mass or space-occupying lesion that can compress the nerve and is easily seen on MRI (Fritz et al. 1992) (figure 3.6). Inokuchi and colleagues (1998) used MRI of the suprascapular region to

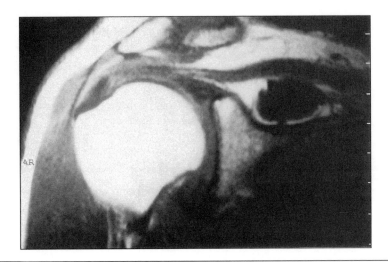

Figure 3.6 Coronal oblique T2-weighted image of the shoulder, demonstrating a ganglion cyst in the region of the suprascapular notch.

aid in the diagnosis of injury to the nerve. There were 22 subjects with suprascapular nerve palsy as diagnosed by EMG and clinical exam: 12 had MRI examinations with T1- and T2-weighted images. Nine of 12 demonstrated a ganglion cyst at the spinoglenoid notch. The ganglion cyst characteristics were low-signal intensity on T1 and high-signal on T2. Muscle changes showed high signal on T1 in four infraspinatus muscles, indicating chronic denervation and fatty atrophy (figure 3.7, a-b). There was a high signal on T2 in six infraspinatus muscles, indicating a more acute muscle edema pattern. One of the six patients with high signal on T2 in the infraspinatus also demonstrated high signal in the supraspinatus. Two patients had EMG electrically silent muscles and high signal on T2, but normal muscle signal returned with recovery of nerve function (Inokuchi et al. 1998). In denervated muscles, high signal on T2 is seen approximately 15 days after injury and may return to normal two to three months after surgical decompression of the nerve. The increased signal is believed to be from muscle edema caused by a decrease in intracellular fluid and a relative increase in extracellular fluid (Polak et al. 1988). Since these changes occur at about the same time that EMG abnormalities develop, both may be related to the change in muscle membrane stability.

There are many reports of suprascapular neuropathies in athletes (Biundo and Harris 1993, Liveson et al. 1991, Vastamaki and Goransson 1993, Zuckerman et al. 1993). Compression can result from an anomalous transverse scapula ligament (Alon et al. 1988), a hypertrophied ligament (Aiello et al. 1982, Ferretti et al. 1987, Garcia 1981), a ganglion cyst (Hadley

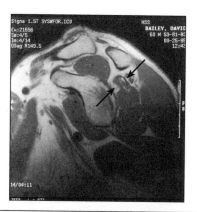
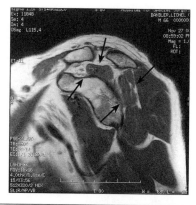

Figure 3.7 *(a)* T1-weighted sagittal image of scapula, demonstrating isolated atrophy of the infraspinatus in a patient with a suprascapular neuropathy involving only the branch to the infraspinatus. *(b)* T1-weighted sagittal image of scapula, demonstrating atrophy of the supraspinatus and infraspinatus in a patient with a suprascapular neuropathy involving the suprascapular nerve proximally.

et al. 1986, Hirayama and Takemitsu 1981, Neviaser et al. 1988, Takagishi et al. 1991, Thompson et al. 1982,), a malignant tumor (Fritz et al. 1992), or from a number of biomechanical factors (Clein 1975, Jackson et al. 1995, Kopell 1959, Kukowski 1993, Rengachary et al. 1979). Traction of the suprascapular nerve occurs as it passes beneath the transverse scapula ligament during shoulder abduction and external rotation as well as during other actions that require extreme scapular motion (Rengachary et al. 1979). Traction of the nerve by the suprascapular ligament has been described as the "sling effect."

Compression at the suprascapular notch has been reported in backpackers (Hadley et al. 1986), weightlifters (Agre et al. 1987), and baseball pitchers (Ringel et al. 1990). Compression at the spinoglenoid notch has occurred in volleyball players (Ferretti et al. 1998), racquet sport players (Thompson et al. 1982), weightlifters (Ganzhorn et al. 1981), baseball pitchers (Bryan and Wild 1989, Liveson et al. 1991, Smith 1995), a football player (Jackson et al. 1995), a gymnast (Laulund et al. 1984), and a dancer (Kukowski 1993). Use of an arm pulley on weight machines has also produced a suprascapular neuropathy (Goodman 1983). A suprascapular neuropathy involving only the branch to the infraspinatus was identified by EMG in 12 of 96 asymptomatic elite volleyball players (Ferretti et al. 1987); compression was thought to be caused by traction on the nerve at the spinoglenoid notch as the infraspinatus eccentrically contracted to decelerate the glenohumeral internal rotation during the serve. Ferretti and colleagues (1998) found that entrapment of the suprascapular nerve at the spinoglenoid notch is usually painless in volleyball players. Holzgraefe and colleagues (1994) also reported on elite volleyball players, finding suprascapular neuropathy in 33% and all players—in every case on the side of their smashing arm. Time duration of training (greater than 20 hours) was felt to be the most important factor, suggesting repetitive stretch of the nerve. Suprascapular neuropathies have also been reported with shoulder dislocations (Liveson 1984, Zoltan 1979).

AXILLARY NEUROPATHY

The axillary nerve is the last nerve to be given off by the posterior cord before it becomes the radial nerve. Axillary nerve fibers originate from the upper trunk and from cervical roots C5 and C6 (see figure 2.4, page 22). The axillary nerve innervates the deltoid and teres minor. It provides sensation to a small area, about the size of a silver dollar, just inferior to the lateral border of the acromion. The nerve courses posteriorly through the quadrangular space before innervating the deltoid and teres minor. Anatomic variations do exist and the nerve may divide before passing through the quadrangular space. The branch innervating the teres minor may also innervate the posterior deltoid separately.

Diagnosis

Patients with axillary nerve injuries have weakness in arm abduction, flexion, and extension—and, if the teres minor is involved, in shoulder external rotation. While isolated injury to the branch innervating the teres minor has also been identified (figure 3.8) (Potter 2000), the etiology and clinical significance of this observation is not yet established. Patients often do not notice the small area of decreased sensation along the proximal lateral aspect of the arm: Sometimes it is detected only in a careful sensory exam. The axillary nerve is injured in 9-18% of anterior shoulder dislocations (Artico 1991, Brown 1972, Hoyt 1967, Liveson 1984, Neviaser et al. 1988, Pasila et al. 1978).

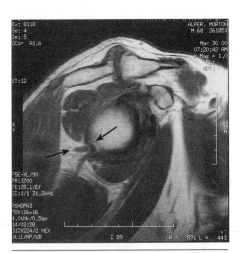

Figure 3.8 Sagittal T1-weighted image of the scapula, demonstrating isolated atrophy of the teres minor.

Hertel and colleagues (1998) devised the "deltoid extension lag sign" for diagnosis and grading of axillary nerve injuries. With the patient seated and the examiner behind her, the examiner elevates both arms nearly to full passive shoulder extension. The patient then relaxes her shoulders to a position of subacromial extension and is instructed to actively maintain the position of extension. A positive sign is a lag (or angular loss), which is quantified in five-degree increments. It can be beneficial to compare the contralateral limb. Using the deltoid extension lag sign to evaluate five individuals after traumatic injury from anterior shoulder dislocation, Hertel's group found that the magnitude of drop was negatively correlated with the functional status and recovery of the deltoid. In the "arm drop test" (as described in Hoppenfeld 1976), an individual actively abducts the arm to ninety degrees and then slowly adducts the arm. If there is a rotator cuff tear, the arm will not lower slowly or smoothly. If the person is able to hold the arm at 90 degrees of abduction, gentle pressure inferiorly on the forearm will cause the arm to drop to the side. The arm drop test (figure 3.9) may indicate injury to the axillary or suprascapular nerve or may represent rotator cuff pathology.

Tuckerman and Devlin (1996) performed MRI of the axillary nerve on three post-traumatic anterior shoulder dislocations. All three had Hill-Sachs lesions, two had labral abnormalities, and two had supraspinatus tendinitis. One patient demonstrated normal T1-weighted images and increased signal in the T2-weighted images of the deltoid and teres minor. The second demonstrated focal increased intensity of the T2-weighted images and normal proton-dense images. The third demonstrated severe atrophy of the teres minor and a normal deltoid, indicating an axillary

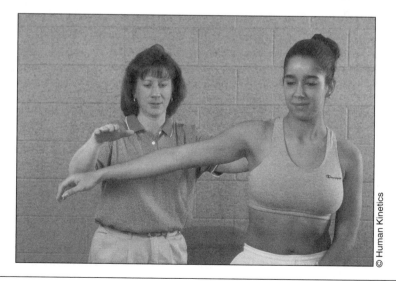

© Human Kinetics

Figure 3.9 The arm drop test.

nerve injury involving only the branch to the teres minor. Tuckerman and Devlin (1996) described MRI findings with denervation of the axillary nerve. Acutely, T1-weighted and proton-dense images are normal, and T2-weighted images demonstrate increased signal. Chronic injuries demonstrate increased intensity on standard spin-echo sequences because muscle is replaced by fat. MR images can also demonstrate fibrous bands in the quadrilateral space. Caution is warranted because neuritis and other neural abnormalities give similar findings.

Vascular compression syndromes can simulate axillary nerve injuries. One study of a thrower found that quadrilateral space compression of the posterior humeral circumflex artery during full abduction and external rotation of the shoulder led to weakness, numbness, and pain (Redler et al. 1986). EMG studies of the muscles innervated by the axillary nerve were normal.

Etiology

The quadrangular space formed by the teres minor, teres major, long head of the triceps, and humeral shaft is a common site of injury. Such injury may be caused by a direct blow to the posterior aspect of the shoulder/ upper-back region in wrestling or football (Bateman 1967). Axillary nerve injury has been reported in a football player hit in the shoulder by a helmet (Kessler and Uribe 1994); a boxer with blunt trauma to the axillary region; and an arm wrestler, probably from muscle compression (Goodman 1983). The axillary nerve can be constricted by fibrous bands (either idiopathic or from microtrauma) within the quadrangular space (Cahill and Palmer 1983), or by thickened hypertrophied muscles that form the quadrangular space (Kirby and Kraft 1972). Paladini and colleagues (1996) observed two volleyball players who had axillary neuropathies in their dominant arms without trauma—apparently resulting from repeated microtrauma and stretching of the nerve. A genetically small quadrilateral space and/or muscle hypertrophy could be predisposing factors. Chronic irritation of the axillary nerve by osteophytes at the posterior inferior glenoid margin has been reported in professional baseball players (Bennett 1941).

Perlmutter (1997) observed direct injury to the axillary nerve of football players as a result of their tackling opposing players, and in hockey players as a result of direct blows. Some athletes had associated contralateral cervical spine flexion and ipsilateral shoulder depression. Long-term follow-up of 11 of the athletes revealed no improvement in 3, moderate improvement in 2, and major improvement in 6. None had full recovery, but all had excellent shoulder function.

Neuralgic amyotrophy is another cause of an axillary neuropathy (Lancet 1980).

MUSCULOCUTANEOUS NEUROPATHY

The musculocutaneous nerve originates from the lateral cord of the brachial plexus and receives contribution from the C5 and C6 nerve roots. The nerve passes through and innervates the coracobrachialis muscle, a potential site of entrapment, and continues to the biceps and brachialis muscles before it becomes the lateral antebrachial cutaneous nerve. The lateral antebrachial cutaneous nerve courses distally to the elbow, runs under the bicipital aponeurosis, and then provides sensation to the lateral forearm.

Diagnosis

Injuries to the musculocutaneous nerve proximally (at about the level of the coracobrachialis) produce weakness of elbow flexion and forearm supination as well as loss of sensation in the lateral forearm. Distal injuries, at the level of the bicipital aponeurosis, usually cause only loss of sensation; however, with significant traction to the nerve at the elbow, there can be more proximal motor involvement.

Etiology

The musculocutaneous nerve can be injured by a stretch with anterior shoulder dislocations (Blom and Dahlback 1970, Corner et al. 1990, Jerosch et al. 1989, Liveson 1984) or by blunt injury (Liveson 1984), or it can be compressed within a hypertrophied coracobrachialis in weightlifters (Braddom 1978). Injury has been reported in a competitive rower (Mastaglia 1986). The lateral antebrachial cutaneous nerve is susceptible to stretch or compression within the coracobrachialis, or under the bicipital aponeurosis with elbow extension and forearm pronation (Davidson et al. 1998). These symptoms can be misdiagnosed as lateral epicondylitis—as reported in a tennis player (Bassett and Nunley 1982), a racquetball player (Felsenthal et al. 1984), and a swimmer doing the backstroke (Bassett and Nunley 1982), all of whom experienced only sensory abnormalities. Similar traction on the lateral antebrachial cutaneous nerve from throwing a football resulted in both sensory loss and motor deficits (Kim and Goodrich 1984).

CONCLUSION

Because most peripheral nerve injuries are uncommon, it is important to keep them in mind when evaluating an injured athlete and to always perform a neurologic examination. Athletes not wanting to be removed from participation may not divulge their entire history or symptoms. This can leave them at greater risk of reinjury or may impair potential neurologic recovery.

A 36-year-old right-handed amateur male golfer complained of right shoulder pain and weakness.

Over four weeks after a weekend golf game, he awoke with severe right-sided shoulder pain that was not related to neck position or shoulder motion and that was worse at night. The pain lasted 10 days. Once it began to subside, the patient noticed weakness, particularly with overhead motion. His wife observed the shoulder blade "sticking out." Although there was no recurrence of the pain, weakness in the shoulder persisted. There was no history of prior neck or shoulder injuries or pain. The patient denied any numbness or tingling.

Medical history: Negative.

Surgical history: Appendectomy.

Medications: None.

Social history: Denied use of tobacco, drank occasionally on weekends, worked as an attorney.

Family history: Negative for neuromuscular disorders.

Physical exam: Gross inspection revealed no focal muscle atrophy. Muscle bulk was symmetric. There were no muscle fasciculations. Passive range of motion in the shoulders was normal and symmetric. Active range of motion demonstrated reduced abduction in the right shoulder by 45 degrees compared to the left. Scapula lateral rotation was very limited with attempts to abduct. There was prominent medial scapula winging with arm flexion and/or abduction (see figure 3.3, page 44). Neck range of motion was normal. Spurling maneuver was negative. Strength was 4/5 with shoulder abduction. All other muscles 5/5. Reflexes 2+ in biceps, triceps, and brachioradialis. Sensory function was fully intact.

Radiographs: Neck and shoulder normal.

Electrodiagnostic studies: Nerve conduction studies were normal, including normal and symmetrical lateral antebrachial sensory amplitudes. EMG demonstrated complete denervation with 4+ fibrillation potentials and positive sharp waves in the serratus anterior. No motor units present.

Diagnosis: Long thoracic neuropathy as a variant of Parsonage-Turner Syndrome or brachial neuritis with complete denervation of the serratus anterior.

Management: Physical therapy to maintain motion in the glenohumeral joint. Strengthening of the rhomboids, levator scapula, and trapezius muscles while manually stabilizing the scapula and preventing scapular winging. No electrical stimulation was recommended initially but would be reconsidered at 3-4 months follow-up if there were no signs of reinnervation.

A 48-year-old right-handed female tennis player complained of right shoulder pain and weakness.

The patient, who played recreational tennis two or three times per week, noticed slowly progressive pain since she started playing more regularly outdoors two months previous to her visit. During that time she also noticed progressive weakness in the right shoulder that was most notable when serving and with overheads. Pain was worse with the same activities, but there was also pain when reaching behind her back and when she slept on the right shoulder at night. The patient denied any history of trauma, neck pain, or numbness and tingling. Her husband had noticed a difference in her shoulders from behind and believed there was a scalloped appearance around the right shoulder blade.

Medical history: Negative.

Surgical history: C-section.

Medications: Ibuprofen for shoulder pain.

Social history: Did not smoke; drank socially.

Family history: Negative for neuromuscular diseases.

Physical exam: There was focal atrophy of the supraspinatus and infraspinatus in the suprascapular and infrascapular fossa (see figure 3.5b, page 47). There were no muscle fasciculations. Passive range of motion was normal and symmetric in the shoulders. Active range of motion demonstrated loss of 60 degrees of abduction, associated with pain in the shoulder. Neck range of motion was normal. Spurling maneuver was negative. Strength was 3/5 in the external rotators of the shoulder and 4/5 in the supraspinatus. All other muscles were 5/5. Reflexes were 2+ in the biceps, brachioradialis, triceps, and pronator teres. Sensory function was fully intact. Neer and Hawkins impingement signs were both positive. Apprehension sign was negative. Shrug sign was negative. Stability exam of glenohumeral was normal and symmetric.

Radiographs: Neck and shoulder were normal.

Electrodiagnostic studies: Suprascapular nerve distal latencies to the supraspinatus and infraspinatus were prolonged and amplitudes were reduced. All other nerve conduction studies, including bilateral lateral antebrachial cutaneous sensory responses, were normal. There were 2+ fibrillation potentials and 3+ positive sharp waves in the supraspinatus and infraspinatus. Both had reduced recruitment but no polyphasics. All other muscles including the deltoid, rhomboid, biceps, and the cervical paraspinals were normal.

MRI of the shoulder demonstrated a ganglion in the suprascapular notch (see figure 3.6, page 48). There was denervation atrophy with

(continued)

Case Report 2 *(continued)*

fatty infiltration of the supraspinatus and infraspinatus seen on sagittal views of the scapula (see figure 3.7b, page 49).

Diagnosis: Suprascapular neuropathy secondary to compression of the suprascapular nerve in the suprascapular notch by a ganglion cyst. There was a secondary supraspinatus impingement syndrome.

Management and outcome: The patient was referred to an orthopedic surgeon for surgical decompression of the suprascapular nerve. The patient was sent for physical therapy postoperatively. At the 4-week follow-up the patient had no residual shoulder pain, but still had weakness in the supraspinatus and infraspinatus. At the 8-week follow-up the patient had normal strength in all muscles. At the 12-week follow-up the patient had resumed playing tennis and was pain-free.

REFERENCES

Agre J, Ash N, Cameron MC, House J. Suprascapular neuropathy after intensive progressive resistive exercise: case report. Arch Phys Med Rehabil 1987; 68(4):236-238.

Aiello I, Serra G, Traina GC, Tugnoli V. Entrapment of the suprascapular nerve at the spinoglenoid notch. Ann Neurol 1982; 12(3):314-316.

Alon M, Weiss S, Fishel B, Dekel S. Bilateral suprascapular nerve entrapment syndrome due to an anomalous transverse scapular ligament. Clin Orthop 1988; 234:31-33.

Antoniadis G, Richter H, Rath S, Braun V, Moese G. Suprascapular nerve entrapment: experience with 28 cases. J Neurosurg 1996; 85:1020-1025.

Artico M. Isolated lesion of the axillary nerve. Neurosurg 1991; 29:697-700.

Barnes R. Traction injuries of the brachial plexus in adults. J Bone Joint Surg Br 1949 Feb; 31(1):10-16.

Bassett F, Nunley J. Compression of the musculocutaneous nerve at the elbow. J Bone Joint Surg Am 1982; 64(7):1050-1052.

Bateman JE. Nerve injuries about the shoulder in sports. J Bone Joint Surg Am 1967; 49(4):785-792.

Bennett G. Shoulder and elbow lesions of the professional baseball pitcher. JAMA 1941; 117:510-514.

Bennett JB, Mehloff TL. Thoracic outlet syndrome. In: DeLee JL, Drez D (eds), *Orthopedic sports medicine: principles and practices,* volume I. Philadelphia: Saunders, 1994:794.

Biundo J, Harris M. Peripheral nerve entrapment, occupation-related syndromes and sports injuries, and bursitis. Curr Opin Rheumatol 1993; 5:224-229.

Blom S, Dahlback L. Nerve injuries in dislocations of the shoulder joint and fractures of the neck of the humerus. Acta Chirurg Scand 1970; 136:461-466.

Braddom R. Musculocutaneous nerve injury after heavy exercise. Arch Phys Med Rehabil 1978; 59:290.

Brown JT. Nerve injuries complicating dislocation of the shoulder. JBJS(Br) 1972; 34:526.

Bryan WJ, Wild JJ. Isolated infraspinatus atrophy: a common cause of posterior shoulder pain and weakness in throwing athletes. Am J Sports Med 1989; 17:130-131.

Cahill B, Palmer R. Quadrilateral space syndrome. J Hand Surg Am 1983; 8(1):65-69.

Callahan J, Scully T, Shapiro SA,Worth RM. Suprascapluar nerve entrapment. J Neurosurg 1991; 74:893-896.

Chen D, Gu Y, Lao J, Chen L. Dorsal scapular nerve compression. Atypical thoracic outlet syndrome. Chin Med J(Engl)1995; 108(8):582-585.

Clein LJ. Suprascapular entrapment neuropathy. J Neurosurg 1975; 43:337-342.

Corner NB, Milner SM, Macdonald R, Jubb M. Isolated musculocutaneous nerve lesion after shoulder dislocation. J R Army Med Corps 1990 Jun; 136(2):107-108.

Davidson JJ, Bassett FH, Nunley JA. Musculocutaneous nerve entrapment revisited. J Shoulder Elbow Surg 1998; 7:250-255.

Demirhan M, Imhoff A, Debski R, Patel P, Fu F, Woo S. The spinoglenoid ligament and its relationship to the suprascapular nerve. J Shoulder Elbow Surg 1998; 7:238-243.

England J, Tiel R. Costoclavicular mass syndrome. Muscle Nerve 1999; 22:412-418.

Fardin P, Negrin P, Daines R. The isolated paralysis of the serratus anterior muscle: clinical and electromyographical follow-up of 10 cases. Electromyogr Clin Neurophysiol 1978; 18:379-386.

Felsenthal G, Mondell D, Reischer M, Mack RH. Forearm pain secondary to compression syndrome of the lateral cutaneous nerve of the forearm. Arch Phys Med Rehabil 1984; 65:139-141.

Ferrante MA, Wilbourn AJ. The utility of various sensory nerve conduction responses in assessing brachial plexopathies. Muscle Nerve 1995 Aug; 18(8):879-889.

Ferretti A, Cerullo G, Russo G. Suprascapular neuropathy in volleyball players. J Bone Joint Surg Am 1987; 69:260-263.

Ferretti A, De Carli A, Fontana M. Injury of the suprascapular nerve at the spinoglenoid notch: the natural history of infraspinatus atrophy in volleyball players. Am J Sports Med 1998; 26(6):759-763.

Flaggman PD, Kelly JJ. Brachial plexus neuropathy. Arch Neurol 1980 Mar; 37:160-164.

Foo CL, Swann M. Isolated paralysis of the serratus anterior. J Bone Joint Surg Br 1983 Nov; 65(5):552-556.

Fritz R, Helms C, Steinbach LS, Genant HK. Suprascapular nerve entrapment: evaluation with MR imaging. Radiology 1992; 182:437-444.

Ganzhorn RW, Hocker JT, Horowitz M, Switzer HE. Suprascapular nerve entrapment. J Bone Joint Surg Am 1981; 63:492-494.

Garcia G, McQueen D. Bilateral suprascapular nerve entrapment syndrome. J Bone Joint Surg Am 1981; 63:491-492.

Glennon T. Isolated injury of the infraspinatus branch of the suprascapular nerve. Arch Phys Med Rehabil 1992; 73:201-202.

Goodman CE. Unusual nerve injuries in recreational activities. Am J Sports Med 1983; 11(4):224-227.

Goodman CE, Kenrick MM, Blum MV. Long thoracic nerve palsy: a follow-up study. Arch Phys Med Rehabil 1975 Aug; 56(8):352-355.

Goss CJ, (ed). *Gray's anatomy,* 29th edition. Philadelphia: Lea and Febiger, 1973:960-964.

Gregg JR, Labosky D, Harty M, Lotke P, Ecker M, DiStefano V, Das M. Serratus anterior paralysis in the young athlete. J Bone Joint Surg Am 1979; 61:825-832.

Hadley M, Sonntag V, Pittman H. Suprascapular nerve entrapment. J Neurosurg 1986; 64:843-848.

Hauser C, Martin W. Two additional cases of traumatic winged scapula occurring in the armed forces. JAMA 1943:667-668.

Henlin J, Rousselot J, Monnier G, Sevrin P, Bady B. Suprascapular nerve entrapment at the spinoglenoid notch [in French]. Rev Neurol (Paris) 1992; 148(5):362-367.

Hertel R, Lambert SM, Ballmer FT. The deltoid extension lag sign for diagnosis and grading of axillary nerve palsy. J Shoulder Elbow Surg 1998 Mar-Apr; 7(2):97-99.

Hirasawa Y, Sakakida K. Sports and peripheral nerve injury. Am J Sports Med 1983; 11:420-426.

Hirayama T, Takemitsu Y. Compression of the suprascapular nerve by a ganglion at the suprascapular notch. Clin Orthop 1981; 155:95-96.

Holzgraefe M, Kukowski B, Eggert S. Prevalence of latent and manifest suprascapular neuropathy in high-performance volleyball players. Br J Sports Med 1994; 28:177-179.

Hoppenfeld S. *Physical examination of the spine and extremities.* East Norwalk, CT: Appleton-Century-Crofts, 1976.

Hoyt W. Etiology of shoulder injuries in athletes. J Bone Joint Surg Am 1967 Jun; 49:755-766.

Ilfeld F, Holder H. Winged scapula: case occurring in soldier from knapsack. JAMA 1942 Oct:448-449.

Inokuchi W, Ogawa K, Horiuchi Y. Magnetic resonance imaging of suprascapular nerve palsy. J Shoulder Elbow Surg 1998; 7:223-227.

Jackson DL, Farrage J, Hynninen BC, Caborn DN. Suprascapular neuropathy in athletes: cases reports. Clin J Sports Med 1995; 5(2):134-137.

Jerosch J, Castro EH, Colemont J. A lesion of the musculocutaneous nerve: a rare complication of anterior shoulder dislocation. Acta Orthop Belg 1989; 55(2):230-232.

Jerosch L, Castro EH, Geske B. Damage of the long thoracic and dorsal scapular nerve after traumatic shoulder dislocation: case report and review of the literature [review]. Acta Orthop Belg 1990; 56(3-4):625-627.

Johnson DC. The upper extremity in swimming. In: Pettrone FA (ed), *Symposium on upper extremity injuries in athletes.* St. Louis: Mosby, 1986:36-46.

Johnson JTH, Kendall HO. Isolated paralysis of the serratus anterior muscle. J Bone Joint Surg Am 1955; 37(3):567-574.

Kaplan P. Electrodiagnostic confirmation of long thoracic nerve palsy. J Neurol Neurosurg Psychiatry 1980; 43:50-52.

Karas S. Thoracic outlet syndrome. Clin Sports Med 1990; 9:297-310.

Kessler K, Uribe J. Complete isolated axillary nerve palsy in college and professional football players: a report of six cases. Clin J Sports Med 1994; 4(4):272-274.

Khalili AA. Neuromuscular electrodiagnostic studies in entrapment neuropathy of the suprascapular nerve. Ortho Rev 1974; 3:27-28.

Kim S, Goodrich A. Isolated proximal musculocutaneous nerve palsy: case report. Arch Phys Med Rehabil 1984; 65:735-736.

Kirby J, Kraft G. Entrapment neuropathy of anterior branch of axillary nerve: report of case. Arch Phys Med Rehabil 1972; 53(7):338-340.

Kiss G, Komar J. Suprascapular nerve compression at the spinoglenoid notch. Muscle Nerve 1990; 13:556-557.

Kopell H, Thompson W. Pain and the frozen shoulder. Surg Gynecol Obstet 1959; 109:92-96.

Kukowski B. Suprascapular nerve lesion as an occupational neuropathy in a semiprofessional dancer. Arch Phys Med Rehabil 1993 Jul; 74(70):768-769.

Lancet. Neuralgic amyotrophy: still a clinical syndrome [editorial]. 1980; II(8197):729-730.

Laulund T, Fedders O, Sogaard I, Kornum M. Suprascapular nerve compression syndrome. Surg Neurol 1984; 22:308-312.

Leffert RD. Thoracic outlet syndrome and the shoulder. Clin Sports Med 1983; 2:439.

Liveson J. Nerve lesions associated with shoulder dislocation: an electrodiagnostic study of 11 cases. J Neurol Neurosurg Psychiatry 1984; 47:742-744.

Liveson J, Bronson M, Pollack M. Suprascapular nerve lesions at the spinoglenoid notch: report of three cases and review of the literature. J Neurol Neurosurg Psychiatry 1991; 54:241-243.

Logigian EL, McInnes JM, Berger AR, Busus NA, Lehrich JR, Shahani BT. Stretch-induced spinal accessory nerve palsy. Muscle Nerve 1988 Feb; 11(2):146-150.

Mastaglia F. Musculocutaneous neuropathy after strenuous physical activity. Med J Aust 1986; 145:153-154.

Mestdagh H, Drizenko A, Ghestem P. Anatomical basis of suprascapular nerve syndrome. Anat Clin 1981; 3:67-71.

Neviaser R, Neviaser T, Neviaser J. Concurrent rupture of the rotator cuff and anterior dislocation of the shoulder in the older patient. J Bone Joint Surg Am 1988; 70:1308-1311.

Osterman AL, Babhulkar S. Unusual compressive neuropathies of the upper limb. Orthop Clin of North Am 1996; 27(2):389-408.

Overpeck D, Ghormley R. Paralysis of the serratus magnus muscle. JAMA 1940; May: 1994-1996.

Paladini D, Dellantonio R, Cinti A, Angeleri F. Axillary neuropathy in volleyball players: report of two cases and literature review. J Neuro, Neurosurg, Psych 1996; 60:345-347.

Parsonage MJ, Turner JWA. Neuralgic amyotrophy: the shoulder-girdle syndrome. Lancet 1948; I:973-978.

Pasila M, Jaroma H, Kiviluoto O, Sundholm A. Early complications of primary shoulder dislocations. Acta Orthop Scand 1978; 49(3):260-263.

Perlmutter GS, Leffert RD, Zarins B. Direct injury to the axillary nerve in athletes playing contact sports. Am J Sports Med 1997; 25(1):65-68.

Polak JF, Jolesz FA, Adams DA. Magnetic resonance imaging of skeletal muscle. Prolongation of T1 and T2 subsequent to denervation. Invest Radiol 1988; 23:365-369.

Post M, Mayer J. Suprascapular nerve entrapment: diagnosis and treatment. Clin Orthop 1987; 223:126-136.

Potter H. Personal communication 2000.

Prescott MU, Zollinger RW. Alar scapula: an unusual surgical complication. Am J Surg 1944; 65:98-103.

Redler M, Ruland L, McCue F. Quadrilateral space syndrome in a throwing athlete. Am J Sports Med 1986; 14(6):511-513.

Rengachary S, Burr D, Lucas S, Hassanein KM, Mohn MP, Matzke H. Suprascapular entrapment neuropathy: a clinical, anatomical, and comparative study. Neurosurg 1979; 5(4):447-451.

Ringel S, Treihaft M, Carry M, Fisher R, Jacobs P. Suprascapular neuropathy in pitchers. Am J Sports Med 1990; 18(1):80-86.

Schultz J, Leonard J. Long thoracic neuropathy from athletic activity. Arch Phys Med Rehabil 1992; 73:87-90.

Smith AN. Suprascapular neuropathy in a collegiate pitcher. J Athl Train 1995; 30(1):43-46.

Steinman I. Painless infraspinatus atrophy due to suprascapular nerve entrapment. Arch Phys Med Rehabil 1988; 69:641-643.

Strukel R, Garrick J. Thoracic outlet compression in athletes. Am J Sports Med 1978; 6(2):35.

Sunderland S. The anatomy and physiology of nerve injury. Muscle Nerve 1990; 13:771-784.

Takagishi K, Maeda K, Ikeda T, Itoman M, Yamamoto M. Ganglion causing paralysis of the suprascapular nerve. Acta Orthop Scand 1991; 62(4):391-393.

Thompson R, Schneider W, Kennedy T. Entrapment neuropathy of the inferior branch of the suprascapular nerve by ganglion. Clin Orthop 1982 Jun; 166:185-187.

Torres-Ramos F, Biondo J. Suprascapular neuropathy during progressive resistive exercises in a cardiac rehabilitation program. Arch Phys Med Rehabil 1992; 73:1107-1111.

Travlos J, Goldberg I, Boome R. Brachial plexus lesions associated with dislocated shoulders. J Bone Joint Surg Br 1990; 72:68-71.

Tsairis P. Peripheral nerve injuries in athletes. In: Jordan BD, Tsairis P, Warren RF (eds), *Sports neurology*. Rockville, MD: Aspen 1989:180.

Tsairis P, Dyck P, Mulder D. Natural history of brachial plexus neuropathy. Arch Neurol 1972; 27:109-117.

Tuckerman G, Devlin T. Axillary nerve injury after anterior glenohumeral dislocation: MR findings in three patients. Am J Radiology 1996; 167:695-697.

Vastamaki M, Goransson H. Suprascapular nerve entrapment. Clin Orthop Relat Res 1993 Dec; 297:135-143.

White S, Witten C. Long thoracic nerve palsy in a professional ballet dancer. Am J Sports Med 1993; 21(4):626-628.

Wilbourn AJ. Electrodiagnostic testing of neurologic injuries in athletes. Clin Sports Med 1990; 9(2):229-245.

Woodhead A. Paralysis of the serratus anterior in a world class marksman. Am J Sports Med 1985; 13(5):359-362.

Wright TA. Accessory spinal nerve injury. Clin Orthop 1975; 108:15-18.

Zoltan J. Injury to the suprascapular nerve associated with anterior dislocation of the shoulder: case report and review of the literature. J Trauma 1979; 19(3):203-206.

Zuckerman J, Polonshy L, Edelson G. Suprascapular nerve palsy in a young athlete. Bull Hosp Jt Dis 1993; 53(2):11-12.

4

Distal
Upper-Extremity
Nerve Injuries

Scott F. Nadler, DO

Upper-extremity nerve injuries at the level of the elbow—particularly of the ulnar nerve—are well documented in sports medicine. Most are the result of improper biomechanics, overexertion, local trauma, or an unknown congenital anomaly. Early neurologic symptoms may initially be ignored until there is an alteration or impairment in performance and function. An understanding of the anatomy and kinesiology of the structures within the elbow, forearm, and wrist is essential for proper diagnosis and treatment.

MEDIAN NERVE

The median nerve is the most commonly injured nerve in the wrist. This injury must be carefully differentiated from injuries within the forearm, which also may occur in competitive athletes.

Anatomy and Etiology

The median nerve receives contributions from both medial (C8-T1 roots) and lateral cords (C5-C7 roots) (figure 4.1). The nerve travels distally across the medial aspect of the arm and enters the forearm between the two heads of the pronator teres. The median nerve then travels underneath the flexor digitorum superficialis—usually giving off the anterior interosseous nerve, a purely motor branch, as it passes. Occasionally, the anterior interosseous branch can branch off the median nerve either above the elbow or further

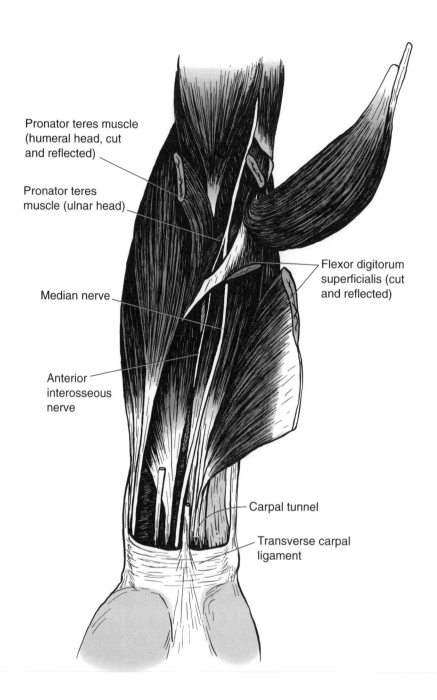

Pronator teres muscle
(humeral head, cut
and reflected)

Pronator teres
muscle (ulnar head)

Median nerve

Anterior
interosseous
nerve

Flexor digitorum
superficialis (cut
and reflected)

Carpal tunnel

Transverse carpal
ligament

Figure 4.1 Median nerve anatomy.

distal in the forearm. The main trunk of the median then travels distally down the forearm and through the carpal tunnel. The carpal tunnel is an enclosed space formed dorsally by the carpal bones of the wrist and medially/laterally by the overlying transverse carpal ligament.

A bony spur arising 3-6 cm from the medial epicondyle, along with an attached fibrous or fibro-osseus ligament (ligament of Struthers), is found in 0.7% to 2.7% of the general population (Hrdlicka 1923) and is the usual cause of median nerve compression in this region of the arm. Entrapment of the median nerve at the ligament of Struthers produces pain with repetitive flexion and extension of the elbow (Bilge et al. 1990, Suranyi 1983).

The pronator syndrome includes three potential causes of median nerve entrapment within the proximal forearm. This can occur from thickening of the bicipital aponeurosis (lacertus fibrosus), from fibrous thickening or hypertrophy of the origin of the pronator teres, or from compression by a thickening of the flexor digitorum superficialis (sublimis bridge). The pronator syndrome has been reported in competitive drivers, weightlifters, and tennis players from repetitive pronation/supination or rapid eccentric contractions of the forearm (Regan and Morrey 1994).

The anterior interosseous nerve can also be compressed by the fibrous edge of the flexor digitorum superficialis, by the deep head of the pronator teres, or by the forearm musculature from overuse or external compression, including direct trauma. Entrapment has been reported in a tennis player from an overtight counterforce brace (Enzenauer and Nordstrom 1991).

Carpal tunnel syndrome (CTS), or median nerve compression at the carpal tunnel, is the most common type of peripheral nerve entrapment in the general population. It has been reported in tennis and baseball as a result of repetitive wrist flexion and extension (Pianka and Hershman 1990), and in athletes exposed to excessive pressure over the palmar aspect of the hand. Bilateral CTS has been reported in a competitive cyclist, caused by compression against the handlebars or from hyperextension of the wrist (Braithwaite 1992). Carpal tunnel entrapment of the median nerve occurred in 46% of 28 wheelchair athletes (Burnham and Steadward 1994). The carpal tunnel syndrome produces symptoms localized to the hand.

A disorder called "bowler's thumb" results from compression of the palmar digital nerve of the thumb and is an infrequent source of distal median nerve entrapment. Dobyns and colleagues (1972) reviewed 17 cases of bowler's thumb caused by compression of the digital nerve by the thumbhole of the bowling ball. Bowler's thumb has also been described in baseball players secondary to a direct contusion to the digital nerve (Belsky and Millender 1980). Entrapment of the median digital nerve to the index finger has also been described in tennis players from compression of the racquet handle (Naso 1984).

Diagnosis

Nocturnal symptoms are common in patients with CTS and are relieved by shaking of the hand. This is referred to as a "flick sign" and is positive in 93% of those with CTS (Pryse-Phillips 1984). Weakness of the abductor pollicis brevis (APB) appears a variable amount of time after sensory loss and may lead to atrophy of the *thenar* eminence. Several tests have been used to help diagnose CTS. Tinel's sign entails tapping over the carpal canal to cause a reproduction of numbness and tingling. Phalen's test, in which both hands are maximally flexed downward and held together, also reproduces symptoms (figure 4.2). Tinel's sign and Phalen's test are positive in about 60-80% of those with CTS. Heller and colleagues (1986) found Tinel's and Phalen's to have a sensitivity of 60-67% and a specificity of 59-77%. The carpal compression test, in which the examiner presses over the tunnel for 30 seconds, is positive in up to 90% of people with CTS (Durkham 1991) (figure 4.3).

thenar—Related to the fleshy mass on the lateral side of the palm.

The pronator syndrome occurs via entrapment of the median nerve in three locations that often can be differentiated on physical examination. Symptoms from entrapment at the ligament of Struthers and the lacertus fibrosus can be accentuated by resisted full-elbow flexion or resisted supination. Compression from the pronator teres and the flexor digitorum superficialis can be accentuated with resisted forearm pronation and resisted middle-finger flexion, respectively (Eversmann 1992, Hartz et al. 1981, Martinelli et al. 1982). Symptoms of the pronator syndrome include hyperesthesia and *paresthesia* of the hand in a median nerve distribution,

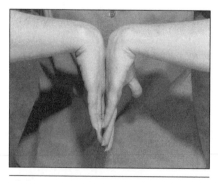

Figure 4.2 Phalen's test.

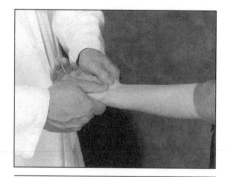

Figure 4.3 Carpal compression test.

weakness of the median and anterior interosseous innervated muscles distal to the entrapment, and pain/tenderness in the proximal forearm (Eversmann 1992, Hartz et al. 1981).

> **paresthesia**—An abnormal touch sensation, such as burning or prickling, in the absence of an external stimulus.

A clinician can isolate digital nerve injury by a careful sensory examination on both radial and ulnar sides of the digits, looking for areas of *hypesthesia* and *dysesthesia*. An unusual cause of median nerve involvement involves emboli being thrown to the vascular arcades of the hand from aneurysms of the axillary artery in major league baseball pitchers (Kee et al. 1995).

> **hypesthesia**—Diminished sensitivity to stimulation.

> **dysesthesia**—A condition whereby disagreeable sensation is produced by ordinary stimulation.

Indications and Applications of Electrodiagnostic Testing

Median nerve entrapment at the carpal tunnel can be identified with electrodiagnostic studies. Antidromic sensory nerve conduction studies are more likely than orthodromic motor nerve conduction studies to reveal abnormalities (Dumitru 1994). Sensory or mixed nerve conduction velocities across the carpal tunnel are slowed. Clinicians often compare median distal latencies to the digital ulnar or superficial radial nerve distal latency. There may be diminution or absence of median sensory nerve action potentials (SNAPs). Reduced amplitude of the compound muscle action potential (CMAP) to the abductor pollicis brevis can be found in more severe injury (Dumitru 1994). Needle electromyography can help ascertain whether axonal injury has occurred. In CTS, the finding of fibrillations or positive sharp waves in the APB would be considered prognostically poor for successful conservative management. Electrodiagnostic studies can help differentiate between median entrapment at the wrist and pronator syndrome, where the nerve is entrapped in the proximal forearm. Segmental motor nerve conduction studies allow isolation of median nerve compression when it occurs at the level of the pronator teres. Fibrillations or positive sharp waves in the forearm flexors localize the median nerve injury proximal to the wrist.

Prevention and Rehabilitation

Because most athletes can't participate with restricted wrist motion, it is difficult to prevent injury to the median nerve. Compression occurs secondary to several factors—including vibration, awkward positioning of the wrist and hand (hyperflexion or extension), local pressure at the base of the palm, and forceful hand motions (Ekenvall et al. 1989). Symptoms are produced not by direct mechanical trauma, but by pressures within the enclosed space that lead to intraneural ischemia. Gelberman and colleagues (1981) found normal pressures within the canal to be 2.5 mm Hg with 90 degrees of wrist flexion or extension. In people with CTS, pressure was 32 mm Hg in the neutral plane and increased to 94 mm Hg with 90 degrees of wrist flexion and 110 mm Hg with 90 degrees of extension. Pressures greater than 30 mm Hg slow intraneural blood flow.

Treatment initially focuses on reducing inflammation and the concomitant swelling-associated *tendinitis* of the long and short finger flexors that may narrow the canal. Oral nonsteroidal anti-inflammatories or local steroid injection into the carpal tunnel may greatly reduce pain and swelling. Protective splinting in neutral to 15 degrees of extension can also help prevent intraneural ischemia. Goodman and Gilliat (1961) reported that 67% of 51 patients treated with splinting alone were free of symptoms in a 6-30 month follow-up. Giannini and colleagues (1991) reported that therapeutic steroid injection relieved symptoms in 90% of CTS patients within 45 days; six months postinjection there was still 93% relief. Gelberman and colleagues (1980) found only 40% to be symptom-free 18 months after therapeutic steroid injection. Criteria proposed for conservative management include

- symptoms present for less than one year,
- no weakness or atrophy,
- lack of denervation noted on electrodiagnostic studies, and
- mild prolongation of distal latency on nerve conduction studies (McGrath 1984).

Characteristics predictive of poor outcome from conservative measures include

- symptoms present longer than one year,
- complaints of weakness and constant numbness in digits 1, 2, and 3,
- objective weakness of the abductor pollicis brevis,
- thenar atrophy,
- two-point discrimination greater than 6 mm,

- marked delay of distal median motor and sensory latency, and
- electromyographic evidence of fibrillation potentials in the abductor pollicis brevis (Gelberman et al. 1980).

Electrodiagnostic testing should be considered to make a definitive diagnosis, to quantify severity, and to prognosticate outcome. When conservative treatment fails, surgical decompression of the carpal tunnel with division of the transverse carpal ligament should be considered.

The pronator syndrome is not common, but may occur in athletes whose sports require repetitive pronation or supination, and among weightlifters (Eversmann 1992). Treatment requires reduction of inflammation via anti-inflammatories, along with modification of activity to avoid pronation/supination. Stretching and strengthening of the involved forearm musculature may help reduce median nerve compression and prevent further injury. If conservative treatment fails, surgical resection of fascial bands, tendinous arches, or the ligament of Struthers may be necessary.

Digital nerve injury can be limited by protection of the involved digit with a padded glove along with measures to reduce inflammation.

ULNAR NERVE

As it courses around the elbow, the ulnar nerve may be subject to significant traction forces in any overhead sport requiring high velocity use of the arm, such as in baseball, tennis, and volleyball. It is important not to overlook injuries to the ulnar nerve in the hand, where it can be subjected to compressive forces.

Anatomy and Etiology

The ulnar nerve is the terminal direct branch of the medial cord (C8-T1 roots) of the brachial plexus. The nerve travels down the medial aspect of the arm in close proximity to the median nerve. The ulnar nerve courses posteriorly in the distal arm and passes underneath the medial head of the triceps and an overlying fascial structure, the arcade of Struthers, which is anatomically present in about 70% of people (Wadsworth and Williams 1973). The nerve passes behind the medial epicondyle of the elbow in the ulnar groove and enters the forearm under the proximal portion of the flexor carpi ulnaris (FCU). A ligamentous/fibrous arch (the arcuate ligament) between the two heads of the FCU overlies the ulnar nerve, forming the cubital tunnel. The nerve travels down the forearm underneath the FCU, passing over the flexor digitorum profundus (FDP). The ulnar nerve innervates both the FCU and the FDP to digits 4 and 5 proximally in the forearm. The ulnar nerve gives off two sensory branches: the palmar cutaneous nerve approximately 8-10 cm proximal to the wrist, and the dorsal ulnar cutaneous nerve 5-6 cm proximal to the wrist. The ulnar nerve proper then travels through Guyon's canal, a space formed by the hamate and pisiform carpal bones enclosed by the overlying carpal ligament (the floor is formed from the pisohamate ligament and the roof from the aponeurosis of the distal FCU tendon as it attaches to the hamate). It divides into a sensory nerve that supplies sensation to the 4th and 5th digits and two motor branches that innervate muscles of the *hypothenar* eminence, both palmar and dorsal interossei, and the lumbricals to digits 3, 4, and 5 within the hand.

> **hypothenar**—Related to the fleshy mass on the medial side of the palm.

Of the three terminal nerves of the upper extremity, the ulnar nerve is probably the most susceptible to athletic injury (Weinstein and Herring 1992). Injury to the ulnar nerve most commonly occurs at the elbow region. In the proximal arm, ulnar injury is rare. Dangles and Bilos (1980) described compression of the ulnar nerve produced by hypertrophy of the medial head of weightlifters' triceps. Ulnar nerve injury at the medial epicondyle has been described in Little League pitchers—attributed to faulty biomechanics that produce excessive valgus stress at the elbow and traction of the ulnar nerve (Hang 1981). Glousman (1990) described recurrent ulnar nerve subluxation in elbows of overhead athletes. The cubital tunnel has been implicated in baseball pitchers as a potential entrapment site (Jobe and Nuber 1986). Elbow flexion induces stretch in the arcuate ligament as the distance between the olecranon and medial epicondyle increases by 1 cm (Osborne 1970). Repetitive flexion and extension of the elbow may chronically irritate the arcuate ligament, resulting in hypertrophy and further compressing the ulnar nerve (MacNicol 1979). Hypertrophy of the FCU muscle was reported in a golfer as a possible site of ulnar nerve entrapment (Campbell et al. 1988). The ulnar nerve can also be compressed as it passes through Guyon's canal. A variable pattern of motor or sensory loss can occur depending on whether the deep ulnar, superficial ulnar, or hypothenar branch is involved. This compressive neuropathy has been reported in bicycle riders and in paraplegic marathon wheelchair racers (Dozono et al. 1995, Eckman et al. 1975).

Diagnosis

Athletes with cubital tunnel syndrome present with a number of symptoms, including numbness, tingling, or paresthesias to the 4th and 5th digits; weakness of grip strength; wasting of ulnar-innervated hand intrinsics; and later, a "clawing" of the hand. Profound ulnar nerve injury may be identified by Wartenberg's sign—inability of the individual to adduct the fifth digit (figure 4.4). Froment's sign may also be present, in which the individual is barely able to adduct the thumb and cannot hold a piece of paper between thumb and index finger when the paper is tugged by the clinician (figure 4.5). Increased elbow flexion causes the arcuate ligament to become taut, the FCU to tighten, and the ulnar collateral ligament to buckle and encroach into the tunnel (Feindel and Stratford 1958, Vanderpool et al. 1968). Apfelberg and Larson (1973) observed a 55% narrowing of the cubital tunnel during elbow flexion. The elbow flexion test (maintaining the fully flexed elbow for one minute) provokes paresthesias in an ulnar distribution (Rayam et al. 1992). Applying pressure to the ulnar nerve with the elbow fully flexed is a sensitive measure of cubital tunnel syndrome (Novak et al. 1994).

Compression of the ulnar nerve at Guyon's canal may cause variable clinical findings depending on where within the canal the nerve is injured. Such compression can cause sensory loss, motor loss, or both. Focal pressure applied between the pisiform and the hook of the hamate may induce symptoms.

Indications and Applications of Electrodiagnostic Testing

Electrodiagnostic testing is invaluable in localizing pathology. SNAPs obtained from stimulation distal to the site of injury may be normal if the mechanism of injury is conduction block or focal demyelination. Stimulation proximally may help demonstrate a reduced sensory amplitude or temporal dispersion.

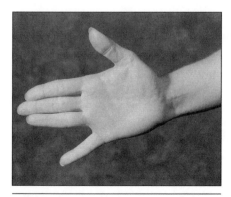

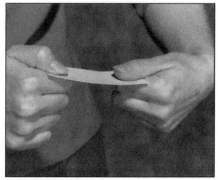

Figure 4.4 Wartenberg's sign (inability to adduct the 5th digit in an individual with an ulnar neuropathy).

Figure 4.5 Froment's sign. In an individual with an ulnar neuropathy, the flexor pollicis longus substitutes for weakness of the adductor pollicis.

Motor nerve conduction studies are the most popular technique for identifying ulnar nerve involvement. CMAPs are recorded from hypothenar muscles in response to stimulation of the ulnar nerve below and above the elbow. Slowing of conduction velocity more than 10 m/s or amplitude drop in excess of 20-30% is diagnostic of ulnar nerve injury (Dumitru 1994). Side-to-side differences in latency, conduction velocity, and amplitude may provide additional information for motor and sensory studies (Chang et al. 1996). The inching technique can be utilized for more specific localization of the site of involvement: The electromyographer performs stimulations at 1-cm increments above and below the elbow, looking for a focal reduction in amplitude, temporal dispersion, or an increase in latency greater than 0.4 ms (Kanakamedala et al. 1988).

In the wrist region, SNAPs can be obtained from the dorsal and palmar cutaneous branches to localize the site of injury in or about the wrist. Normal and symmetric dorsal ulnar cutaneous sensory amplitudes suggest that nerve injury is at a level distal to the wrist. In addition, segmental conduction velocities can be performed across Guyon's canal. Needle electromyography can further assist in localization; it can also identify whether significant axonal injury has occurred and whether there is reinnervation present.

Prevention and Rehabilitation

In the athletic setting, the first step in management is to reduce extrinsic compression of the ulnar nerve via avoidance or padding. In sports requiring repeated elbow flexion, modification of biomechanics may be necessary. It is essential that the athlete avoid valgus overload and strengthen the surrounding musculature in order to stabilize the elbow joint. Nonoperative management includes anti-inflammatory medication and splinting of the elbow at night to prevent elbow flexion greater than 60 degrees. Seror (1993) reported 100% subjective improvement in 22 patients with cubital tunnel syndrome who for six months used a night splint that prevented flexion beyond 60 degrees. Nerve conduction velocity across the elbow at a mean follow-up of 11.3 months was improved by 6.5 m/s in motor nerves and 9.5 m/s in sensory nerves in 16 of 17 patients. Various nerve gliding techniques can also be utilized to improve nerve mobility and reduce traction.

RADIAL NERVE

The radial nerve innervates the wrist extensors, which provide power for the gripping necessary in many sports. Proximal injuries result in significant disability, while injury about the wrist may result in no disability to the competitive athlete.

Anatomy and Etiology

The radial nerve is the continuation of the posterior cord (C5-T1 roots) of the brachial plexus (figure 4.6). The nerve emerges in the upper arm between the long and lateral heads of the triceps, in the posterior aspect of

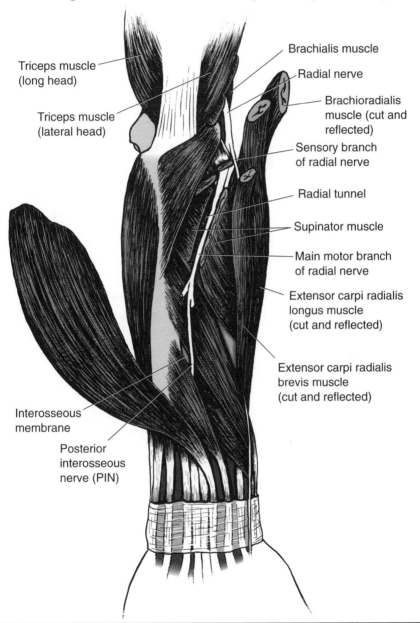

Triceps muscle (long head)

Triceps muscle (lateral head)

Brachialis muscle

Radial nerve

Brachioradialis muscle (cut and reflected)

Sensory branch of radial nerve

Radial tunnel

Supinator muscle

Main motor branch of radial nerve

Extensor carpi radialis longus muscle (cut and reflected)

Extensor carpi radialis brevis muscle (cut and reflected)

Interosseous membrane

Posterior interosseous nerve (PIN)

Figure 4.6 Radial nerve anatomy.

the upper arm. It wraps around the spiral groove of the humerus, traveling medially to laterally to emerge between the brachioradialis and the brachialis on the lateral aspect of the elbow. A sensory branch given off at this point travels distally toward the radial aspect of the wrist. The main motor branch, the posterior interosseous nerve (PIN), passes under the supinator, through the radial tunnel, and courses along the interosseous membrane toward the wrist.

The radial nerve is rarely a site of focal neuropathy in athletes. A proximal entrapment of the radial nerve occasionally occurs at the level of the spiral groove with forceful elbow extension (Manske 1977, Mitsunaga and Nakano 1988, Prochaska 1993). High radial nerve palsy secondary to a fibrous arch from the long head of the triceps has been described in a tennis player after overexertion (Prochaska et al. 1993). Previous studies had demonstrated a similar high radial neuropathy from a fibrous arch at the border of the lateral head of the triceps (Manske 1977, Mitsunaga and Nakano 1988). The precipitating factor in both types of proximal involvement was felt to be forceful elbow extension, as occurs with the overhead serve in tennis.

The PIN can be entrapped at three sites: by fibrous bands from the radiocapitellar joint, at the proximal fibrous origin of the supinator (arcade of Frohse), and at the tendinous origin of the extensor carpi radialis brevis. Roles and Maudsley (1972) demonstrated, via surgical exploration, that entrapment of the posterior interosseous nerve can cause refractory tennis elbow. Repetitive pronation and supination, as well as eccentric contraction of the forearm musculature, were implicated as the precipitating cause. Younge and Moise (1994) reported compression of the PIN by normal enlargement of the supinator or extensor carpi radialis brevis during exercise. The radial nerve sensory branch is an unusual source of focal sensory neuropathy at the wrist that may be involved following blunt trauma to the wrist in contact sports.

Diagnosis

Injury to the radial nerve is fairly uncommon, but can present with a confusing picture. Injury to the radial nerve in the region of the triceps typically causes sensory loss in the dorsal aspect of digits 1-3 and the radial 1/2 aspect of digit 4, in addition to a thin patch in the midline of the dorsal forearm. Motor loss with proximal radial nerve injury typically spares the triceps but causes weakness of the supinator, brachioradialis, wrist extensors, and digital extensors at the metacarpophalangeal (MCP) joint. Involvement of the PIN causes a classic clinical picture. The superficial radial nerve has split from the main trunk of the radial nerve prior to its entrance through the supinator. Injury at this location may produce deep forearm pain as well as wrist pain, since the PIN supplies articular branches to the carpus. Additionally, branches to the extensor carpi radialis brevis (ECRB) and the extensor carpi radialis longus (ECRL) have split prior to the supinator. These two anatomical occurrences help to differentiate injury above or below the elbow. Individuals with injury to the PIN present with no loss of sensation; and when wrist extension occurs, it does so in radial deviation because the extensor carpi ulnaris is no longer active and the ECRL and ECRB go unopposed. Complete wrist drop and lack of sensation to the top of the hand and wrist imply more proximal injury at or about the distal arm or proximal elbow region. Motor loss includes all finger extensors at the MCP joint and the extensor carpi ulnaris, causing the wrist to deviate radially with extension. "Cheiralgia paresthetica," or involvement of the distal superficial radial sensory branch at the wrist, causes numbness alone in the dorsal aspect of digits 1-3 and the radial 1/2 of digit 4.

Indications and Applications of Electrodiagnostic Testing

Involvement of the posterior interosseous nerve results in a normal SNAP when the superficial radial nerve is tested at the wrist. Motor nerve conduction studies show a drop in amplitude when stimulating proximal to the site of injury above the elbow and recording with surface electrodes over the extensor indicis propius. Evaluating the configuration of the waveform may provide additional information, as changes in morphology may indicate focal injury. It may be difficult to accurately assess amplitude drop when using needle pickup in the extensor indicis propius, as needle position in the muscle may vary. Needle position may be confirmed by contracting the muscle while monitoring for needle movement. Despite the limitations on assessment of amplitude, a sharper take-off can be obtained with a needle-recording electrode, making the assessment of conduction velocity more accurate. Needle electromyography may help identify involved musculature and aid in mapping the site of involvement. Involvement of the superficial radial nerve at the wrist can be identified by performing sensory nerve conduction studies and identifying a drop in SNAP amplitude or significant latency changes.

Prevention and Rehabilitation

The initial step in treatment is to limit pain that may be present in the extensor musculature. This can be accomplished with nonsteroidal anti-inflammatory medication, or sometimes with a low-dose antidepressant (amitryptiline). Individuals with involvement of the posterior interosseous nerve should modify their activities appropriately while the nerve is compromised. The wrist extensors bring great power to normal grasping, and injury leads to overuse of the wrist and finger flexors. In addition, compensatory biomechanics may lead to overuse of the rotator cuff and scapular stabilizers. Appropriate splinting in approximately 30 degrees of wrist extension allows for more normal activation of the hand intrinsics. Assuming that no space-occupying lesions exist in the forearm, the clinical picture should be monitored for approximately 8-12 weeks in hopes that spontaneous recovery will occur. If persistent weakness remains, further work-up should be considered, as these entrapments are uncommon. Surgical exploration should be considered in the event of poor response to conservative care.

CONCLUSION

Injury or entrapment of the median, ulnar, or radial nerves may result in significant disability to the competitive athlete. A comprehensive assessment should include a history (including the mechanism of injury), physical examination, and, when appropriate, electrodiagnostic testing to more completely elucidate the injury and prognosticate recovery. While most injuries respond to conservative measures, in rare circumstances surgical exploration is appropriate for those with evidence of focal entrapment causing conduction block and or axonal injury.

Case Report 1

A 19-year-old college wrestler presented with right hand numbness that developed insidiously after a match.

Medical history: The wrestler reported grabbing his opponent's arm and feeling a sharp pain radiating down his forearm toward his 5th finger. He immediately let go and completed the match. He noted a continuation of numbness (that has persisted) into the last two digits. He denied any neck pain.

Surgical history: None.

Medications: None.

Social history: None.

Family history: None.

Physical examination: Neck motion was full in all planes. Shoulder, elbow, and wrist motions were full. Strength was 5/5 in bilateral upper extremities. Sensation was decreased in the ulnar distribution on the right. Reflexes were normal. Tinel's and elbow flexion test were positive on the right.

Radiographs: None.

Electrodiagnostic testing: Consistent with slowing across the cubital tunnel with mild amplitude decrease 2 cm distal to the medial epicondyle. Needle evaluation was negative.

Diagnosis: Cubital tunnel syndrome with probable early subluxation of ulnar nerve.

Management and outcome: The patient was placed on anti-inflammatory medication and was instructed to use an elbow pad during all activities. The numbness and tingling resolved and he had no recurrence of symptoms.

A 45-year-old mountain climber presented with pain, which has come on insidiously over the past several months, in his wrist associated with numbness in the top of his hand.

Medical history: He described increasing his strength-training program in anticipation of an upcoming climbing trip. More specifically, he described adding push-ups and rowing exercises on a daily basis to an already extensive aerobic and conditioning program. He denied neck pain.

Surgical history: None.

Medications: None.

Social history: None.

Family history: None.

Physical examination: Cervical, shoulder, and elbow ranges of motion were full. Wrist and finger extension were weak in the 4/5 range. Reflexes were normal. Sensation was decreased to pin prick on the dorsal aspect of the hand and digits 1-3 in the superficial radial distribution. The ulnar distribution was normal. Spurling's maneuver was negative.

Radiographs: None.

Electrodiagnostic testing: Consistent with conduction block of the radial nerve with stimulation just proximal to the insertion of the lateral triceps and pick-up at the extensor indicis proprius. No axonal involvement was noted on electromyography.

Diagnosis: Radial neuropathy at the lateral head of the triceps.

Management and outcome: The patient was placed on anti-inflammatory medication and instructed to discontinue all triceps strengthening activities. Six weeks later there was a complete resolution of the neuropathy, and conduction block was no longer present on nerve conduction studies.

Case Report 3

A 27-year-old amateur golfer presented with a four-week history of right forearm pain and numbness in the hand.

Medical history: The golfer reported that the pain began after he played in the rain and has subsequently worsened. He noted that two days previous to his appointment, after making a "divot," he had the immediate onset of sharp pain radiating into his hand. He denied weakness and reported that the numbness was present consistently throughout the day.

Surgical history: None.

Medications: None.

Social history: None.

(continued)

Case Report 3 *(continued)*

Family history: None.

Physical examination: Range of motion was full in the cervical, shoulder, elbow, and wrist regions. Strength was full in all muscles tested. Reflexes were normal. Sensation was decreased to pin prick in lateral three 1/2 digits along with the thenar eminence.

Radiographs: None.

Electrodiagnostic testing: Nerve conduction studies were normal. Needle electromyography was consistent with axonal involvement of the median nerve; fibrillations were noted in the abductor pollicis brevis, flexor digitorum superficialis, and flexor digitorum profundus, with sparing of the pronator teres.

Diagnosis: Pronator syndrome.

Management: The patient was placed on a program of occupational therapy to strengthen forearm musculature and to perform nerve gliding exercises. He was instructed to avoid golfing activities during the course of therapy. Over the course of the next six months, the numbness and forearm discomfort abated and he resumed all previous activities.

REFERENCES

Apfelberg DB, Larson SJ: Dynamic anatomy of the ulnar nerve at the elbow. *Plastic Reconstr Surg*, 51:76-81; 1973.

Belsky M, Millender LH: Bowler's thumb in a baseball player. *Orthopedics*, 3:122; 1980.

Bilge T, Yalaman O, Bilge S, Cokneseli B, Barut S: Entrapment neuropathy of the median nerve at the level of the ligament of Struthers. *Neurosurg*, 27(5):787-789; 1990.

Braithwaite IJ: Bilateral median nerve palsy in a cyclist. *Br J Sport Med*, 26(1):27-28; 1992.

Burnham RS, Steadward R: Upper extremity peripheral nerve entrapments among wheelchair athletes: prevalence, location and risk factor. *Arch Phys Med Rehabil*, 75(5): 519-524; 1994.

Campbell WW, Pridgeon RM, Salmi SK: Entrapment neuropathy of the ulnar nerve at its point of exit from the flexor carpi ulnaris muscle. *Muscle Nerve*, 11:467-470; 1988.

Chang AS, Dilingham TR, Yu KF: Statistical methods of computing reference values for side to side differences in nerve conduction studies. *Am J Phys Med Rehabil*, 75(6):437-442; 1996.

Dangles CJ, Bilos ZJ: Ulnar neuritis in a world champions weightlifter. *Am J Sports Med*, 8:443-445; 1980.

Dobyns JH, O'Brien ET, Linschied RL, Farrow GM: Bowler's thumb diagnosis and treatment: a review of seventeen cases. *JBJS (A)*, 54:751; 1972.

Dozono K, Hachisuka K, Hatada K, Ogata H: Peripheral neuropathies in the upper extremities of paraplegic wheelchair marathon racers. *Paraplegia*, 33(4):208-211; 1995.

Dumitru D: *Electrodiagnostic medicine: focal peripheral neuropathies.* Philadelphia: Hanley & Belfus 1994; 851-927.

Durkam JA: New diagnostic test for CTS. *J Bone Joint Surg,* 73A:535-538; 1991.

Eckman PB, Perlstein G, Altrocchi PH: Ulnar neuropathy in bicycle riders. *Arch Neurol,* 32:130-131; 1975.

Ekenvall G, Gemne, Tegne R: Correspondence between neurological symptoms and outcome of quantitative sensory testing in hand-arm vibration syndrome. *Br J Ind Med,* 46:570-574; 1989.

Enzenauer RJ, Nordstrom DM: Anterior interosseous nerve syndrome associated with forearm band treatment of lateral epicondylitis. *Orthopedics,* 14(7):788-790; 1991.

Eversmann WW: Proximal median nerve compression. *Hand Clin,* 8(2):307-315; 1992.

Feindel W, Stratford J: The role of the cubital tunnel in tardy ulnar palsy. *Clin J Surg,* 1:287-300; 1958.

Gelberman RH, Aronson D, Weisman MH: Carpal tunnel syndrome: results of a prospective trial of steroid injection and splinting. *J Bone Joint Surg,* 62:1181-1184; 1980.

Gelberman RH, Hergenroeder PT, Hargens AR, Lundborg GN, Akeson WH: The carpal tunnel syndrome: a study of carpal canal pressures. *J Bone Joint Surg,* 36A:380; 1981.

Giannini F, Passero S, Cioni R, Paradiso C, Battistini N, Giordano N, Vaccai D, Marcolongo R: Electrophysiologic evaluation of local steroid injection in carpal tunnel syndrome. *Arch Phys Med Rehabil,* 72:738-742; 1991.

Glousman RE: Ulnar nerve problems in the athlete's elbow. *Clin Sports Med,* 9:365-377; 1990.

Goodman HV, Foster JB: Effect of local corticosteroid injection on median nerve conduction in carpal tunnel syndrome. *Ann Phys Med,* 6:287-294; 1962.

Goodman HV, Gilliat RW: The effect of treatment on median nerve conduction in patients with the carpal tunnel syndrome. *Ann Phys Med,* 6:137-155; 1961.

Hang YS: Tardy ulnar neuritis in a little league baseball player. *Am J Sports Med,* 9:244-246; 1981.

Hartz CR, Linscheid RL, Gramse RR, Daube JR: Pronator teres syndrome: compressive neuropathy of the median nerve. *J Bone Joint Surg,* 63(A):885-890; 1981.

Heller L, Ring H, Costeff H, Solzi P: Evaluation of Tinel's and Phalen's signs in diagnosis of the carpal tunnel syndrome. *European Neurology,* 25(1):40-42; 1986.

Hrdlicka A: Incidence of the supracondyloid process in whites and other races. *Am J of Anthropology,* 6:405-406; 1923.

Jobe FW, Nuber G: Throwing injuries of the elbow. *Clin Sports Med,* 5:621-636; 1986.

Kanakamedala RV, Simons DG, Porter RW, Zucker RS: Ulnar nerve entrapment at the elbow localized by short segment stimulation. *Arch Phys Med Rehabil,* 69:959-963; 1988.

Kee ST, Dake MD, Wolfe-Johnson B, Semba CP, Zarins CK, Olcott C: Ischemia of the throwing hand in major league baseball pitchers: embolic occlusion from aneurysms of axillary artery branches. *J Vasc Interventional Radiol,* 6(6):979-982; 1995.

MacNicol MF: The results of operation for ulnar neuritis. *J Bone Joint Surg,* 61B:159-164; 1979.

Manske PR: Compression of the radial nerve by the triceps muscle. *J Bone Joint Surg Am,* 59:835-836; 1977.

Martinelli P, Gambellini A, Poppi M, Gallassi R, Pozzati E: Pronator syndrome due to thickened bicipital aponeurosis. *J Neurol Neurosurg Psychiatry,* 45:181-182; 1982.

McGrath M: Local steroid therapy in the hand. *J Hand Surg,* 9(A):915-921; 1984.

Mitsunaga MM, Nakano K: High radial nerve palsy following strenuous muscular activity. *Clin Orthop,* 234:39-42; 1988.

Naso SJ: Compression of the digital nerve: a new entity in tennis players. *Orthop Rev,* 13:47; 1984.

Novak CB, Lee GW, Mackinnon SE, Lay L: Provocative testing for cubital tunnel syndrome. *J Hand Surg,* 19(5A):817-820; 1994.

Osborne GV: Compression neuritis of the ulnar nerve at the elbow. *Hand,* 2:10-13; 1970.

Pianka G, Hershman EB: Neurovascular injuries. In: Nicholas JA, Hershman EB (eds.), *Upper extremity in sports medicine.* St. Louis: Mosby, 1990; 691-722.

Prochaska V, Crosby LA, Murphy RD: High radial nerve palsy in a tennis player. *Orthop Rev,* 22(1):90-92; 1993.

Pryse-Phillips W: Validation of a diagnostic sign in CTS. *J Neurol Neurosurg Psychiatry,* 47:870-872, 1984.

Rayam GM, Jensen C, and Duke J: Elbow flexion test in the normal population. *J Hand Surg,* 17A:86-89, 1992.

Regan WD, Morrey BF: Entrapment neuropathies about the elbow. In: DeLee JC, Drez D (eds.), *Orthopaedic sports medicine.* Philadelphia: Saunders, 1994; 844-859.

Roles N, Maudsley R: Radial tunnel syndrome: Resistant tennis elbow as a nerve entrapment. *J Bone Joint Surg Br,* 54:499-508; 1972.

Seror P: Treatment of ulnar nerve palsy at the elbow with a night splint. *J Bone Joint Surg,* 75(B):322-327; 1993.

Suranyi L: Median nerve compression by Struthers ligament. *J Neurol Neurosurg Psych,* 46:1047-1049; 1983.

Vanderpool SW, Chalmers J, Lamb DW, Whiston TB: Peripheral compression lesions of the ulnar nerve. *J Bone Joint Surg,* 50B:792-803; 1968.

Wadsworth TG, Williams JR: Cubital tunnel external compression syndrome. *Br Med J,* 1:662-666; 1973.

Weinstein SM, Herring SA: Nerve problems and compartment syndromes in the hand, wrist and forearm. *Clin Sport Med,* 11(1):161-188; 1992.

Younge DH, Moise P: The radial tunnel syndrome. *Int Orthop,* 18:268-270; 1994.

5

Lumbar
Radiculopathies

Stephen G. Geiger, MD
Gregory E. Lutz, MD

A lumbar radiculopathy is an injury or irritation to a lumbar spinal nerve. Although Tall and DeVaulty (1993) reviewed numerous reports of the incidence of lumbar spine injuries in athletes, few researchers have addressed the specific issue of lumbar radiculopathy. Carefully designed and executed epidemiologic studies of the true incidence of lumbar radiculopathy in athletes are needed. Quite often these injuries can have not only a profound impact on athletes' abilities to perform sports but also on their abilities to perform basic activities of daily living. A lumbar radiculopathy can be a career-threatening injury that represents a significant management challenge to the sports medicine physician.

The sports most often associated with injuries that may result in a lumbar radiculopathy are football, weightlifting, gymnastics, soccer, golf, tennis, running, rowing, and basketball (Borgesen and Vang 1974, DeOrio and Bianco 1982). The most common cause of lumbar radiculopathy in middle-aged athletes is lumbar disc disease (i.e., disc herniation, protrusion, and extrusion). As athletes age and degenerative changes further narrow the spinal canal, degenerative lumbar spinal stenosis becomes the most common cause. Although rare in young athletes, lumbar radiculopathy can occur and is usually associated with either a disc herniation (Micheli and Yancey 1994) or *spondylolisthesis* (Jackson 1979). Other less common causes are lumbar fracture, infection, tumor, spondyloarthropathies, and metabolic disorders. Baba and colleagues (1996) reported cases of posterior limbus vertebral lesions or osteocartilaginous vertebral corner defects in adolescents who presented with variable degrees of lumbar radiculopathy.

spondylolisthesis—Forward displacement of the body of one vertebra on the vertebra below it, most commonly due to a defect in the pars interarticularis.

Although an athlete may initially present with symptoms and signs of a lumbar radiculopathy that occurred during a sport activity, the problem may not be related to the actual physical activity the person was performing. For example, a bodybuilder presented with radicular symptoms that appeared during weightlifting—but was found to have spinal epidural lipomatosis induced by anabolic steroid abuse (Fiirgard and Madsen 1997).

This chapter focuses on the relevant anatomy of the lumbar spine and how it relates to the degenerative cascade, key clinical findings and diagnostic tests, a discussion of operative versus nonoperative treatment, and finally, the rehabilitation program necessary to return athletes to a level of functioning at or near their previous level.

ANATOMY

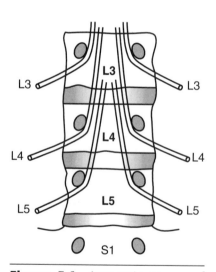

Figure 5.1 Anatomic course of the lumbar spinal nerves.

In order to obtain an accurate diagnosis, provide effective treatment, and prevent recurrent injuries, a clinician needs to understand the relevant anatomy of the lumbar spine and the biomechanical stresses to which it is subject during athletic activities. There are five lumbar vertebrae and five lumbar spinal nerves (figure 5.1). Each nerve is numbered according to the lumbar vertebra beneath which it passes. The L3 spinal nerve passes below the L3 pedicle in the L3-L4 *intervertebral foramen*, the L4 spinal nerve lies below the L4 vertebra in the L4-L5 intervertebral foramen, and so on.

intervertebral foramen—The opening formed by the inferior and superior notches on the pedicles of adjacent vertebrae that transmits the spinal nerve.

Each lumbar spinal nerve attaches centrally to the spinal cord by its segmental dorsal and ventral roots (figure 5.2). The *dorsal root* carries sensory information from the spinal nerve toward the spinal cord. The *ventral root* primarily carries motor information from the spinal cord peripherally to the spinal nerve. The cell bodies of the sensory fibers are located in the *dorsal root ganglion,* an enlargement of the dorsal root located just proximal to its junction with the spinal nerve. The motor cell bodies lie in the ventral horn of the spinal cord. Each dorsal and ventral root converges to form a single trunk that connects to the spinal nerve in the intervertebral foramen. Just distal to the foramen, the spinal nerve divides into a *dorsal* and *ventral ramus.* The dorsal rami innervate the skin, ligaments, and muscles of the lumbar spine as well as the posterior spinal elements. The ventral rami innervate the skin, ligaments, and muscles of the lower limb. Further detail of the innervation of the lumbar spine is described elsewhere (Bogduk 1983, Bogduk et al. 1981).

dorsal root—Sensory branch of a spinal nerve that enters the dorsal part of the spinal cord.

ventral root—Motor branch of a spinal nerve that enters the ventral part of the spinal cord.

dorsal root ganglion—Collection of nerve cell bodies in the dorsal root.

dorsal ramus—A branch of a spinal nerve that supplies the posterior area of the body.

ventral ramus—A branch of a spinal nerve that supplies the anterior area of the body and the extremities.

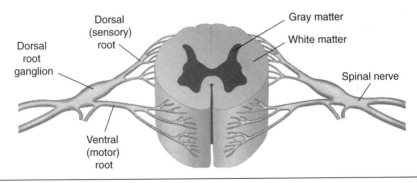

Figure 5.2 Typical spinal nerve.

Reprinted, by permission, from J. Wilmore and D. Costill, 1999, *Physiology of sport and exercise,* 2nd ed. (Champaign, IL: Human Kinetics), 67.

In order to permit movement yet remain stable while bearing weight, the lumbar spine requires complex interaction between the lumbar vertebral bodies, intervertebral discs, posterior spinal elements, and associated muscles and ligaments. The primary weightbearing portions of the lumbar spine are the vertebral bodies and the intervertebral discs. Strong but lightweight, the vertebral body comprises a hard outer shell of cortical bone surrounding *cancellous bone* that contains trabeculae aligned to provide strength and resilience (Bogduk 1997). Each intervertebral disc consists of a centrally located *nucleus pulposus* surrounded by a peripheral *annulus fibrosus*. The nucleus is a semifluid matrix of protein, glycosaminoglycan, and water (Bullough and Boachie-Adjei 1988). The annulus has a similar composition, but with a higher concentration of collagen fibers that are arranged into 10-20 concentric rings (Roberts et al. 1989). The elastic annulus and gelatinous nucleus allow the disc to function as a shock absorber for the spine (figure 5.3, a-b).

cancellous bone—Bone that has a lattice- or spongy-like structure.

nucleus pulposus—A semifluid mass that forms the central portion of an intervertebral disc.

annulus fibrosus—A concentric ring of fibers that forms the outer portion of an intervertebral disc.

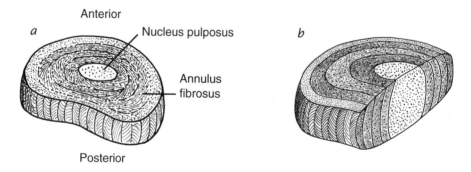

Figure 5.3 (*a*) Concentric bands of annular fibers; (*b*) horizontal section through a disc.

The ability of the nucleus pulposus to absorb and distribute forces is a function of its semifluid properties. The mucopolysaccharide gel of the nucleus deforms under pressure and distributes force in equal directions. The disc's ability to transport water also helps to absorb mechanical loads—when the disc is compressed, it releases water to absorb the load (Virgin 1951). When mechanical pressures are reduced, the nucleus re-absorbs the lost water through the end plates (Kramer et al. 1985). The ability of the disc to move water in and out of the nucleus becomes impaired with aging and signals the beginning of the degenerative lumbar cascade.

THE LUMBAR DEGENERATIVE CASCADE

The natural aging process results in degeneration of the intervertebral disc. With aging, there is a decrease in the proteoglycan content of the disc and an increase in the collagen content (Buckwalter 1995). The net result is loss of water volume and a decrease in the capacity of the disc to bind water. As the nucleus loses its water-binding capacity, the disc becomes less able to absorb forces, and adaptive changes occur throughout the lumbar spine.

Stages of the Lumbar Degenerative Cascade

These adaptive changes have been described by Kirkaldy-Willis and colleagues (Kirkaldy-Willis 1992, Kirkaldy-Willis and Farfan 1982) as the "lumbar degenerative cascade" and are classified into three stages.

The Three Phases of the Degenerative Cascade

- **Stage I:** Dysfunction
- **Stage II:** Instability
- **Stage III:** Stability

- **Stage I: Dysfunction.** The first stage is characterized by the mechanical breakdown of the disc. The cumulative effects of repetitive microtrauma, such as repetitive flexion or torsional loading, result in tears of the outer annulus (Adams and Hutton 1981, Farfan et al. 1970). Tears can be followed by endplate failure, leading to loss of nuclear nutrition and loss of disc water volume (Bernick and Calliet 1982). Further torsional loading leads to further annular weakening as annular tears can coalesce to become radial tears (Kirkaldy-Willis et al. 1978). Annular weakening allows progressive migration of nuclear material toward the periphery of the annulus. When the annulus fails, there is herniation of nuclear material through the annulus into the spinal canal. If the herniated nucleus pulposus (HNP) is central or paracentral, the patient can experience radicular pain and symptoms consistent with the exiting nerve root at that segment (i.e., L4-L5 HNP causes L5 radiculopathy). If the disc herniation is lateral, there will be compromise of the descending nerve root from the superior segment (i.e., L4-L5 lateral HNP causes L4 radiculopathy).

• **Stage II: Instability.** The second stage is characterized by mechanical instability. With the loss of disc hydrostatic pressure, the disc height decreases, vertebral bodies come closer together, ligaments become lax, and the whole stability of the spine is compromised (Borenstein 1996). Loss of stability results in excessive joint motion in all planes. Facet joints are subjected to greater weightbearing loads and undergo cartilage degeneration and capsular laxity.

• **Stage III: Stability.** The final stage is characterized by reestablishing the stability of the spine. The disc is stabilized by progressive narrowing, fibrosis, and osteophyte formation around its periphery. Facet joint subluxation, hypertrophy, and capsular fibrosis stabilize the posterior elements (McCulloch and Transfeldt 1997). Further proliferation of bone—including pedicle thickening, traction spurs, and osteophyte formation—stabilizes the spine. The combination of all these adaptive changes in spinal stenosis often progresses to nerve root compression.

Causes of the Degenerative Cascade

The degenerative cascade leading to lumbar radiculopathy is not only an aging process but is also related to repeated mechanical stresses applied to the spine. Athletes place great demand on the spine with the rapid and repetitive flexion, extension, torsional, and compressive loading associated with many sports. The repetitive flexion and rotation needed to field a ground ball or kick a soccer ball increases the tension on the posterior annulus fibers and can progress to annular tears with overuse (Watkins 1995). Axial compression injuries can occur in any sport that calls for repetitive jumping, running, or player contact, causing annular disruption and possible endplate fracture (Steinkamp 1995). The rapid and repetitive rotational and compressive movements required to play golf, tennis, and baseball can lead to an overuse lumbar spine injury. Axial torsion can cause circumferential tears in the annulus, which with repeated microtrauma can progress to radial tears. Repetitive hyperextension maneuvers performed by gymnasts, football players, and wrestlers can cause traumatic spondylosis or spondylolisthesis and subsequent nerve root compression

(Dreyer et al. 1995). Football linemen have the highest incidence of lower back pain associated with athletic activity (Saal 1988a, Saal 1988b, Semon and Spengler 1981). The flexed position during the three-point stance causes compression and narrowing of the disc anteriorly, and the drive forward and upward and extension of the lumbar spine during collisions of blocking and tackling create shear forces at the facet joints (Gatt et al. 1997). All of these sporting activities place large potential loads on the lumbar spine and may accelerate degeneration of the spine (Videman et al. 1997).

Are athletes more at risk than the general population for developing lumbar spine injuries and radiculopathy? The answer to this question remains unclear. In a three-year longitudinal study of adolescent athletes, Kujula and colleagues (1996) found that athletes participating in ice hockey, soccer, figure skating, and gymnastics had a significantly higher incidence of disabling low back pain than did age-matched controls. In contrast, Mundt et al. (1993), in another epidemiologic study of middle-aged and older athletes, found that baseball, softball, golf, bowling, swimming, jogging, aerobics, and racquet sports were not associated with increased risk for disc herniation—in fact, these activities may even be protective. Magnetic resonance imaging (MRI) studies also do not definitively identify athletes at a higher risk for lumbar spine injury. Sward et al. (1991) compared the incidence of MRI abnormalities in 19- to 29-year-old male elite gymnasts to male nonathletes matched for age. Certain high-risk sports, such as gymnastics and football, were associated with a higher incidence of MRI abnormalities in the elite gymnasts compared to the male nonathletes. Yet when Videman and colleagues (1997) studied the effects of lifetime endurance exercise on the lumbar discs of monozygotic twins ages 35-69, they found no signs of either harmful or beneficial effects of exercise on disc degeneration. Videman et al. (1995), comparing 50-year-old elite athletes with controls, found that maximal weightlifting and soccer were associated with greater degeneration of the lumbar discs on MRI. However, this did not correlate with a greater incidence of symptoms in the athletes—a finding consistent with other reports that degenerative changes seen on imaging do not necessarily correlate with symptoms (Boden et al. 1990, Jensen et al. 1994).

Despite the large potential loads that certain sporting activities place on the spine, the incidence of disc herniation and radiculopathy is low in young athletes. While the true incidence is unknown, most reports state that only 0.8% to 3.8% of all disc herniations occur in the adolescent population (Epstein et al. 1984, Garrido et al. 1978). In contrast to older athletes, disc tissue in adolescents is firm, well hydrated, and without degenerative changes (Micheli and Yancey 1994). DeOrio and Bianco (1982) suggested that a herniated disc in this age group is more likely to result from cumulative microtrauma to the spine than from a large single, momentary force. Some studies have also suggested that adolescent athletes are at higher risk for injury if sudden excessive stresses are applied to the lumbar spine during the adolescent growth spurt (Micheli 1979, Micheli and Yancey 1994). The most common cause of lumbar radiculopathy in young athletes is related to the *pars interarticularis* of the lumbar spine (Jackson 1979). The cumulative microtrauma from repetitive bending and twisting in certain sports can lead to vertebral slippage and lumbar radiculopathy secondary to spondylolisthesis (Jackson 1979).

pars interarticularis—The segment of bone between the superior and inferior articular processes of a lumbar vertebra.

KEY CLINICAL FINDINGS AND DIAGNOSTIC TESTS

Detailed histories followed by thorough physical examinations will lead physicians to the correct diagnosis in the majority of athletes who present with symptoms of a lumbar radiculopathy. Pain drawings and pain scores that athletes complete prior to evaluation can reveal the quality, location, and intensity of the pain (Ransford et al. 1976). Diagnostic tests can confirm the clinical diagnosis, rule out other potential causes, assess the severity of the injury, and provide a prognosis of the expected clinical outcome.

Assessing Signs and Symptoms

An athlete presenting with a lumbar radiculopathy may complain of classic radicular pain in a *dermatomal* distribution associated with numbness and weakness. However, in our experience, many cases can initially present with thigh or calf pain in a nondermatomal distribution not associated with other neurologic symptoms.

dermatome—The area of skin supplied by a single posterior nerve root.

Athletes often think initially that their pain is a result of a muscle strain. It is usually after weeks to months of refractory pain that they present for medical evaluation, because their symptoms do not appear to be improving. There are many variations on the theme of pain referral with a lumbar radiculopathy, depending on the degree of neural compromise and the etiology. Athletes may at first have only hip or groin pain, which later radiates down the thigh into the calf and then into the foot. Usually they will give a years-long history of episodic axial low back pain that responded to conservative care. It is only when the pain quality changes in location or intensity to a point that it interferes with their athletic ability that they seek medical attention.

It is important to assess not only the location, quality, and intensity of pain but also aggravating and alleviating factors. Typically, patients with lumbar disc herniations complain of increased pain during activities that load the spine with compressive and torsional stresses (hitting, throwing, kicking, lifting, and running). Usually the pain is relieved by positions that decrease intradiscal pressure, such as lying supine with the knees bent. Athletes with lumbar spinal stenosis usually present with an inability to walk or stand for prolonged periods due to leg pain and weakness. Sitting or recumbency relieves their pain. They can swing to hit a golf ball, but they cannot walk the course.

On physical examination, the patient with a lumbar disc herniation usually cannot flex the spine forward. If there is a foraminal disc herniation or spinal stenosis, extension of the spine may aggravate the radicular pain. Focal neurologic findings such as sensory loss, reflex loss, or motor weakness in a *myotomal* pattern may or may not be present.

> **myotome**—A group of muscles innervated from a single spinal segment.

Dural tension signs are common in individuals with lumbar disc herniation but rare in those with degenerative lumbar spinal stenosis. In general, athletes with severe radicular pain with extension and a positive crossed straight-leg raise and a scoliotic list toward the side of their pain usually have an *extruded/sequestered disc* that deforms normal neuromeningeal dynamics (Kosteljanetz et al. 1988). In our experience, these athletes tend to fare poorly with nonsurgical care targeted to decrease nerve root inflammation. The extreme mechanical deformation of the nerve root by the extruded or sequestered disc is the primary cause of the athlete's pain and warrants early surgical intervention. These patients are usually selected out early for surgical intervention. In contrast, patients whose radicular pain decreases with spinal extension (centralization), and who have no contralateral dural tension signs, tend to have a favorable prognosis with nonsurgical treatment (Donelson et al. 1990).

> **extruded disc**—A type of disc herniation in which the nucleus pulposus protrudes through the annulus fibrosus and the nuclear material remains attached to the disc.

> **sequestered disc**—A type of disc herniation in which a free fragment is in the spinal canal outside of the annulus fibrosus and the nuclear material is no longer attached to the disc.

Diagnostic Tests

There is a wide variety of diagnostic tests to choose from when assessing an athlete with lumbar radiculopathy (see below). Electrodiagnostic studies can be useful in diagnosing radiculopathy (Ellenberg et al. 1994). Electromyography can help distinguish nerve root dysfunction from other common referred pain patterns that are unclear from a physical exam. It is also a valuable way to determine the distribution and overall prognosis for a peripheral nerve injury. A comprehensive review of the various imaging techniques available for assessing spinal pathology is beyond the scope of this chapter and can be found elsewhere (Davis and Feinberg 1997, Weinstein and Herring 1997). If the practitioner suspects that acute dynamic overload or chronic repetitive overexertion have lead to fracture or instability of the spine, plain radiographs are advisable. In most cases, however, a magnetic resonance imaging (MRI) for detailed anatomic imaging and electromyography (EMG) for neurophysiologic testing should provide enough information for the clinician to arrive at the correct diagnosis. Note that the pathology seen on imaging studies does not always correlate with the athlete's symptoms—asymptomatic patients can also exhibit disc herniation on computer tomography (CT) or MRI (Boden et al. 1990, Jensen et al. 1994, Wiesel et al. 1984). Any abnormalities seen on diagnostic imaging must be strictly correlated with clinical signs and symptoms before treatment is initiated.

Common Diagnostic Tests for Evaluating Lumbar Radiculopathy

- Plain X ray
- Magnetic resonance imaging (MRI)
- Computer tomography (CT)
- Myelogram

Finally, there are many disease processes that may initially present with spinal symptoms. Clinicians must be aware of any concomitant nonmechanical symptoms such as fever, chills, weight loss, or night pain. If an athlete presents with the signs and symptoms of a lumbar radiculopathy along with one or more of these associated constitutional symptoms, a thorough medical evaluation is mandatory to rule out nonmechanical causes.

OPERATIVE VERSUS NONOPERATIVE TREATMENT

The decision whether to operate on an athlete with a lumbar radiculopathy can be perplexing unless the clinician is aware of the natural history of the underlying disease process, the potential risks of the surgical procedure performed, the prognosis for recovery of function, and the state of the art of nonsurgical treatment for that specific condition. There are certain clinical scenarios for which surgical intervention is the appropriate first step in treatment for lumbar radiculopathy— including lumbar fracture with instability, lumbar cauda equina syndrome, rapidly progressive weakness due to a single level radiculopathy, and severe intractable pain not responding to nonsurgical care. Numerous reports in the literature have demonstrated that, for the majority of cases of lumbar disc herniation, spontaneous reduction of disc material occurs over time without surgical intervention (Ellenburg et al. 1993, Maigne et al. 1992, Saal et al. 1990). In fact, improvement of clinical symptoms often precedes any appreciable morphologic change on anatomic imaging studies (Saal et al. 1990). Larger disc herniations, which normally are the most responsive to surgery, often show the greatest reduction in size.

There are certain issues to consider when dealing with an athlete with a lumbar radiculopathy. One of the main considerations is whether or not she can return to her previous level of athletic activity—and if yes, how quickly can she do so? Does surgery offer any advantage over nonsurgical treatment? This question has not been answered with prospective, blinded, randomized, controlled studies in the athletic population. In acute or subacute stages, surgery appears to resolve radicular pain more quickly than conservative treatment; but over time (greater than one year), there is no significant difference in functional outcome (Weber 1983). Conservative treatment in these studies did not include the current recommended nonoperative treatment—that is, fluoroscopically guided, contrast-enhanced transforaminal epidural steroid injections, combined with goal-directed medically supervised rehabilitation (Lutz et al. 1998). Ambiguities continue in the management of athletes with lumbar radiculopathy, and well-designed studies are needed to assess outcomes more clearly. Until there is clear evidence favoring surgical over nonsurgical treatment, the majority of our athletes with lumbar radiculopathy are initially managed with aggressive nonsurgical treatment. If the athlete has progressive neurologic signs and symptoms or severe intractable pain unresponsive to nonsurgical care, then surgical intervention is warranted.

STAGES OF REHABILITATION

Rehabilitation of athletes with lumbar radiculopathy is a comprehensive process that begins with accurate diagnosis and a decision to embark on a nonsurgical treatment path. Our rehabilitation program is divided into five stages based on rehabilitation and biomechanical principles. We discourage "cookbook" protocols: Each athlete's rehabilitation program is designed to meet his disease process and athletic goals. These stages are meant only to provide a general guideline, not to replace regular physician follow-up. The time frame for each stage varies depending on the individual athlete, the severity of the injury, response to treatment, and the final goal.

Stages of Spine Rehabilitation

- **Stage I:** Early protected mobilization
- **Stage II:** Lumbar stabilization training
- **Stage III:** Spine-safe strengthening and conditioning
- **Stage IV:** Return to sports
- **Stage V:** Maintenance program

Stage I: Early Protected Mobilization

The first goals of this stage are to control pain and inflammation and to promote healing of the injured lumbar segment. The proper combination of patient education, oral medications, selective spinal injection procedures, and bracing will help reduce pain and allow early therapeutic exercise, thus preventing the harmful effects of prolonged immobilization.

Patient Education

Our athletes with symptomatic lumbar radiculopathy are first instructed in proper body mechanics and positioning. They are given reading material and personal instruction in the basic biomechanics of the spine and are taught how to perform transfers and low-level activities safely during the healing process. Prolonged periods of bed rest are discouraged, and early mobilization is encouraged after the athlete is taught how to maintain a neutral spine-safe posture.

A neutral spine-safe posture can be defined as that position of the spine where there are minimal or no symptoms. Maintaining an extension-biased posture is important for athletes with disc herniations, as is maintaining a flexion-biased posture in athletes with posterior element-generated pain. Our patients are also instructed in the use of superficial modalities that may be beneficial in managing pain from muscle spasm: Ice application is useful in acute injury to reduce muscle spasm; superficial heat helps in treating chronic recurrent paraspinal spasm and stiffness.

Oral Medications

If there are no contraindications, our athletes are initially given a trial of nonsteroidal anti-inflammatory drugs (NSAIDs). If there is no improvement within 7-14 days, a different class of NSAID is used. Opiate analgesics are used judiciously in selected cases for breakthrough pain in the short term. McCormack (1994) reported that some NSAIDs, in addition to their inhibitory effect on prostaglandin synthesis, block the synthesis and activity of other neuroactive substances believed to have key roles in processing afferent nociceptive input.

Selected Spinal Injection Procedures

If there is no improvement in pain or if NSAIDs are contraindicated, selective spinal injections are considered. These procedures involve the injection of a preparation of corticosteroid and anesthetic into the epidural space. Spinal injections should be used only as adjuvant treatment to facilitate the rehabilitation process and not simply as a means of providing short-term pain relief. These procedures should be performed by skilled physicians using fluoroscopic guidance (Dreyfuss 1993). Needle misplacement has been reported in up to 40% of caudal and 30% of translaminar injections performed without fluoroscopy (El-Khoury et al. 1988, Mehta and Salmon 1985, Renfrew et al. 1991).

The rationale for using corticosteroids in treating radicular symptoms is to decrease pain by suppressing the inflammatory reaction. Corticosteroids suppress both the early vasodilatory and late fibrotic phases of the inflammatory response. While corticosteroids may be given systemically, drug delivery may be inadequate and systemic side effects more prevalent. The advantage of spinal injections is delivery of medication directly into the epidural space, thus allowing a higher concentration of steroid to reach the target tissue.

Biochemical Factors Involved in the Inflammatory Response

Administration of high concentrations of corticosteroids via spinal injections decreases the inflammatory response by neutralizing inflammatory mediators and stabilizing neuronal membranes. There is now strong evidence that radicular pain may be explained by inflammation caused by biochemical factors (Saal 1995).

Experimental models have suggested that homogenized nucleus pulposus acts as a chemical or immunological irritant in producing the inflammatory response. McCarron et al. (1987) found that homogenized nucleus pulposus from dogs provoked an acute inflammatory response when injected into the lumbar epidural space. Similarly, epidural application of autologous nucleus pulposus in pigs induced profound changes in nerve root structure and function, and these effects were dramatically reduced by high doses of methylprednisolone (Olmarker et al. 1993, Olmarker et al. 1994). An immunohistologic study by Doita and colleagues (1996) concluded that inflammatory cells found near extruded discs might induce neovascularization and persistence of inflammation.

A number of studies have looked at the role of inflammatory mediators and their effects on the neural structures (Weinstein et al. 1995). Saal et al. (1990) showed that the nucleus pulposus contains high amounts of the inflammatory mediator phospholipase A2 (PLA2). They identified high levels of PLA2 in perineural tissues of human subjects with a herniated nucleus pulposus: PLA2 appears to disseminate from the nucleus pulposus after annular injury, sensitizing annular nerve endings and the dorsal root ganglion (DRG) by causing an inflammatory reaction. Franson and colleagues (1992) have more recently shown that PLA2 has a powerful inflammatory activity in vivo. Ozaktay et al. (1998) report that PLA2 in herniated human discs may be neurotoxic to immediately adjacent neural tissues: It appears that extrusion of herniated nucleus pulposus may cause sensitization of *nociceptors* in the DRG and dorsal nerve roots adjacent to the herniation site, causing paresthesias and pain. Lee and colleagues (1998) suggest that nerve root irritation is caused in part by a high level of PLA2 activity initiated by inflammation, and that steroids inhibit PLA2 activity.

> **nociceptor**—A receptor that responds to tissue damage, or the chemical mediators associated with tissue damage. They signal the sensation the brain interprets as pain.

Neurophysiologic experiments have shown that nociceptors previously chemically sensitized or inflamed can transmit painful ectopic impulses. Compressing normal nerve roots evokes only paresthesias and numbness, but compression of previously sensitized nociceptors in the dorsal nerve roots can cause a shooting, lancinating pain of radicular quality (Macnab 1972). The concept is that nociceptors in the DRG or dorsal nerve roots already sensitized by an inflammatory mediator are more likely to transmit painful ectopic discharges when mechanically compressed by disc protrusion, herniation, or canal stenosis.

Routes of Administration

There are three basic routes of epidural administration of medication:

- Translumbar (translaminar)
- Transsacral (caudal)
- Transforaminal

The benefits of the caudal approach are that it is easy to perform and there is a low risk of inadvertent dural puncture. The main disadvantage is the large volume of medication needed to reach the target tissue. Injectates of larger volume dilute out the potential therapeutic effects of the corticosteroids.

In the translaminar approach, the needle is directed much closer to the target tissue. A perceived benefit of this approach is that less volume of medication is needed than with caudal techniques. There is a higher chance of dural puncture with a translaminar injection, but the risk is low in the hands of an experienced injectionist.

Neither the conventional lumbar nor caudal approach, however, guarantees that the injectate will reach the inflamed target nerve. If the perceived target site in patients with lumbar radiculopathy is the interface between the posterior intervertebral disc and the ventral dural sac, then it would seem unlikely that a translaminar injection into the dorsal epidural space or a transsacral injection to the inferior epidural space would reliably reach the target site. Moreover, epidural ligaments, scarring, or compressive spinal lesions can further limit the amount of medication reaching the target tissue.

Transforaminal techniques have been developed in an attempt to deliver the injectate directly around the inflamed target tissue. A higher concentration of injectate can be delivered to the ventral epidural space with this technique. The procedure has been described by Derby et al. (1993) and allows the injectionist to reliably guide the flow of medication specifically to the level and side of the patient's clinical findings.

The technique at the L5 level or above involves a double-needle paramedian approach in which a 25-gauge needle is curved through a 20-gauge introducer needle into the so called "safe triangle" (figure 5.4). This triangle

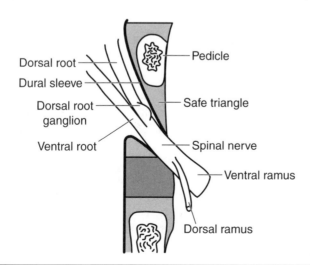

Figure 5.4 The "safe triangle" is composed of the inferior border of the pedicle, the lateral border of the vertebral body, and the exiting nerve root.

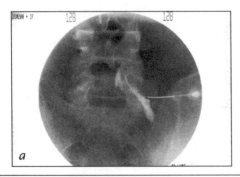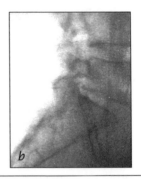

Figure 5.5 *(a)* Anteroposterior fluoroscopic image of a right L5 transforaminal epidural steroid injection. Note contrast dye outlining the exiting L5 nerve. *(b)* Lateral fluoroscopic image of an L5 transforaminal injection. Note ventral position of needle tip.

comprises the inferior border of the pedicle, the lateral border of the vertebral body, and the exiting nerve root. This technique reliably allows flow to the ventral epidural space and posterior disc region (figure 5.5, a-b).

Two recent studies assessed the potential benefit of transforaminal epidural steroids. Lutz et al. (1998) prospectively followed 69 patients with lumbar disc herniations and lumbar radiculopathy. Each patient received a transforaminal epidural injection (2 ml 2% Xylocaine and 6 mg Celestone) at the presumed level of involvement under fluoroscopic guidance, with preinjection of contrast to confirm spread to the target area. Follow-up data, after an average of 20 months, showed that 75.4% of the patients reported at least a greater than 50% reduction between preinjection and postinjection pain scores. The average number of injections to achieve this effect was 1.8 per patient. Weiner and Fraser (1997) studied 30 patients with severe lumbar radiculopathy secondary to foraminal and extraforaminal disc herniation. Treatment consisted of foraminal injection of local anesthetic and steroids. The authors reported immediate pain relief in 27 patients after injection and sustained pain relief in 22 of 28 patients available for follow-up (average follow-up 3.4 years).

A transforaminal epidural steroid injection is the procedure of choice for an athlete with persistent unilateral radicular pain that does not respond to conventional rehabilitation protocols. If symptoms are bilateral or generated from multiple segments, a caudal or translaminar approach is used. The athlete's response to the injection is usually evaluated after one to two weeks. If there is persistent disabling radicular pain, a second epidural is administered. More than three epidurals in a six-month period is not recommended. If the athlete's pain persists despite these efforts, surgical evaluation should be considered.

Bracing

Lumbosacral orthoses have a limited role during the healing period in selected athletes with symptomatic lumbar radiculopathy. Use of a lumbosacral corset is an effective short-term treatment of acute disc herniation and has been found to decrease intradiscal pressure by 25% when the wearer is standing (Nachemson et al. 1983). Antilordotic and modified Boston braces have been recommended for symptomatic spondylolisthesis (Bell et al. 1988, Steiner and Micheli 1985). Selected individuals may use a lumbosacral orthosis as an adjunct to protect the injured lumbar segment so that they can begin early spine-safe exercise.

Early Exercise

Once athletes have achieved a sustained reduction of pain—either through oral medication, selective spinal injections, or bracing—they can begin early therapeutic exercise. Early mobilization should be done in a protected fashion to allow controlled loading of healing structures. If a pool is available, aqua therapy allows for early active exercise in a controlled environment. The advantages of aquatic spine programs are directly related to the intrinsic properties of water (Cole et al. 1994). Water buoyancy decreases joint compression and supports the body, facilitating stretching, transfers, and spine stabilization exercises. We have found aqua therapy to be most beneficial in the early healing stage of rehabilitation. Low-impact aerobic conditioning such as walking should also be initiated early. Remind athletes to maintain a neutral spine-safe posture at all times during the workout.

After athletes have had adequate time for healing and pain reduction, they can begin restoring range of motion via gradual, progressive passive/active stretching exercises. These exercises must be performed in a spine-safe manner, and design of the exercises must take into account the patient's specific pathology. For example, repetitive extension exercises in a patient with spondylolisthesis will only lead to increased pain and prolong disability. Athletes should avoid aggressive stretching of the hamstrings and neural elements until radicular pain and signs of dural tension have disappeared. The key areas to be stretched are the thoracolumbar fascia; the hip flexors, abductors, and rotators; the knee flexors and extensors; and the ankle dorsiflexors. Stretching exercises are important in restoring range of motion so that the athlete with lumbar radiculopathy can safely begin the next stage of rehabilitation.

For Further Reading on . . .

Exercises for Treating Lumbar Radiculopathies
   Saal JA. Dynamic muscular stabilization in the nonoperative treatment of lumbar pain syndromes. Orthop Rev 19(8):691-700, 1990.

Stage II: Lumbar Stabilization Training

A properly designed spine stabilization exercise program minimizes repetitive stress to the injured lumbar segment in order to restore optimum function. Saal (1990) popularized dynamic muscular lumbar stabilization, which has proven successful in patients with lumbar disc herniations and radiculopathy. Lumbar spine stabilization involves active exercise and improved muscular control. Enhanced muscular and ligamentous control allows protected loading of the spine, which lessens the effect of repetitive microtrauma and sudden large, momentary loads.

A spine stabilization program begins with simple nonweightbearing exercises. All exercises are performed in the neutral spine-safe posture learned in stage I. The intensity of the exercises gradually rises by increasing the number of repetitions, sets, or weights, and/or by decreasing the rest period. Exercises are initially performed in the prone position and gradually progressed through prone, quadruped, and ball exercises. Each level becomes more challenging and requires more neuromuscular control. The athlete must emphasize proper form in all exercises.

During stage II, the athletes begin isometric strengthening, and they further progress the range-of-motion and aerobic conditioning exercises begun in stage I. They focus on strengthening their abdominal, oblique, and extensor muscles, because these are used to maintain the neutral spine-safe position. They continue low-impact aerobic conditioning with walking, stepping, or swimming, while applying stabilization concepts. They maintain and then gradually increase their spinal segmental mobility and limb flexibility through continued controlled stretching exercises. At the end of stage II, athletes are instructed in a 15-20 minute routine of *isometric* strengthening, flexibility, and stabilization exercises.

> **isometric exercise**—One in which the muscle is activated without change in the joint angle (i.e., the muscle does not shorten with activation).

Stage III: Spine-Safe Strengthening and Conditioning

This stage is characterized by more advanced exercises to provide the athlete with greater strength, coordination, and endurance. *Isotonic exercises* can create reinjury if performed too early or progressed too quickly. Athletes should perform these exercises only after they have mastered basic stabilization exercises, have had an adequate period of healing, and their pain is under control. A knowledge of spinal biomechanics is essential in selecting spine-safe isotonic exercises. Individuals with lumbar injury should avoid heavy squats, overhead military presses, and unsupported bent-over rows.

> **isotonic exercise**—One in which a muscle shortens and moves a load (maintains constant tension).

Initially, athletes should use machines rather than free weights. Machines provide increased spine support and are easier to learn because balance of the weight is not as difficult. The training routine should begin with submaximal high-repetition exercises that strengthen large muscle groups such as the legs and back. It should then progress to include the muscle groups of the chest, shoulders, and arms. Total body strengthening is essential for symmetry and enhancement of functional activities. Free-weight isotonic exercises are added once machine exercises are mastered. Examples of safe exercises to perform after lumbar injury are latissimus pull-downs, bodyweight squats, and lunges.

At the end of stage III, athletes have achieved significant gains in muscular strength, endurance, and flexibility—the goal is at least 20-30 minutes of aerobic exercise two to three times a week. They also should perform 30 minutes of isotonic strengthening exercises and flexibility stretching three times per week.

Stage IV: Return to Sports

The criteria for return to sports are

- full pain-free range of motion,
- demonstrated spine stabilization during sport-specific agility exercises, and
- restoration of adequate muscular strength, endurance, and control to prevent reinjury (Lutz et al. 1996).

The clinician must educate athletes regarding spine-safe and appropriate sporting activities. Athletic goals need to be realistic. Almost all of our athletes can return to some level of athletic activity if it is chosen properly and performed with moderation. If athletes' radicular pain reoccurs and does not resolve quickly, or if it progresses after the sporting activity, they should stop the activity and be reassessed.

Stage V: Maintenance Program

Athletes suffering from lumbar radiculopathy need to realize that the gains of the rehabilitation program are short-lived if they stop their exercises.

Our recommendations are that before discharge from a supervised physical therapy program, athletes be given an outline of the key exercises they should perform to maintain gains in flexibility, strengthening, and endurance. They should perform these exercises at least two or three times a week. If they are feeling well and want to progress to higher levels of exercise, intermittent follow-up to review their program is helpful.

CONCLUSION

Injury to the lumbar nerve roots in athletes can be devastating and career-threatening.

The first step in effective management is an accurate and timely diagnosis—which is facilitated when coaches and trainers are educated about the early signs and symptoms of a lumbar radiculopathy. With early medical intervention, potentially career-ending injuries often can be treated effectively without surgery, allowing athletes to return to levels at or near their previous levels of functioning (Nelson et al. 1999). Our treatment approach involves the judicious use of diagnostic tests, followed by the aggressive nonsurgical treatment approach outlined in this chapter. Patient involvement and motivation are keys to a successful outcome. Many times the physician's role is similar to that of a "medical coach," educating and motivating athletes to progress through the various stages of rehabilitation in order to reach their final goal of athletic competition.

Case Report 1

A 38-year-old male runner presented with a chief complaint of low back pain with radiation into the left leg. He had a preexistent history of intermittent low back pain, which was treated conservatively with exercise, but the leg pain was new and had come on after a long run six weeks prior to his initial evaluation. His pain was aggravated by sitting, forward bending, coughing, and sneezing, and it was associated with some weakness and numbness in the left leg. He denied any bowel or bladder changes. Prior to his initial consultation he was treated with a combination of oral anti-inflammatories, activity modification, chiropractic care, and physical therapy, with no relief of his symptoms.

Medical history: Significant for overall excellent health.

Surgical history: None.

Medications: Naproxen.

Social history: No smoking or alcohol use.

Family history: Noncontributory.

Physical examination: Patient was a well-developed male in a moderate amount of distress. His lumbar spine range of motion was restricted and painful with flexion past 30 degrees, and extension reduced his pain. He had a positive straight-leg raise at 30 degrees on the left side. His hip active range of motion was full and pain-free. Neurologic examination revealed decreased sensation in the lateral aspect of his left foot with an absent left ankle jerk; weakness in his gastrocnemius, as well as his gluteus maximus, graded 4 out of 4+/5. He also had difficulty with toe walking on the left side.

Radiographs: MRI of the lumbar spine revealed a moderate to large extruded disc herniation at the L5-S1 segment, creating compromise for the space of the exiting left S1 nerve root (figure 5.6, a-b).

Diagnosis: Left S1 radiculopathy secondary to a L5-S1 disc herniation.

Management and outcome: The patient underwent a fluoroscopically guided, contrast-enhanced, S1 transforaminal epidural steroid injection (figure 5.6c). One week after his injection he had a significant reduction in his radicular pain and was able to resume his rehabilitation program, which included a spine stabilization exercise program. He progressed through the rehabilitation over the ensuing four to six weeks, with improvement in his lumbar range of motion and strength and sensation in his left leg. He eventually was able to resume his previous level of athletic activity.

At his one-year follow-up, the patient remained asymptomatic, continued to be active, and was running on a regular basis.

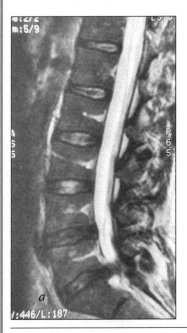
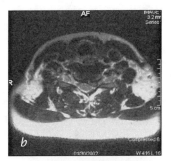
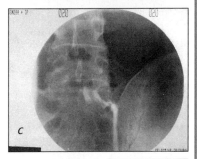

Figure 5.6 *(a)* Sagittal MRI image revealing an L5-S1 disc herniation. *(b)* Axial MRI image revealing left paracentral L5-S1 disc herniation. *(c)* Example of a left S1 transforaminal epidural steroid injection. Note outline of the left S1 nerve.

A 60-year-old tennis player presented with acute onset of low back pain with radiation into the left leg.

Medical history: Prior to his initial consultation, he had a two-year history of chronic, intermittent low back pain, which was aggravated by athletic activity, particularly golfing and tennis. He had no prior history of leg pain and attributed the onset of his pain to a vigorous tennis match two weeks prior to his initial consultation. The pain was aggravated by standing or walking and usually improved with sitting and recumbency. He denied any progressive weakness but noticed numbness in the left foot. He had been seen by his internist and was placed on oral anti-inflammatories, with little relief of his pain. He came in for further recommendations.

Surgical history: None.

Social history: No smoking or alcohol use.

Family history: Noncontributory.

Physical examination: Patient was a well-developed male who was in no acute distress. His thoracolumbar motion was restricted and painful with extension and lateral bending, which reproduced back pain, as well as radiating pain into the left leg in an L5-dermatomal distribution; flexion reduced this pain. Hip active range of motion was full and pain-free. Distal vasculature was intact. Neurologic examination revealed decreased sensation in the left L5 dermatome with weakness in the left extensor hallucis longus and gluteus medius muscle, graded 4/5. His deep tendon reflexes were physiologic and symmetric with downgoing plantar responses.

Radiographs: Radiographs of the lumbar spine showed evidence of grade I degenerative spondylolisthesis at the L4-5 segment, associated disc space narrowing, and facetal sclerosis.

MRI of the lumbar spine (figure 5.7, a-c) revealed degenerative spondylolisthesis at the L4-5 segment, with a large facet cyst off of the left L4-5 facet extending into the spinal canal, creating compromise for the exiting left L5 nerve root.

Management and outcome: Under direct fluoroscopic vision, the left L4-5 facet cyst was aspirated percutaneously with concomitant injection of lidocaine and Celestone. Postinjection the patient reported considerable relief of his left leg pain. He began a comprehensive spine rehabilitation program emphasizing judicious use of therapeutic modalities, postural reeducation, and a gradual progressive, neutral-spine lumbar stabilization program. After six weeks, he regained strength in his left leg and was able to return to his previous level of athletic activity.

At one-year follow-up, the patient still had residual mild low back pain, which was treated with occasional oral anti-inflammatories. He was on a regular exercise program; he had no recurrent leg pain and was able to return to both golf and tennis.

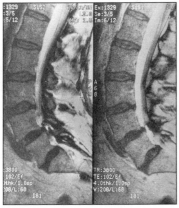

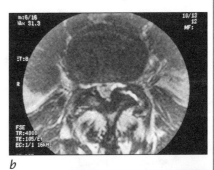

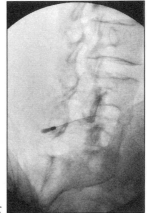

b

a

c

Figure 5.7 *(a)* Sagittal MRI image revealing degenerative spondylolisthesis of L4-L5 with large facet cyst. *(b)* Axial MRI image reveals degenerative left facet cyst compromising the space for the exiting left L5 nerve. *(c)* Fluoroscopic lumbar facet joint aspiration and injection with arthrogram.

REFERENCES

Adams M, Hutton WC: The relevance of torsion to the mechanical derangement of the lumbar spine. Spine 6:241-248, 1981.

Baba H, Uchida K, Furusawa N, Maezaawa Y, Azuchi M, Kamitanik, Annen S, Imura S, Tomita K: Posterior limbus vertebral lesions causing radiculopathy and the cauda equina syndrome. Spinal Cord 34:427-434, 1996.

Bell DF, Ehlich MG, Zaleske DJ: Brace treatment for symptomatic spondylolisthesis. Clin Orthop 236:192-198, 1988.

Bernick S, Calliet R: Vertebral end-plate changes with aging of human vertebrae. Spine 7:97-102, 1982.

Boden SD, Davis DO, Dina TS, Patronas NJ, Wiesel SW: Abnormal magnetic resonance scans of the lumbar spine in asymptomatic subjects. A prospective investigation. J Bone Joint Surg 72A:403-408, 1990.

Bogduk N: The innervation of the lumbar spine. Spine 8:286-293, 1983.

Bogduk N, ed.: *Clinical anatomy of the lumbar spine and sacrum*, 3rd edition. New York: Churchill Livingstone, 6, 1997.

Bogduk N, Tynan W, Wilson AS: The nerve supply to the intervertebral discs. Anat 132:39-56, 1981.

Borenstein DG, Lane, NE, Wolfe F: Chronic lower back pain. In: *Rheumatic disease clinics of North America*. Philadelphia: WB Saunders Company, 22:439-463, 1996.

Borgesen SE, Vang PS: Herniation of the lumbar intervertebral disk in children and adolescents. Acta Orthop Scand 45:540-549, 1974.

Buckwalter JA: Spine update. Aging and degeneration of the intervertebral disc. Spine 20:1307-1314, 1995.

Bullough PG, Boachie-Adjei O: *Atlas of spinal disease*. Philadelphia: Lippincott, 94-105, 1988.

Cole AJ, Moschetti ML, Eagleston RE: Spine pain: aquatic rehabilitation strategies. J Back Musculoskel Rehabil 4:273-286, 1994.

Davis BA, Feinberg JH: Anatomic localization: imaging techniques. In: Gonzalez EG, Materson PS (eds.): *The nonsurgical management of acute low back pain: cutting through the AHCPR guidelines*. New York: Domos Vermande, 31-57, 1997.

DeOrio JK, Bianco AJ: Lumbar disc excision in children and adolescents. J Bone Joint Surg 64A:991-995, 1982.

Derby R, Bogduk N, Kine G: Precision percutaneous blocking for localizing spinal pain. Part 2. The lumbar neuroaxial compartment. Pain Digest 3:175-188, 1993.

Doita M, Kanatani T, Harada T, Mizuno K: Immunohistologic study of the ruptured intervertebral disc of the lumbar spine. Spine 21:235-241, 1996.

Donelson R, Silva G, Murphy K: Centralization phenomenon. Its usefulness in evaluating and treating referred pain. Spine 15:211-213, 1990.

Dreyer SJ, Falco FJE, Lester JP, Windsor RE: Weight lifting. In: White AH (ed.): *Care: diagnosis and conservative treatment*, Vol I. St. Louis: Mosby, 746-761, 1995.

Dreyfuss P: Epidural steroid injections. A procedure ideally performed with fluoroscopic control and contrast media. International Spinal Injection Society Newsletter 1:34-40, 1993.

El-Khoury G, Ehara S, Weinstein JN: Epidural steroid injection: a procedure ideally with fluoroscopic control. Radiology 168:554-557, 1988.

Ellenberg MR, Honet JC, Treanor WJ: Cervical radiculopathy. Arch Phys Med Rehabil 75:342-352, 1994.

Ellenberg MR, Ross ML, Honet JC, Schwartz M, Chodoroff G, Enochs S: Prospective evaluation of the course of disc herniations in patients with proven radiculopathy. Arch Phys Med Rehabil 74:3-8, 1993.

Epstein JA, Epstein NE, Marc J, Rosenthal AD, Lavine LS: Lumbar intervertebral disk herniation in teenage children: recognition and management of associated anomalies. Spine 9:427-432, 1984.

Farfan HF, Cossette JW, Robertson GH, Wells RV, Kraus H: The effects of torsion on the lumbar intervertebral joints: the role of torsion in the production of disc degeneration. J Bone Joint Surg 52A: 468-497, 1970.

Fiirgard B, Madsen FH: Spinal epidural lipomatosis. Case report and review of the literature. Scand J Med Sci Sports 7:354-357, 1997.

Franson RC, Saal JS, Saal JA: Human disc phospholipase A2 is inflammatory. Spine 17 (suppl): 129-132, 1992.

Garrido E, Humphreys RP, Hendrick EB, Hoffman HJ: Lumbar disc disease in children. Neurosurgery 2:22-26, 1978.

Gatt CJ, Hosea TM, Palumbo RC, Zawadsky JP: Impact loading of the lumbar spine during blocking. Am J of Sports Med 25:317-320, 1997.

Jackson DW: Low back pain in young athletes: evaluation of stress reaction and discogenic problems. Am J Sports Med 7:364-366, 1979.

Jensen MC, Brant-Zawadzki MN, Obuchowski N, Modic MT, Malkasian D, Ross JS: Magnetic resonance imaging the lumbar spine in people without back pain. NEJM 331:69-73, 1994.

Kirkaldy-Willis WH: Pathology and pathogenesis of low back pain. In: Kirkaldy-WH, Burton CV (eds.): *Managing low back pain,* 3rd edition. New York: Churchill-Livingstone, 49-79, 1992.

Kirkaldy-Willis WH, Wedge JH, Yong-Hing K, Reilly J: Pathology and pathogenesis of lumbar spondylosis and stenosis. Spine 3:319-328, 1978.

Kirkaldy-Willis WH, Farfan HF: Instability of the lumbar spine. Clin Orthop 165:110-123, 1982.

Kosteljanetz M, Bang F, Schmidt-Olsen S: The clinical significance of straight-leg raising (Lasegue's sign) in the diagnosis of prolapsed lumbar disc. Interobserver variation and correlation with surgical finding. Spine 13:393-395, 1988.

Kramer J, Kolditz D, Gown R: Water and electrolyte of human intervertebral discs under variable load. Spine 10:69-71, 1985.

Kujala UM, Taimela S, Erkintalo M, Salminen JJ, Kaprio J: Low back pain in adolescent athletes. Med Sci Sports Exerc 28:165-170, 1996.

Lee H, Weinstein JN, Meller ST, Hayashi N, Spratt KF, Gebhart GF: The role of steroids and their effects on phospholipase: an animal model of radiculopathy. Spine 23:1191-1196, 1998.

Lutz GE, Vad VB, Wisneski RJ: Segmental instability: rehabilitation considerations. Seminars in Spine Surgery 8:332-338, 1996.

Lutz GE, Vad VB, Wisneski RJ: Fluoroscopic transforaminal lumbar epidural steroids: an outcome study. Arch Phys Med Rehabil 79:1362-1366, 1998.

Macnab I: The mechanism of spondylogenic pain. In: Hirsch C, Zotterman Y (eds.): *Cervical pain.* Oxford: Pergamon Press, 89-95, 1972.

Maigne J-Y, Rime B, Deligne B: Computed tomographic follow-up study of forty-eight cases of nonoperatively treated lumbar intervertebral disc herniation. Spine 17:1071-1074, 1992.

McCarron RF, Wimpee MW, Hudkins PG, Laros GS: The inflammatory effect of nucleus pulposus. A possible element in the pathogenesis of low-back pain. Spine 12:760-764, 1987.

McCormack K: Non-steroidal anti-inflammatory drugs and spinal nociceptive processing. Pain 59:9-43, 1994.

McCulloch JA, Transfeldt EE (eds.): *Macnab's backache,* 3rd edition. Baltimore: Williams & Wilkins, 417, 1997.

Mehta M, Salmon N: Extra dural block. Confirmation of the injection site by x-ray monitoring. Anesthesia 40:1009-1012, 1985.

Micheli LJ: Low back pain in the adolescent: differential diagnosis. Am J Sports Med 7:362-364, 1979.

Micheli LJ, Yancey RA: Thoracolumbar spine injuries in pediatric sports. In: Stanitski CL, DeLee JC, Drez D (eds.): *Pediatric and adolescent sports medicine* Vol 3. Philadelphia: WB Saunders Company, 162-174, 1994.

Mundt DJ, Kelsey JL, Golden AL Panjabi MM, pastides H, Berg AT, Sklar J, Hosea T: An epidemiologic study of sports and weightlifting as possible risk factors for herniated lumbar and cervical discs. The Northeast Collaborative Group on Low Back Pain. Am J Sports Med 21:854-860, 1993.

Nachemson A, Schiltz A, Andersson G: Mechanical effectiveness studies of lumbar spinal orthoses. Scand J Rehabil Med 9:139-149, 1983.

Nelson BW, Carpenter DM, Dreisinger TE, Mitchell M, Kelly CE, Wegner JA: Can spinal surgery be prevented by strengthening exercises? A prospective study of cervical and lumbar patients. Arch Phys Med Rehabil 80:20-25, 1999.

Olmarker K, Byrod G, Cornefjord M, Nordborg C, Rydevik B: Effects of methylprednisolone on nucleus pulposus induced nerve root injury. Spine 19:1803-1808, 1994.

Olmarker K, Rydevik B, Nordborg C: Autologous nucleus pulposus induces neurophysiologic and histologic changes in porcine cauda equina nerve roots. Spine 18:1425-1432, 1993.

Ozaktay AC, Kallakuri S, Cavanaugh JM: Phospholipase A2 sensitivity of the dorsal and dorsal root ganglion. Spine 23:1297-1306, 1998.

Ransford AD, Cairns D, Mooney V: The pain drawing as aid to the psychologic evaluation of patients with low back pain. Spine 1:127-134, 1976.

Renfrew DL, Moore TE, Kathol MH, El-Khoury GY, Lemke JH, Walker CW: Correct placement of epidural steroid injections: fluoroscopic guidance and contrast administration. Am J Neuroradiol 12:1003-1007, 1991.

Roberts S, Menage J, Urban PG: Biochemical and structural properties of the cartilage end plate and its relation to the intervertebral disc. Spine 14:166-174, 1989.

Saal JA: Rehabilitation of football players with lumbar spine injury. Part 1. Physician Sportsmed 16:61-68, 1988a.

Saal JA: Rehabilitation of football players with lumbar spine injury. Part 2. Physician Sportsmed 16:117-125, 1988b.

Saal JA: Dynamic muscular stabilization in the nonoperative treatment of lumbar pain syndromes. Orthop Rev 19(8):691-700, 1990.

Saal JA, Saal JS: Nonoperative treatment of herniated lumbar intervertebral disc with radiculopathy: an outcome study. Spine 14:431-437, 1989.

Saal JA, Saal JS, Herzog RJ: The natural history of lumbar intervertebral disc extrusions treated nonoperatively. Spine 15:683-686, 1990.

Saal JS: The role of inflammation in lumbar pain. Spine 20:1821-1827, 1995.

Saal JS, Franson RC, Dobrow R, Saal JA, White AH, Goldthwaite N: High levels of inflammatory phospholipase A2 activity in lumbar spine disc herniations. Spine 15:674-678, 1990.

Semon RL, Spengler D: Significance of lumbar spondylosis in college football players. Spine 6:172-174, 1981.

Steiner ME, Micheli LJ: Treatment of symptomatic spondylolysis and spondylolisthesis with modified Boston brace. Spine 10:937-943, 1985.

Steinkamp L. Soccer. In: White AH (ed.): *Spine care: diagnosis and conservative treatment*, Volume 1. St. Louis: Mosby, 721-726, 1995.

Sward L, Hellstrom M, Jacobsson B, Nyman R, Peterson L: Disc degeneration and associated abnormalities of the spine in elite gymnasts. A magnetic resonance imaging study. Spine 16:437-443, 1991.

Tall RL, DeVaulty W: Spinal injury in sport: epidemiologic considerations. In: Sinston JT, Wiesel SW (eds.): *Clinics in sports medicine: spine problems in athletes*. Philadelphia: Saunders, 441-448, 1993.

Videman T, Battie MC, Gibbons LE, Manninen H, Gill K, Fisher LD, Koskenvus M: Lifetime exercise and disk degeneration: a MRI study of monozygotic twins. Med Sci Sports Exerc 29:1350-1356, 1997.

Videman T, Sarna S, Battie MC, Koskinen S, Gill K, Paananen H, Gibbons L: The long term effects of physical loading and exercise lifestyles on back-related symptoms, disability, and spinal pathology among men. Spine 20:699-709, 1995.

Virgin WJ: Experimental investigations into the physical properties of the intervertebral disc. J Bone Joint Surg 33B:607-611, 1951.

Watkins RG: Baseball. In: White AH (ed.): *Spine care: diagnosis and conservative treatment*, Volume 1. St.Louis: Mosby, 608-626, 1995.

Weber H: Lumbar disc herniation: a controlled, prospective study with ten years of observation. Spine 8:131-140, 1983.

Weiner BK, Fraser RD: Foraminal injection for lateral lumbar disc herniation. J Bone Joint Surg 79B:804-807, 1997.

Weinstein SM, Herring SA: Principles and practice of imaging athletic injuries to the cervical, thoracic and lumbar spine. In: Halpern B, Herring SA, Altchek D, Herzog R (eds.): *Imaging in musculoskeletal sports medicine.* Cambridge, MA: Blackwell Scientific, 58-81, 1997.

Weinstein SM, Herring SA, Derby R: Contemporary concepts in spine care: epidural steroid injections. Spine 20:1842-1846, 1995.

Wiesel SW, Tsourmas N, Feffer HL, Citrin CM, Patronas N: A study of computer-assisted tomography: the incidence of positive CAT scans in an asymptomatic group of patients. Spine 9:549-551, 1984.

6

Lower-Extremity Nerve Injuries

Lisa S. Krivickas, MD

Although sports injuries themselves are common, injuries that involve peripheral nerves are relatively rare. In 1995, 5.4 million sports injuries in the United States required emergency room care. Of these, less than 1% were nerve injuries. Nevertheless, severe nerve injuries can have a lasting impact on athletes' careers as well as on their ability to perform nonathletic activities. All physicians practicing sports medicine need to be familiar with the anatomy of the peripheral nervous system and with common patterns of nerve injury. The majority of nerve injuries sustained by athletes involve nerves of the brachial plexus and the upper extremity rather than nerves of the lower extremity.

In the largest series of sports-related nerve injuries reported to date, only 24 of 216 (11%) were to lower-extremity nerves (Krivickas and Wilbourn 2000)—including 17 peroneal, 3 tibial, 2 sciatic, and 1 saphenous nerve injury. In addition to nerve injuries directly caused by sporting activity, athletes may develop nerve injuries as complications of the treatment of sports injuries. Treatments most commonly associated with nerve injury are cast application and arthroscopic surgery. Athletes are also susceptible to nerve injuries not related to sports—see Stewart (2000) for a review of such injuries.

This chapter summarizes the literature on sports injuries affecting the nerves that originate from the lumbosacral plexus.

NEUROPATHIES OF THE LUMBAR PLEXUS

Neuropathies involving nerves that originate from the lumbar plexus include femoral, lateral femoral cutaneous, saphenous, and obturator neuropathies.

Femoral Neuropathy

The femoral nerve is formed from the posterior portions of the ventral rami of the L2, L3, and L4 nerve roots and passes between the psoas and iliacus muscles (figure 6.1). The nerve is prone to compression as it enters the thigh deep to the inguinal ligament, which is the upper border of the femoral triangle (Peri 1991). The other boundaries of the femoral triangle are the sartorius laterally and the adductor longus medially. In the triangle, the femoral nerve divides into motor branches—to the four quadriceps muscles, the sartorius muscle, and the pectineus; and into three sensory branches—the saphenous (supplying the skin of the medial leg) and the intermediate and medial cutaneous nerves of the thigh (supplying the skin of the anterior thigh) (figure 6.2). The femoral nerve is not commonly entrapped at any particular site along its course.

Diagnosis

Signs and symptoms of a femoral nerve lesion include pain, paresthesias, and numbness of the anterior thigh and medial leg. Hip flexor and knee extensor weakness may present as knee buckling or difficulty climbing stairs. With severe injuries, atrophy of the quadriceps muscles occurs and is usually first observed in the distal portion of the vastus medialis. The knee jerk reflex may be diminished or lost. Patients with a femoral neuropathy from an iliacus hematoma usually experience upper-thigh ecchymoses, pain, and swelling in the iliac fossa and inguinal area and are most comfortable with the hip in a flexed position.

The differential diagnosis of a suspected femoral neuropathy includes lumbar radiculopathy (L3 or L4) and lumbar plexopathy. *Electrodiagnostic studies (EDXs)* can help differentiate between these entities. Nerve conduction studies can be performed for both the femoral motor nerve and the saphenous nerve, but the needle electrode examination is most important in attempting to narrow the differential diagnosis. A thorough needle electrode examination should assess the iliopsoas, at least two of the quadriceps muscles, the adductor longus (supplied by the obturator nerve), and the lumbar paraspinal muscles. A lesion at or proximal to the femoral triangle will affect all four of the quadriceps muscles. Denervation in the adductor longus suggests either a plexopathy or a radiculopathy, and denervation in the paraspinal muscles suggests a radiculopathy.

> **electrodiagnostic study (EDX)**—The clinical electromyographic (EMG) study performed to diagnose a peripheral nerve injury. This study should include both a set of nerve conduction studies and a needle electrode examination of selected muscles in order to be considered complete.

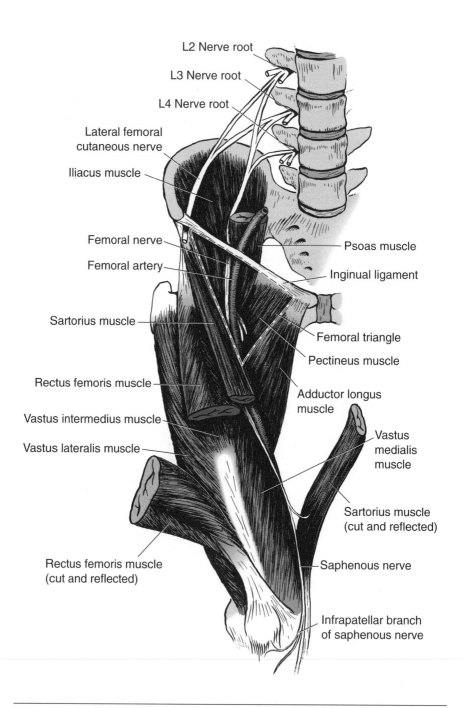

Figure 6.1 Anatomic course of the femoral nerve.

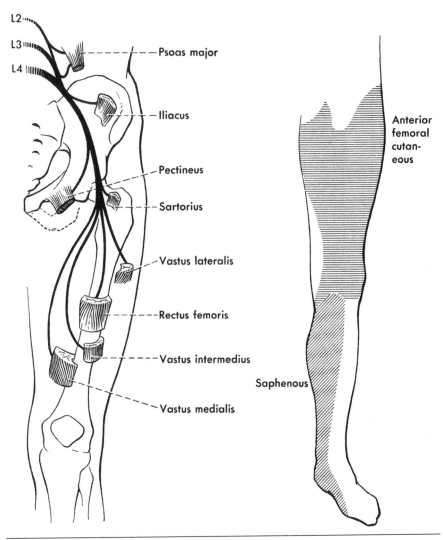

Figure 6.2 Distribution of the femoral nerve.

Reprinted, by permission, from D.B. Jenkins, 1991, *Hollinshead's functional anatomy of the limbs and back*, 4th ed. (Philadelphia, PA: W.B. Saunders).

Femoral motor nerve conduction studies performed within one month of injury provide useful prognostic information. In a study of 32 unilateral femoral neuropathies produced by a variety of causes, a compound motor action potential (CMAP) amplitude (a rough estimate of percentage of axon loss) greater than or equal to 50% that of the unaffected side was the single best prognostic indicator; 90% of such patients demonstrated clinical improvement within one year of injury (Kuntzer et al. 1997).

Any athlete presenting with an isolated femoral nerve injury probably warrants an MRI of the pelvis to rule out the presence of a hematoma or other mass lesion. If no acute history of injury is given, a brief neurologic examination should be performed to rule out other sites of focal weakness that might indicate a mononeuritis multiplex.

Etiology

The femoral nerve is rarely injured in sports. The literature contains case reports of a femoral neuropathy that developed in a male gymnast following a workout (Brozin et al. 1982) and in two female modern dancers (Miller and Benedict 1985, Sammarco and Stephens 1991). None of these neuropathies involved trauma, and the purported mechanism of injury was described in only one case. One of the dancers experienced the acute onset of quadriceps muscle weakness and anterior thigh numbness while performing a "hinge" maneuver, which involves hyperextension of the hip while in a kneeling position. Based on this history, the mechanism was thought to be a stretch injury. The femoral nerve crosses over the pubic ramus before passing under the inguinal ligament and can be stretched over the pubic bone with extreme hip extension. The injury most likely occurred in a very thin individual. All three of these femoral nerve injuries affected all portions of the quadriceps, indicating that the lesions were at or proximal to the femoral triangle.

Carter et al. (1995) described a case of idiopathic distal femoral neuropathy involving incomplete axon loss, affecting only the motor branch to the vastus lateralis, in a 16-year-old female track athlete. In this particular case, short T1 inversion recovery (STIR) magnetic resonance imaging (MRI) was used, in conjunction with EMG, to delineate the area of pathology. Needle electrode examination found denervation only in the vastus lateralis muscle, and this was confirmed by the MRI. With the STIR/MRI sequence, acutely denervated muscle has a higher signal intensity than normal muscle.

Severe trauma that tears the iliopsoas muscle or fractures the femur can produce an anterior thigh compartment syndrome or hematoma, injuring either the main trunk of the femoral nerve or one of its more distal branches. Acute compartment syndromes are surgical emergencies requiring *fasciotomy* and hematoma removal.

fasciotomy—Surgical incision of the fascia overlying muscle, generally performed to release excessive pressure build up.

Lateral Femoral Cutaneous Neuropathy

The lateral femoral cutaneous nerve is a pure sensory nerve formed from the posterior portions of the ventral rami of the L2 and L3 nerve roots. It enters the lower extremity by passing slightly medial and inferior to the anterior superior iliac spine (ASIS), inferior to the inguinal ligament, and superior to the sartorius muscle. The nerve is prone to entrapment and compression at the fibromuscular ring outlined by the inguinal ligament and the iliopsoas and more distally within the femoral fascia (Peri 1991). The nerve supplies sensation to the anterolateral thigh. Injury causes burning, pain, or numbness in its region of innervation—collectively known as the "meralgia paresthetica syndrome." Standing or walking often aggravates the pain, and sitting improves or relieves it. In some individuals, placing the hand in the ipsilateral front trouser pocket produces *allodynia.*

allodynia—Pain produced by nonnoxious stimulation of the skin in the territory of a damaged nerve.

It is difficult to perform nerve conduction studies of the lateral femoral cutaneous nerve, and responses often cannot be obtained in normal individuals; thus, the diagnosis of lateral femoral cutaneous neuropathy is usually made clinically. EDX evaluation helps to exclude other entities in the differential diagnosis; these include L2 radiculopathy, femoral neuropathy, and lumbar plexopathy. The evaluation should be similar to that described for a femoral neuropathy.

A "hip pointer" is a contusion to the ASIS that can injure the lateral femoral cutaneous nerve, usually with a *neurapraxic* lesion; this injury may occur in football, hockey, soccer, and basketball players. Skipping rope, using uneven parallel bars in gymnastics, and wearing a tight weightlifting belt also have caused meralgia paresthetica (Hirasawa and Kisaburo 1983, Spindler and Pappas 1995). Lateral femoral cutaneous neuropathy has been reported in two female gymnasts, ages 14 and 18 (Macgregor 1977). The injuries were produced by "beating" the low bar, a movement performed in uneven parallel bar routines that involves extreme flexion of the body around the low bar while the hands grasp the high bar. Because of advances in uneven parallel bars technique, which require a wider separation between the low and high bars, "beats" are no longer performed by advanced- or elite-level gymnasts. (Note: A hip pointer must involve a contusion; not all lateral femoral cutaneous neuropathies are "hip pointers.")

neurapraxia—Mild nerve injury in which only the myelin sheath, and not the axon, is damaged.

Saphenous Neuropathy

The saphenous nerve provides sensation to the medial aspect of the leg, distal to the medial femoral condyle, and to the proximal medial side of the foot. The saphenous nerve exits from the adductor canal (Hunter's canal), travels behind the sartorius muscle, and becomes subcutaneous between the tendons of the sartorius and gracilis.

Diagnosis

Injury to this nerve may produce a sensory deficit or pain with minimal sensory deficit. The pain may be localized to the medial aspect of the knee (Edwards et al. 1989), mimicking pes anserine bursitis or even internal derangement of the knee joint such as a meniscal tear. Pain may also be localized to the distal medial tibia, mimicking medial tibial stress syndrome or a stress fracture (Hemler et al. 1991). The differential diagnosis of an athlete presenting with pain or a sensory deficit in this distribution must include a partial femoral neuropathy and an L4 radiculopathy.

An EDX examination assists the clinician primarily by excluding other entities in the differential diagnosis. Saphenous nerve conduction studies may be performed, but they are one of the most difficult lower-extremity sensory responses for the electromyographer to obtain. An absent saphenous response is significant only when a response is present on the contralateral side. The electrodiagnostic evaluation of a saphenous neuropathy should include femoral nerve conduction studies and a needle electrode examination. The tibialis anterior is an important muscle to study because denervation in this muscle suggests an L4 radiculopathy rather than a saphenous neuropathy.

Etiology

There are few reports of sports-related saphenous nerve injuries. Surfers have developed them, presumably from holding the surf board between their knees while waiting for a wave to approach (Fabian et al. 1987). Hemler et al. (1991) described a runner who developed a saphenous neuropathy from compression by a swollen pes anserine bursa; he was initially misdiagnosed as having a stress fracture. Patella dislocation has been associated with saphenous neuropathy in a rugby player (Gleeson and Kerr 1996). Many athletes undergo knee surgery or arthroscopy for sports-related meniscus and ligament injuries; saphenous nerve injury has been reported as a complication of medial knee arthroscopy or arthrotomy (Logue and Drez 1996, Worth et al. 1984). Ankle arthroscopy can injure the saphenous nerve at the ankle (Ferkel et al. 1996).

Obturator Neuropathy

The obturator nerve is formed within the psoas major muscle from the anterior divisions of the ventral primary rami of L2, L3, and L4. The nerve enters the obturator canal, where it divides into anterior and posterior branches and ultimately exits the pelvis via the obturator foramen. It supplies motor function to the thigh adductors (except the posterior portion of the adductor magnus, which is innervated by the sciatic nerve), gracilis, and obturator externus. In addition, it supplies sensation to a small patch of skin on the upper medial thigh. The nerve may become entrapped (either in the obturator canal or distal to the canal) between two muscles—for example, the pectineus and obturator externus, the adductor longus and brevis, or the obturator externus and adductor magnus.

Diagnosis

Obturator neuropathy may produce a generalized sense of "leg weakness" that the athlete has difficulty localizing to the adductor muscles, or it may produce a sensory deficit on the inner thigh. An L3 or L4 radiculopathy and a lumbar plexopathy are included in the differential diagnosis. The diagnosis of an obturator neuropathy is made primarily by EDX. Since nerve conduction studies of the obturator nerve are not practical, the diagnosis is made by demonstrating denervation, on needle electrode examination, in the adductor muscles and by excluding involvement of muscles not innervated by the obturator nerve.

Etiology

Only one group of authors has reported sports-related obturator nerve injuries. Bradshaw and colleagues (1997) reported 31 cases of obturator neuropathy in athletes, 26 of whom were Australian-rules football players. These athletes presented with chronic groin pain, postexercise medial thigh pain, adductor muscle weakness, or paresthesias in the distribution of the obturator nerve. All patients reportedly had EDX evidence of denervation in obturator-innervated muscles. The authors felt that these cases of obturator neuropathy were focal entrapments by fascial and vascular structures overlying the obturator externus and short adductors at the level of the obturator foramen. Stating that conservative treatment approaches often fail, they advocated the confirmatory use of a diagnostic local anesthetic block followed by surgical release of the nerve entrapment. The mechanism by which Australian footballers develop this entrapment is unclear; it does not appear to have a preference for the kicking versus the nonkicking leg. Until this nerve entrapment is reported by additional investigators, it should be viewed with caution as an explanation for groin pain in athletes.

NEUROPATHIES OF THE SACRAL PLEXUS

Neuropathies involving nerves that originate from the sacral plexus include sciatic, peroneal, tibial, and pudendal neuropathies.

Sciatic Neuropathy

The anterior and posterior ventral rami from L4-S2 and the anterior ventral ramus of S3 combine to form the sciatic nerve as these roots leave the lumbosacral plexus. The anterior rami contribute the fibers that become the tibial nerve, and the posterior rami contribute the peroneal fibers (figures 6.3 and 6.4). The peroneal fibers are lateral to the tibial fibers, are arranged in fewer, larger funiculi, and are tethered at the knee. All of these factors predispose the peroneal fibers to more severe damage when the sciatic nerve is injured. Series of sciatic nerve injuries have consistently

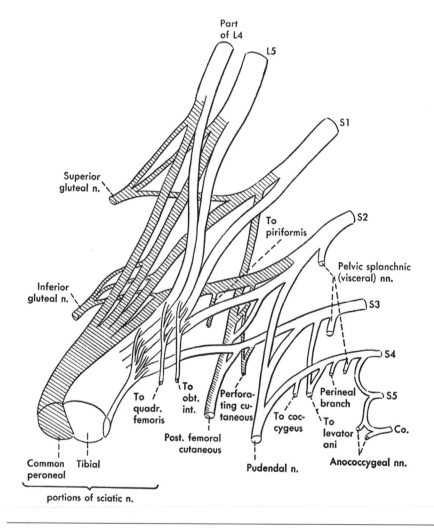

Figure 6.3 Diagram of the sacral plexus. The posterior parts of the plexus are shaded.

Reprinted, by permission, from D.B. Jenkins, 1991, *Hollinshead's functional anatomy of the limbs and back*, 4th ed. (Philadelphia, PA: W.B. Saunders).

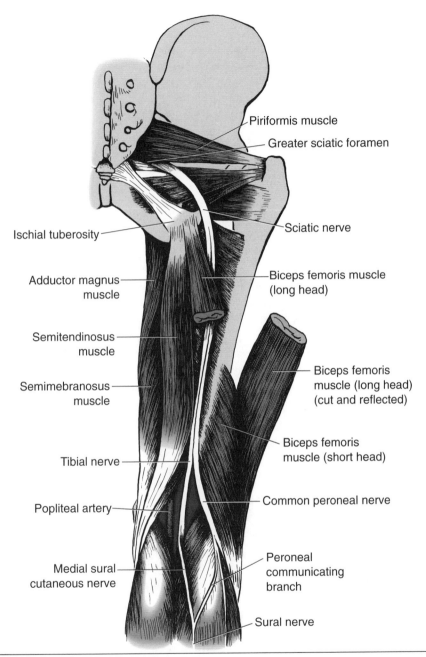

Piriformis muscle

Greater sciatic foramen

Sciatic nerve

Ischial tuberosity

Adductor magnus muscle

Biceps femoris muscle (long head)

Semitendinosus muscle

Semimebranosus muscle

Biceps femoris muscle (long head) (cut and reflected)

Biceps femoris muscle (short head)

Tibial nerve

Popliteal artery

Common peroneal nerve

Medial sural cutaneous nerve

Peroneal communicating branch

Sural nerve

Figure 6.4   Anatomic course of the sciatic nerve.

demonstrated that the peroneal fibers typically are injured more severely than the tibial fibers (Fassler et al. 1993, Yuen et al. 1994). The sciatic nerve exits the pelvis via the greater sciatic foramen just lateral to the ischial tuberosity; it usually exits from beneath the piriformis muscle. In rare instances, either the common peroneal portion of the nerve or the entire nerve pierces the piriformis muscle and emerges from it. The sciatic nerve can divide into its separate tibial and common peroneal branches anywhere between the piriformis muscle and the popliteal fossa. Branches to the four hamstring muscles are usually given off prior to the bifurcation of the tibial and common peroneal nerve fibers. The peroneal fibers in the sciatic nerve innervate the short head of the biceps femoris; all other hamstring muscles and the posterior portion of the adductor magnus are innervated by the tibial fibers. Involvement of the short head of the biceps femoris allows differentiation between a peroneal nerve lesion at the knee and a sciatic nerve lesion above the knee.

Diagnosis

Injury to the sciatic nerve produces pain, paresthesia, and numbness anywhere in the leg below the knee—except along the medial aspect of the leg, which is innervated by the saphenous nerve. If the injury is in the region of the buttock or proximal thigh, pain may radiate distally from the site of injury, mimicking a lumbosacral radiculopathy; a positive *straight-leg raising test* may also be present. The motor fibers most frequently affected are those in the peroneal division of the nerve, producing a foot drop, toe extensor weakness, and evertor weakness. Injury to the tibial portion produces weakness in ankle plantar flexion, impairing the athlete's ability to run and jump. Although hamstring weakness may also occur, it often is less apparent clinically. When a severe injury affects the tibial fibers, the ankle jerk is lost.

> **straight-leg raising test**—Physical examination maneuver in which the examiner passively lifts the supine patient's leg by flexing the hip with the knee extended. If this maneuver produces back pain radiating into the leg, it is suggestive of a lumbosacral radiculopathy.

The differential diagnosis of a sciatic neuropathy includes the differential diagnosis of foot drop as well as that of tibial neuropathy. The etiology of foot drop due to a peripheral nerve lesion, from most to least prevalent, is common peroneal neuropathy, L5 radiculopathy, polyneuropathy, sciatic neuropathy, lumbosacral plexus lesion, and cauda equina lesion (Langenhove et al. 1989). EDX is extremely useful for localizing the lesion. Tibial, peroneal, and sural nerve conduction studies may all be abnormal with a sciatic nerve lesion. Key muscles to examine with a needle electrode are the biceps femoris short head, which will assist with distinguishing a peroneal from a sciatic lesion, and the glutei, which help distinguish a plexus or root lesion from a sciatic neuropathy.

Etiology

Because only major trauma can damage it, the sciatic nerve is rarely injured in sports. A severe fall on the buttocks, a posterior hip dislocation, or a femur fracture all potentially can injure the sciatic nerve. This author has seen sciatic injuries associated with a fall from a bicycle, also resulting in a proximal tibia fracture; with a softball sliding injury, also producing a combined tibia-fibula fracture and ligamentous disruption of the knee (Krivickas and Wilbourn 1998); and with a blow to the buttock from a football helmet. A transient sciatic neuropathy has been reported following use of a stationary exercise bicycle (Haig 1989) and from prolonged sitting in the lotus position, with the feet tucked under the thighs, during a yoga retreat (Vogel et al. 1991). The posterior femoral cutaneous nerve, which receives nerve fibers from the S1-S4 nerve roots and provides sensation to the posterior thigh, runs parallel to the sciatic nerve through the buttock and has been compressed by similar mechanisms (i.e., bicycling and sitting in a yoga position) (Arnoldussen and Korten 1980). *Myositis ossificans*, which occasionally develops following a severe hamstring muscle strain, has produced sciatic neuropathy in both a weightlifter and a football player (Gristina and Horelick 1981, Jones and Ward 1980).

myositis ossificans—Calcification that develops in a muscle after an injury such as a severe contusion or strain.

The prognosis for full functional recovery is better for tibial than for peroneal nerve fibers. In one series of patients with non-sports-related sciatic nerve injuries, residual disability was attributed primarily to peroneal deficits (Fassler et al. 1993). In the series of Yuen et al. (1994), the best predictors of good recovery were a recordable compound motor action potential from the extensor digitorum brevis muscle and incomplete paralysis of the ankle plantar flexors and dorsiflexors. Maximal recovery may take two to three years because of the length of the sciatic nerve.

Some physicians believe that *piriformis syndrome* is a form of sciatic compression neuropathy, but this remains to be proven conclusively from an electrodiagnostic standpoint. Two forms of piriformis syndrome are possible. The first is "true" piriformis syndrome in which the sciatic nerve, or one of its two divisions, is damaged by compression from the piriformis muscle. An extensive review of the literature has identified only two patients with EDX evidence of a sciatic neuropathy and what appeared at surgery to be sciatic nerve compression by the piriformis muscle; neither of these patients had an anatomic anomaly in which the nerve pierced the muscle (Nakano 1987, Stein and Warfield 1983). Many more cases of "disputed" or nonneurogenic piriformis syndrome have been described. These patients experience pain in the buttock and in the distribution of the sciatic nerve but do not have neurologic deficits or abnormal EDXs. They are often slender individuals, and external compression of the nerve while sitting may produce some of their symptoms.

Common Peroneal Neuropathy

The common peroneal nerve is a continuation of the sciatic nerve and is derived from the L4-S2 nerve roots, although the main nerve root contribution is from L5 (figure 6.5). After passing through the lateral aspect of the popliteal fossa, the common peroneal nerve passes behind the fibular head, winds around the neck of the fibula, and descends the leg superficially in close proximity to the fibula for approximately 10 cm. It then passes through the peroneus longus muscle and divides into the superficial and deep peroneal branches.

Diagnosis

An injury to the common peroneal nerve produces paresthesias, numbness, and pain on the dorsum of the foot. Weakness occurs in the ankle evertors, ankle dorsiflexors, and toe extensors, often producing a foot slap when walking on a hard floor.

EDX evaluation is the most important diagnostic test for a suspected peroneal nerve injury, as it allows other diagnoses to be excluded and identifies the pathophysiology of the nerve injury, thus determining the prognosis. The differential diagnosis of a common peroneal neuropathy includes L5 radiculopathy, sciatic neuropathy, and a lumbosacral plexopathy. The EDX should include peroneal motor nerve conduction studies (recording from both the extensor digitorum brevis and the tibialis anterior muscles) and superficial peroneal sensory studies. Katirji and Wilbourn (1988) found that the motor nerve conduction study recording from the tibialis anterior muscle is the most sensitive study for assessing the degree of *conduction block* versus axon loss (Katirji and Wilbourn 1988, Wilbourn 1986). The distinction between axon loss and conduction block allows a clinician to provide the athlete with an accurate prognosis. On needle electrode examination, the short head of the biceps femoris is a crucial muscle because it allows one to distinguish a sciatic neuropathy primarily affecting the peroneal fibers from a common peroneal neuropathy.

> **conduction block**—Failure of action potential propagation along a nerve, caused by demyelination or damage to the myelin sheath. Conduction block occurs in neurapraxic injuries. Conduction is possible, however, below the point of the block.

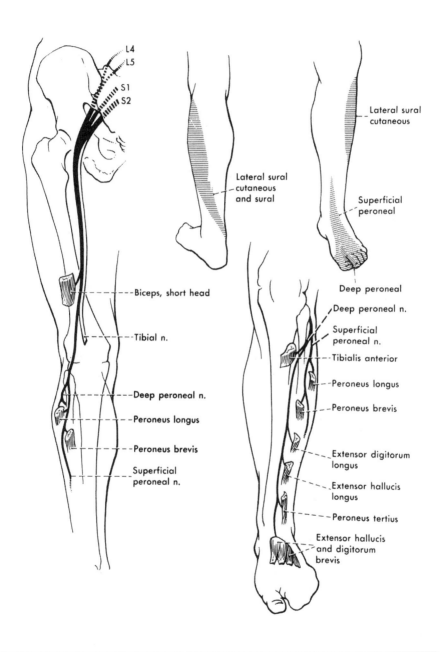

Figure 6.5 Distribution of the common peroneal nerve.

Reprinted, by permission, from D.B. Jenkins, 1991, *Hollinshead's functional anatomy of the limbs and back,* 4th ed. (Philadelphia, PA: W.B. Saunders).

Etiology

The common peroneal nerve is injured more frequently than either of its branches in isolation. In fact, common peroneal neuropathy is the most frequent lower-extremity mononeuropathy. The common peroneal nerve can be injured by a stretch injury or by direct compression, usually from a blow to the lateral aspect of the leg near the fibular head. Occasionally, it is compressed by a constricting fascial band. Stretch injuries are associated with both inversion ankle injuries and knee injuries.

We have seen peroneal nerve injuries associated with isolated tears of the anterior cruciate ligament (ACL) or with ACL tears in combination with tears in either the lateral collateral ligament (LCL) or posterior cruciate ligament (PCL). These injuries have occurred without associated fractures in football players, soccer players, and in a broad jumper (Krivickas and Wilbourn 1998). Peroneal nerve injury has also been reported in a basketball player in association with injury to the ACL, LCL, and popliteus tendon resulting from a varus blow to the knee with the foot planted (McMahon and Craig 1994). A similar mechanism occasionally injures the peroneal nerve without concomitant ligament injury (Seckler and DiStefano 1996, Streib 1983). Peroneal nerve injuries in skiers have been reported in association with combined tibia and fibula fractures and with knee dislocations (Myles et al. 1992, Nobel 1966).

The orthopedic literature suggests that 20-30% of knee dislocations are associated with peroneal nerve injury (Malizos et al. 1997, Montgomery et al. 1995, Wascher et al. 1997). When the tibial nerve is injured, there is always a peroneal nerve injury. Most knee dislocations result from high-energy trauma such as motor vehicle accidents, but Wascher and colleagues (1997) reported 10 knee dislocations associated with recreational sports activities. Many sports medicine specialists now consider complete bicruciate knee ligament injuries to be dislocations that have spontaneously reduced.

Hockey pucks, soccer kicks, and football helmets may deliver direct blows to the fibular head (Lorei and Hershman 1993). A dancer's fall on a maximally flexed knee, causing posterolateral subluxation of the superior tibiofibular joint, has produced a peroneal nerve injury (Gillham and Villar 1989). An unusual case of a closed rupture of the nerve has been reported in a cricket player who wore a set of poorly fitting pads with a tight leather strap around the upper calf; the strap presumably produced traction that caused the nerve to rupture when the calf muscles contracted (Holt et al. 1996). Peroneal nerve injury, known as "dead foot," has also been reported in bungee jumpers; the mechanism is thought to be traction related to the use of a harness around the ankle (Torre et al. 1993, Vanderford and Meyers 1995).

A rare entity associated with tibia and fibula fractures is a peroneal nerve injury caused by a peroneal nerve sheath hematoma; the hematoma produces nerve ischemia and excruciating pain similar to that of an acute compartment syndrome (Nobel 1966). A ruptured vasa nervorum produces the hematoma, and immediate surgical evacuation of the hematoma is imperative to prevent permanent neurologic damage.

Inversion ankle sprains, as mild as grade I, have also been associated with peroneal nerve injuries which, surprisingly, are almost always localized to the fibular head, not the ankle (Hyslop 1941, Meals 1977); the mechanism is most likely a traction injury as the nerve passes around the fibular head. In one study, 17% of patients with grade II sprains and 86% of those with grade III sprains had fibrillation potentials in their peroneal innervated leg muscles, despite the lack of clinical signs and symptoms of nerve injury, suggesting a subclinical mild axonal injury (Nitz et al. 1985).

Chronic repetitive activity can also compress the peroneal nerve. Attributed to a variety of causes, this type of injury is reported most frequently in runners. Runners with peroneal nerve compression were found to have a tight fascial band at the edge of the peroneus longus muscle (Leach et al. 1989). The athletes reported the onset of pain, paresthesias, or foot drop with prolonged running but not with walking; most had relief of symptoms with surgical release of a fascial band at the edge of the peroneus longus. Chronic entrapment of the nerve can also be caused by mechanical irritation due to hypermobility of the fibular head (Moller and Kadin 1987) or the presence of an accessory ossicle in the lateral gastrocnemius muscle *(fabella syndrome)*.

fabella syndrome—Entrapment of the common peroneal nerve by an accessory ossicle in the lateral gastrocenemius.

Sports-related peroneal nerve injuries may occur indirectly, as a result of treatment for another injury that was caused by sports participation. Most of these indirect injuries are surgical complications. The peroneal nerve has been injured during arthroscopic lateral meniscus repair by a misplaced suture, transected during diagnostic arthroscopy, and injured during knee ligament reconstruction (Miller 1988, Peicha et al. 1998, Putukian et al. 1995). Cryotherapy to treat a lower-extremity injury can also injure the peroneal nerve, as in the case of a football player who developed a foot drop after icing a hamstring muscle strain; athletes should be careful not to apply ice directly over the fibular head where the nerve is very superficial (Moeller et al. 1997).

Deep and Superficial Peroneal Nerves

The superficial peroneal nerve innervates the peroneus longus and brevis and supplies sensation to the dorsum of the foot. The deep peroneal nerve supplies the tibialis anterior, peroneus tertius, and all toe extensor muscles. It supplies sensation to the first web space of the foot.

Diagnosis

Injury confined to the deep peroneal nerve will produce a foot drop without evertor weakness and a sensory deficit only in the first web space of the foot. Occasionally, injury to the deep peroneal nerve causes "toe drop" or toe extensor weakness without a foot drop (Streib et al. 1982). When injury to the superficial peroneal nerve causes only evertor weakness, it is easy to miss the injury as a factor contributing to recurrent inversion ankle sprains. Muscle stretch reflexes are unaffected by injury to the peroneal nerve.

Chronic compartment syndromes affecting the anterior or lateral compartments of the leg cause symptoms referable to the deep and superficial peroneal nerves, respectively. Chronic compartment syndromes present with exercise-induced tightness, aching, and pain in the involved compartment; while paresthesias often accompany these symptoms, motor deficits occur only in extreme cases. The symptoms are produced by muscle swelling in a restricted fascial space, which compresses the vascular supply to the peroneal nerve. Symptoms resolve after a period of rest, the length of which depends on the degree of pressure increase within the compartment. Diagnosis requires compartment pressure measurement using a wick or slit catheter technique while the patient is symptomatic.

Occasionally, *acute compartment syndromes* develop as a result of athletic activity (Lipscomb and Ibrahim 1977). Severe pain develops and persists in the involved compartment, then worsens within hours after activity ends. The muscles in the involved compartment become rock hard, eventually becoming completely paralyzed. Acute compartment syndromes are surgical emergencies caused by both muscle and nerve ischemia. They require immediate fasciotomy to prevent permanent paralysis of the involved muscles. Partial acute compartment syndromes may selectively involve a single muscle; in the anterior compartment of the leg, the tibialis anterior or extensor hallucis longus are most often involved in partial compartment syndromes. After fasciotomy, the presence of fibrillation potentials in a muscle is a good prognostic sign indicating that complete ischemic muscle necrosis has not occurred.

> **compartment syndrome**—Elevated pressure in a fascial compartment, caused by swelling or hemorrhage of the contents; it can produce nerve injury and/or muscle necrosis.

Etiology

Anterior compartment syndromes are more than three times as common as lateral compartment syndromes (Detmer et al. 1985). However, superficial peroneal neuropathy has been reported in association with anterior compartment syndromes and as a complication following anterior compartment fasciotomy (Styf 1989); the proposed mechanism is nerve compression by muscles of the anterior compartment that bulge through a fascial defect to impinge on the superficial peroneal nerve. In one case, a neuroma was found just proximal to the distal end of a fascial defect in the lateral compartment fascia through which the peroneus brevis bulged (Garfin et al. 1977).

Few sports-related injuries to the superficial peroneal nerve have been reported other than those caused by compartment syndrome. Compression at the ankle by an overly tight roller skate has been described (Dewitt and Greenberg 1981). An infrequent indirect cause of injury is ankle arthroscopy. In one series, injury to the superficial peroneal nerve accounted for more than half of the nerve injuries complicating ankle arthroscopy; all of these injuries were produced by portal or distractor pin placement (Ferkel et al. 1996).

Isolated injury of the deep peroneal nerve has been reported as a complication of knee arthroscopy when the bifurcation of the common peroneal nerve is unusually high and proximal to the popliteal fossa (Esselman et al. 1993).

The deep peroneal nerve may be compressed at the ankle by tight ski boots (Lindenbaum 1978) or by skates, or by repetitively kicking a soccer ball. Ballet dancers can also compress the nerve by stretching it over the bony prominences of the anterior ankle when en pointe (Schon 1994). Symptoms and signs include paresthesias on the dorsum of the foot radiating to the big toe and inability to voluntarily contract the extensor digitorum brevis. Toe extension is not weak, because the extensor hallucis longus and extensor digitorum longus are innervated proximal to the site of compression. These injuries are often referred to as anterior tarsal tunnel syndrome, because it is thought that the deep peroneal nerve is compressed beneath the inferior extensor retinaculum of the ankle (Marinacci 1968). The electrodiagnostic findings are (1) a prolonged peroneal distal latency when recording from the extensor digitorum brevis (EDB), (2) normal nerve conduction velocity proximal to the ankle, and (3) minimal denervation in the EDB muscle (Wilbourn 1992). Modification of footwear often can prevent these mild injuries. Few of these lesions have been demonstrated electrodiagnostically, and their existence is somewhat controversial (Gessini et al. 1984). Compression of the deep peroneal nerve distal to the anterior tarsal tunnel, under the extensor hallucis brevis muscle, has also been reported (Kanbe et al. 1995). This lesion causes paresthesias and pain radiating to the big toe, but no motor weakness.

Tibial Neuropathy

Like the common peroneal nerve, the posterior tibial nerve is a continuation of the sciatic nerve. It is derived from the L4-S3 nerve roots (figure 6.6).

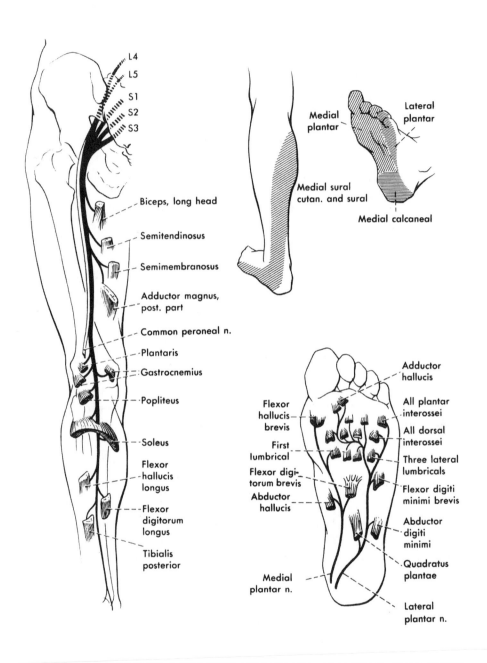

Figure 6.6 Distribution of the tibial nerve.

Reprinted, by permission, from D.B. Jenkins, 1991, *Hollinshead's functional anatomy of the limbs and back*, 4th ed. (Philadelphia, PA: W.B. Saunders).

The tibial nerve travels from the popliteal fossa into the deep posterior compartment of the leg, where it is well protected by overlying muscle until it reaches the tarsal tunnel posterior to the medial malleolus. At the level of the medial malleolus, the posterior tibial nerve divides into three main branches: the lateral plantar, medial plantar, and medial calcaneal nerves. The posterior tibial nerve innervates the soleus, gastrocnemius, flexor digitorum longus, flexor hallucis longus, tibialis posterior, and intrinsic foot muscles. It also provides sensation to the sole of the foot.

Diagnosis

Tibial nerve injuries can be quite painful, producing burning paresthesias on the sole of the foot; loss of sensation and numbness may also occur on the posterior calf. The plantar flexors, toe flexors, and intrinsic foot muscles lose strength and impair the push-off phase of gait. With long-standing injury, clawing of the toes develops because of weakness and atrophy of the foot intrinsic muscles.

Differential diagnosis of a tibial nerve injury consists of partial sciatic nerve injury, sacral plexopathy, and S1-S2 radiculopathy. The electrodiagnostic study should be planned to allow differentiation among these possibilities. Nerve conduction studies should include the tibial, peroneal, and sural nerves. If a low amplitude is recorded from the abductor hallucis with stimulation of the tibial nerve, it may be helpful to record motor amplitudes from the abductor digiti quinti pedis or soleus muscles. The needle examination should include evaluation of the paraspinal muscles, gluteal muscles, and hamstrings in addition to muscles innervated by the tibial nerve.

The tarsal tunnel is a fibro-osseous canal formed by the flexor retinaculum and the bones of the foot posterior to the medial malleolus. It contains the posterior tibial nerve, artery, and vein; and the tibialis posterior, flexor digitorum longus, and flexor hallucis longus tendons. Entrapment of the tibial nerve or one of its terminal branches in the tarsal tunnel is referred to as "tarsal tunnel syndrome." Tarsal tunnel syndrome produces burning, sharp pain, paresthesias, and numbness at the medial malleolus or on the sole of the foot. Weightbearing often aggravates the symptoms. The pain also tends to be worse at night and least in the morning (Jackson and Haglund 1992). A *Tinel's sign* may be elicited by tapping over the tunnel. Tenderness proximal or distal to the tunnel may be present, and this is known as a *Valleix sign*. An unusual clinical presentation of tarsal tunnel syndrome is the "syndrome of painful legs and moving toes," in which spontaneous, involuntary toe flexion occurs (Pla et al. 1996). The fibers belonging to the lateral plantar branch of the tibial nerve are injured more frequently than those belonging to the medial plantar branch. In athletes, the differential diagnosis for tarsal tunnel syndrome includes plantar fasciitis, heel spurs, plantar callosities, a tibial or sciatic neuropathy with selective plantar fascicle involvement, *Morton's neuroma*, and plantar neuropathy. From the viewpoint of the electromyographer, tarsal tunnel syndrome is vastly overdiagnosed. Although several nerve conduction techniques are available for assessing tarsal tunnel syndrome, the EDX is almost always normal.

> **Tinel's sign**—Electric shock sensation produced in the territory of a nerve when the nerve is tapped or palpated.

> **Morton's neuroma**—Mechanically induced degenerative neuropathy of the interdigital nerves of the foot, most commonly in the second or third web space.

Etiology

Because it is so well protected by overlying muscles, the tibial nerve is much less prone than the peroneal nerve to injury by trauma. Tibial nerve injuries have occurred with severe trauma such as a tibia fracture sustained while sliding into a base or a deep calf laceration from a skate blade in a figure skater (see case report 2, page 134). Knee injuries resulting in disruption of the posterior capsule or frank dislocation may also injure the tibial nerve. Injuries severe enough to produce a tibial neuropathy are likely to produce a concomitant vascular injury.

In runners, entrapment of the proximal tibial nerve by the tendinous arch of the origin of the soleus muscle has been reported (Peri 1991). Surgical decompression may relieve this entrapment. Tibial nerve injury has resulted from compression by a Baker's cyst (Kashani et al. 1985). A *Baker's cyst* is a synovial cyst in the popliteal fossa formed by accumulation of fluid in a noncommunicating bursa or by distension of a bursa by fluid from the knee joint. Baker's cysts are associated with meniscal tears, a common sports injury. Distal tibial nerve injury has been reported in a rugby player who sustained a distal fibula fracture and disruption of both the deltoid ligament and the syndesmosis (O'Sullivan et al. 1992).

Tibial nerve injury may also occur as a complication of surgically treating other sports injuries. A complete tibial nerve injury has been reported as a complication of a thigh tourniquet used during ACL reconstruction (Guanche 1995). The tibial nerve has also inadvertently been resected in place of a plantaris tendon graft for use in the repair of an Achilles tendon rupture; this surgical error produced permanent loss of tibial nerve function (McGeorge et al. 1992).

Entrapment of the main trunk of the tibial nerve or of one of its branches in the tarsal tunnel has been described in mountain climbers (Hirasawa and Kisaburo 1983), runners (Jackson and Haglund 1991, 1992), skiers

(Jackson and Haglund 1991, Yamamoto et al. 1995), and other athletes. The most common cause of electrophysiologically documented tarsal tunnel syndrome in athletes is a space-occupying lesion—such as a synovial or ganglion cyst (Mann 1995) or an accessory flexor digitorum longus muscle (Sammarco and Stephens 1990) or soleus muscle (Pla et al. 1996). An os trigonum has been found compressing the tibial nerve at the tarsal tunnel in runners (Murphy and Baxter 1985). A fracture of the medial tubercle of the posterior process of the talus (Cedell fracture), which occurred in conjunction with a grade II lateral ankle sprain sustained while playing basketball, has also been reported as a source of compression of the tarsal tunnel contents (Stefko et al. 1994). In skiers, poorly fitting ski boots have compressed the tibial nerve in the tarsal tunnel (Jackson and Haglund 1991, Yamamoto et al. 1995). Many believe that excessive pronation stretches the tibial nerve in runners, making it more vulnerable to other sources of compression or trauma (Schon 1994). Other proposed mechanisms of tibial nerve compression include repetitive flexion and extension of the ankle, causing tenosynovitis in the tarsal tunnel and fibrosis of the tunnel following recurrent ankle sprains (Lorei and Hershman 1993).

Plantar and Digital Neuropathies

As stated previously, the tibial nerve divides into three branches in or slightly distal to the tarsal tunnel. The medial calcaneal nerve supplies sensation to the sole of the heel. The medial plantar nerve, which passes beneath the abductor hallucis muscle origin and under a fibrous arch formed by the flexor hallucis brevis, provides sensation to the medial sole of the foot and innervation to the abductor hallucis, first lumbrical, flexor hallucis brevis, and flexor digitorum brevis. The lateral plantar nerve, which also passes under the abductor hallucis and then runs between the flexor digitorum brevis and quadratus plantae muscles, provides sensation to the lateral sole of the foot and innervation to the abductor digiti minimi, flexor digiti minimi, adductor hallucis, lumbrical, and interosseous muscles. The medial plantar nerve divides into the medial plantar proper digital nerve, which supplies sensation to the medial side of the big toe, and three interdigital nerves, which supply sensation to the first three web spaces. The lateral plantar nerve terminates in an interdigital nerve supplying the fourth web space.

Diagnosis and Etiology of Entrapment Neuropathies

A variety of entrapment neuropathies in runners' and other athletes' feet, distal to the tarsal tunnel, have been reported but cannot be well localized electromyographically. Motor nerve conduction studies of the medial and lateral plantar nerves may be performed, recording from the abductor hallucis and abductor digiti quinti pedis muscles, respectively. These two muscles may also be examined with a needle electrode to look for fibrillation potentials indicating denervation; but since these muscles are difficult for patients to voluntarily activate, recruitment of motor units cannot be well assessed. Other intrinsic foot muscles are difficult and painful to examine with a needle electrode.

Medial plantar nerve and medial calcaneal nerve entrapment may occur at the border of the abductor hallucis muscle, just proximal to the navicular tuberosity (Henricson and Westlin 1984, Rask 1978). Because medial calcaneal nerve entrapment produces pain over the anterior medial aspect of the heel and the abductor hallucis belly, it may mimic plantar fasciitis. Medial plantar nerve entrapment causes burning pain in the heel, aching in the longitudinal arch of the foot, and sensory loss. Distance running with the foot pronated or in excessive valgus may predispose to this entrapment, which has been named "jogger's foot."

Lateral plantar neuropathy producing diffuse heel pain has been reported in an elite competitive gymnast (Fredericson et al. 2001). At surgery, scar tissue was found surrounding the nerve. The etiology of the scar tissue was hypothesized to be trauma produced by the gymnast's striking her heel on the uneven bars and subsequently aggravated by repetitive barefoot running and jumping.

Continuous weightbearing activities (i.e., those requiring constant stance phase), such as using cross-country ski or stair stepper exercise machines, may compress the interdigital nerves and cause paresthesias of the toes during exercise; the paresthesias subsequently disappear with rest (Schon 1994).

Diagnosis and Etiology of Neuromas

Neuroma formation in the interdigital nerves is an additional source of foot pain in athletes. The term Morton's neuroma refers to what is believed to be a mechanically induced degenerative neuropathy of the interdigital nerves, most commonly in the third or second web space. Morton's neuroma is typically considered a problem of middle-aged women, but it can occur in athletes. The primary symptom is pain in the forefoot; the pain may radiate to the toe and is aggravated by weightbearing, especially bearing weight on the ball of the foot. The diagnosis is generally made clinically by the web space compression test, performed by squeezing the metatarsal heads together with one hand and simultaneously compressing the involved web space with the thumb and index finger of the opposite hand (Wu 1996). Electrodiagnostic studies are usually not performed to make the diagnosis of an interdigital neuroma. Oh and colleagues (1984) have described a near nerve conduction technique that may be used to document conduction abnormalities of the digital nerves, but this technique is not commonly used in clinical practice. Conservative treatment of Morton's neuroma involves the use of metatarsal pads, orthotics, nonsteroidal anti-inflammatory medications, and injection of corticosteroid and local anesthetic into the involved web space. If these treatments are not successful at relieving the foot pain, surgery may be considered.

Sural Neuropathy

A branch from the tibial nerve (medial sural nerve) and another from the common peroneal nerve (lateral sural nerve) fuse just inferior to the popliteal fossa to form the sural nerve. The nerve travels in a groove between the two heads of the gastrocnemius muscle until it reaches the lower third of the leg, where it becomes subcutaneous and travels laterally to course behind the lateral malleolus and terminate on the side of the foot. It supplies sensation to the lateral aspect of the ankle and the lateral border of the foot. The primary root supplying the sural nerve is S1. In a rare anatomic variant, the sural nerve is derived entirely from the common peroneal nerve and is thus susceptible to all of the previously described mechanisms of common peroneal nerve injury (Phillips and Morgan 1993).

Diagnosis

The differential diagnosis of a sural nerve injury includes S1 radiculopathy and partial sciatic, peroneal, and tibial neuropathies. Thus, the EDX should be similar to those described previously for evaluation of suspected peroneal and tibial neuropathies. Sural nerve conduction studies should be performed bilaterally to allow side-to-side comparison of amplitudes.

Etiology

Few sports-related sural nerve injuries have been reported. It may be that these injuries are unreported because they do not produce a functional deficit, and the chief symptom is paresthesia. At the knee, the nerve may be injured by compression from a Baker's cyst (Nakano 1978) or inadvertently during knee arthroscopy. In the leg, external pressure from a tight ski boot, skating boot, or other boot may compress the nerve. The ankle is the most common site of injury; in athletes, the injury is usually caused by a fracture or by a severe sprain, or iatrogenically during reconstructive ankle surgery. In the foot, the nerve may be injured when the base of the fifth metatarsal sustains an avulsion fracture (Gould and Trevino 1981). The nerve runs beneath the base of the fifth metatarsal and may become tented over the avulsed fragment; treatment is surgical and consists of removal or internal fixation of the bony fragment.

Pudendal Neuropathy

The pudendal nerve contains fibers from the S2-S4 roots and is the lowest branch of the sacral plexus. It supplies sensation to the anal and genital areas. Two large series of cyclists participating in multiday touring races have documented an 11% and a 22% incidence of penile numbness or hypesthesia, which persisted anywhere from hours to more than one month after completion of the race (Andersen and Bovine 1997, Weiss 1985). In the study by Andersen and Bovine, 13% of the riders also complained of temporary impotence lasting anywhere from days to more than a month after the race. Because of the complex neurologic pathways involved in erection, the exact mechanism of nerve compression or ischemia leading to impotence in cyclists is unclear. Interventions that help alleviate both numbness and impotence include correction of low handlebars or a high saddle, maintaining the saddle in a horizontal position, and frequent weight shifts from a sitting to a standing position. Goodson (1981) described a man who lost sensation over the penile shaft after a 180-mile bicycle ride, presumably as a result of pudendal nerve compression between a hard, narrow bicycle seat and the pubis. His symptoms resolved over a four-week period and did not recur once he switched from a narrow racing seat to a wider padded one. In another case report, a 55-year-old man developed impotence from riding an exercise bicycle only 20 minutes per day; his symptoms resolved within a month of stopping this form of exercise (Solomon and Cappa 1987). Although electrodiagnostic techniques are available for assessment of the pudendal nerve, only one report of pudendal neuropathy and impotence in a cyclist has included electrodiagnostic data (Desai and Gingell 1989). History and physical examination findings are usually sufficient for diagnosis.

CONCLUSION

Sports-related injury to the lower-extremity nerves, originating from the lumbosacral plexus, is rare but may have serious consequences. Injuries to the common peroneal nerve are by far the most frequent lower-extremity nerve injuries, followed in a distant second place by injuries to the tibial nerve. Common peroneal neuropathies are often associated with knee and ankle ligament injuries; they also may be caused by a blow to the lateral aspect of the leg, near the head of the fibula. Tibial nerve injuries generally accompany only the most severe traumatic knee and ankle injuries. However, entrapment of the distal branches of the tibial nerve (the plantar and digital nerves) can be a source of chronic foot pain in athletes. This chapter also reviews uncommon neuropathies that affect athletes' femoral, saphenous, lateral femoral cutaneous, obturator, sciatic, sural, and pudendal nerves.

A 23-year-old recreational soccer player complained of a foot drop two months after an injury to the ipsilateral knee. He had collided with another player during a match and sustained a hyperextension injury of the right knee. He almost immediately developed a prominent effusion. On initial physical examination, the Lachman test had been positive, and an MRI confirmed the presence of an ACL tear without any other intra-articular pathology. The athlete opted for a trial of nonsurgical treatment. He used crutches to ambulate for the next two months. When he was ready to abandon the crutches, he noted for the first time a foot drop on the right.

Medical history: Negative.

Surgical history: Negative.

Medications: None.

Physical examination: Unable to dorsiflex the ankle or evert the foot. Inversion and plantar flexion strength were normal. A sensory deficit was noted over the dorsum of the right foot, but sensation was intact on the sole of the foot and elsewhere in the lower extremity.

Radiographs: None.

Electrodiagnostic studies: An electrodiagnostic evaluation was ordered to assess a probable peroneal nerve injury. Table 6.1 gives the results of the nerve conduction studies, and table 6.2 shows the results of the needle electrode examination. No sensory response could be obtained from the right superficial peroneal nerve. With stimulation of the right deep peroneal nerve, no response was obtained from the extensor digitorum brevis, and only a low amplitude response was obtained from the tibialis anterior. All other nerve conduction studies were normal. Severe denervation, as indicated by profuse fibrillation potentials and an absence of voluntary motor units, was observed in all muscles innervated by the right common peroneal nerve that were studied. All other muscles studied were normal.

Diagnosis: Severe axon loss lesion of the common peroneal nerve.

Management and outcome: The athlete was fitted with an ankle foot orthosis for management of his foot drop, and he decided to undergo surgical exploration of the peroneal nerve and repair of his torn ACL. The common peroneal nerve was observed to be fibrotic and scarred for a 5-cm segment coursing through the popliteal fossa, presumably from a severe stretch injury. Six months after his ACL reconstruction, this athlete did not have any clinical or electrophysiologic evidence of peroneal reinnervation. At this point, he opted to undergo a tibialis posterior muscle transfer to provide him with ankle dorsiflexion. This procedure allowed him to discard his ankle foot orthosis, but he was unable to return to participation in soccer or other sports that require running.

(continued)

Table 6.1   Nerve Conduction Studies, Case 1

	Amplitude (µV)	Latency (ms)	Velocity (m/s)
Sensory nerves			
R sural	29 (>6.0)	3.1 (<4.4)	
L sural	32	3.3	
R superficial peroneal	NR (>6.0)	NR (<4.4)	
L superficial peroneal	34	2.5	
Motor nerves	**Amplitude (mV)**	**Latency (ms)**	**Velocity (m/s)**
R deep peroneal (extensor dig. brevis)	NR (>3.0)	NR (<5.5)	NR (>40)
L deep peroneal (extensor dig. brevis)	15	3.0	53
R deep peroneal (tibialis anterior)	0.4 (>4.0)	5.5 (<4.0)	
L deep peroneal (tibialis anterior)	11.1	3.3	
R tibial (abductor hallucis)	13 (>6.0)	3.0 (<5.8)	57 (>40)
L tibial (abductor hallucis)	13	3.4	55

Normal values are in parentheses. For motor studies, the name of the muscle from which the CMAP was recorded is below the nerve.

dig. = digitorum; L = left; µV = millivolts; ms = milliseconds; m/s = meters per second; mV = millivolts; NR = no response; R = right.

Table 6.2 Needle Electrode Examination, Case 1

| | | Motor Units | | | |
Muscle	Fibrillation	Amplitude	Duration	Phases	Recruitment
R TA	+++				No units
R per. long.	+++				No units
R EDB	+++				No units
R ADQP	0	N	N	N	N
R AH	0	N	N	N	N
R FDL	0	N	N	N	N
R med. gast.	0	N	N	N	N
R BFSH	0	N	N	N	N
R v. lat.	0	N	N	N	N
R glut. med.	0	N	N	N	N
L TA	0	N	N	N	N
L med. gast.	0	N	N	N	N
L AH	0	N	N	N	N

ADQP = abductor digiti quinti pedis; AH = abductor hallucis; BFSH = biceps femoris, short head; EDB = extensor digitorum brevis; FDL = flexor digitorum longus; glut. med. = gluteus medius; L = left; med. gast. = medial gastrocnemius; per. long. = peroneus longus; R = right; TA = tibialis anterior; v. lat. = vastus lateralis.

Case Report 2

An 11-year-old pairs figure skater was unable to plantarflex her ankle nine months after a severe calf laceration. She had originally fallen while attempting a lift with her partner. Her partner accidentally stepped on her right leg with his skate blade, severely lacerating her calf. She was taken to the hospital and soon thereafter to the operating room. The wound was surgically explored. All vessels and nerves appeared to be intact. After copious irrigation, the wound was closed with several layers of sutures. Postoperatively, the skater noted numbness on the sole of her foot and was unable to plantarflex the ankle or toes. Nine months later, she still had no apparent tibial nerve function.

Medical history: Negative.

Surgical history: As above.

Medications: None.

Physical exam: The patient was unable to plantarflex her right ankle or toes. She was also unable to invert the ankle. Knee flexion, ankle dorsiflexion and eversion, and toe extension strength were all normal. A sensory deficit was present on the sole of the right foot. Neurologic exam was otherwise normal. Vascular exam was unremarkable.

Electrodiagnostic studies: At this point, an EDX evaluation was performed. Table 6.3 gives the results of the nerve conduction studies, and table 6.4 shows the results of the needle electrode examination.

Diagnosis: Complete axon loss lesion of the right tibial nerve.

Management and outcome: Shortly after the EDX study, the patient underwent a right tibial nerve surgery, with neuroma resection and a primary anastamosis of the tibial nerve. Two years after the surgery, she had normal plantar flexor strength in the right leg but had also developed calf hypertrophy. An MRI of the right leg revealed marked hypertrophy of both bone and the posterior compartment muscles. This case demonstrates the unusual phenomenon of limb hypertrophy that occasionally occurs following recovery from an axonal nerve injury (De Beuckeleer et al. 1999).

Table 6.3   Nerve Conduction Studies, Case 2

	Amplitude (µV)	Latency (ms)	Velocity (m/s)
Sensory nerves			
R sural	22 (>6.0)	3.4 (<4.4)	
L sural	30	3.1	
R superficial peroneal	23 (>6.0)	2.8 (<4.4)	
L superficial peroneal	27	2.7	
Motor nerves	**Amplitude (mV)**	**Latency (ms)**	**Velocity (m/s)**
R deep peroneal (extensor dig. brevis)	11 (>3.0)	3.8 (<5.5)	56 (>40)
L deep peroneal (extensor dig. brevis)	10	3.6	58
R tibial (abductor hallucis)	NR (>6.0)	NR (<5.8)	NR (>40)
L tibial (abductor hallucis)	11	3.6	54
R tibial (soleus)	0.5 (>3.0)	4.5	

Normal values are in parentheses. For motor studies, the name of the muscle from which the CMAP was recorded is below the nerve.

dig. = digitorum; L = left; µV = millivolts; ms = milliseconds; m/s = meters per second; mV = millivolts; NR = no response; R = right.

(continued)

Case Report 2 *(continued)*

Table 6.4 Needle Electrode Examination, Case 2

Muscle	Fibrillation	Motor Units Amplitude	Duration	Phases	Recruitment
R TA	0	N	N	N	N
R per. long.	0	N	N	N	N
R EDB	0	N	N	N	N
R ADQP	++				No units
R AH	++				No units
R FDL	++				No units
R med. gast.	++				No units
R BFLH	0	N	N	N	N
R semitend.	0	N	N	N	N
R v. lat.	0	N	N	N	N
R glut. med.	0	N	N	N	N

ADQP = abductor digiti quinti pedis; AH = abductor hallucis; BFLH = biceps femoris, long head; EDB = extensor digitorum brevis; FDL = flexor digitorum longus; glut. med. = gluteus medius; L = left; med. gast. = medial gastrocnemius; per. long. = peroneus longus; R = right; semitend. = semitendinosus; TA = tibialis anterior; v. lat. = vastus lateralis.

For Further Reading on . . .

Neuropathies

Dawson, D.M., M. Hallett, A. J. Wilbourn. 1998. *Entrapment Neuropathies.* Baltimore: Lippincott, Williams & Wilkins.

Dumitru, D., A.A. Amato, and M. Zwarts. 2001. *Electrodiagnostic medicine.* Philadelphia: Hanley and Belfus.

Kline, D.G. and A. R. Hudson. 1995. *Nerve injuries: operative results of major nerve injuries, entrapments, and tumors.* Philadelphia: Saunders.

Logigian, E.L., ed. 1999. *Neurologic clinics: entrapment and other focal neuropathies.* Philadelphia: Saunders.

Rosse, C. and P. Gaddum-Rosse. 1997. *Hollinshead's Textbook of Anatomy.* Baltimore: Lippincott, Williams & Wilkins.

Stewart, J.D. 2000. *Focal peripheral neuropathies.* Baltimore: Lippincott, Williams & Wilkins.

REFERENCES

Andersen, K.V. and G. Bovine. 1997. Impotence and nerve entrapment in long distance amateur cyclists. *Acta Medica Scandinavia* 95:233-240.

Arnoldussen, W. and J. Korten. 1980. Pressure neuropathy of the posterior femoral cutaneous nerve. *Clinical Neurology and Neurosurgery* 82:57-60.

Bradshaw, C., P. McCrory, S. Bell, P. Brukner. 1997. Obturator nerve entrapment: a cause of groin pain in athletes. *American Journal of Sports Medicine* 25(3):402-408.

Brozin, I., J. Martfel, et al. 1982. Traumatic closed femoral nerve neuropathy. *Journal of Trauma* 22(2):158-160.

Carter, G.T., C.M. McDonald, T.T. Chan, A.J. Margherita. 1995. Isolated femoral mononeuropathy to the vastus lateralis: EMG and MRI findings. *Muscle and Nerve* 18:341-344.

De Beuckeleer, L., F. Vanhoenacker, A. DeSchepper, P. Seynaeve. 1999. Hypertrophy and pseudohypertrophy of the lower leg following chronic radiculopathy and neuropathy: imaging in two patients. *Skeletal Radiology* 28(4):229-232.

Desai, K. and J. Gingell. 1989. Hazards of long distance cycling. *British Medical Journal* 298:1072-1073.

Detmer, D.E., K. Sharpe, R.L. Sufit, F.M. Girdley. 1985. Chronic compartment syndrome: diagnosis, management, and outcomes. *American Journal of Sports Medicine* 13(3):162-170.

Dewitt, L.D. and H.S. Greenberg. 1981. Roller disco neuropathy. *Journal of American Medical Association* 246(8):836.

Edwards, J.C., C.T. Green, E. Riefel. 1989. Neurilemmoma of the saphenous nerve presenting as knee pain. *Journal of Bone and Joint Surgery (American)* 71A:1410-1411.

Esselman, P.C., M.A. Tomski, L.R. Robinson, J. Zisfein, S.J. Marks. 1993. Selective deep peroneal nerve injury associated with arthroscopic knee surgery. *Muscle and Nerve* 16:1188-1192.

Fabian, R.H., K.A. Norcross, M.B. Hancock. 1987. Surfer's neuropathy. *The New England Journal of Medicine* 316(9):555.

Fassler, P.R., M.F. Swiontkowski, A.W. Kilroy, M.L. Routt. 1993. Injury of the sciatic nerve associated with acetabular fracture. *Journal of Bone and Joint Surgery (American)* 75-A(8):1157-1166.

Ferkel, R.D., D.D. Heath, J.F. Guhl. 1996. Neurologic complications of ankle arthroscopy. *Arthroscopy* 12(2):200-208.

Fredericson, M., S. Standage, L. Chou, G. Matheson. 2001. Lateral plantar nerve entrapment in a competitive gymnast. *Clinical Journal of Sport Medicine* 11:111-114.

Garfin, S., S. Mubarak, C.A. Owen. 1977. Exertional anterolateral-compartment syndrome. *Journal of Bone and Joint Surgery (American)* 59-A(3):404-405.

Gessini, L., B. Jandolo, A. Pictrangeli. 1984. The anterior tarsal tunnel syndrome. *Journal of Bone and Joint Surgery (American)* 66-A:786-787.

Gillham, N. and R. Villar. 1989. Postero-lateral subluxation of the superior tibio-fibular joint. *British Journal of Sports Medicine* 23(3):195-196.

Gleeson, A. and J. Kerr. 1996. Patella dislocation neurapraxia—a report of two cases. *Injury* 27(6):519-520.

Goodson, J. 1981. Pudendal neuritis from biking. *The New England Journal of Medicine* 304:365.

Gould, N. and S. Trevino. 1981. Sural nerve entrapment by avulsion fracture of the base of the fifth metatarsal bone. *Foot and Ankle* 2(3):153-155.

Gristina, J.A. and M.G. Horelick. 1981. An uncommon location and complication of myositis ossificans: a case presentation. *Contemporary Orthopaedics* 3(11):1035-1037.

Guanche, C.A. 1995. Tourniquet-induced tibial nerve palsy complicating anterior cruciate ligament reconstruction. *The Journal of Arthroscopic and Related Surgery* 11(5):620-622.

Haig, A.J. 1989. Pedal pusher's palsy. *The New England Journal of Medicine* 320(1):63.

Hemler, D.E., W.K. Ward, K.W. Karstetter, P.M. Bryant. 1991. Saphenous nerve entrapment caused by pes anserine bursitis mimicking stress fracture of the tibia. *Archives of Physical Medicine and Rehabilitation* 72:336-337.

Henricson, A.S. and N.E. Westlin. 1984. Chronic calcaneal pain in athletes: Entrapment of the calcaneal nerve. *American Journal of Sports Medicine* 12(2):152-154.

Hirasawa, Y. and S. Kisaburo. 1983. Sports and peripheral nerve injury. *American Journal of Sports Medicine* 11:420-426.

Holt, M., P. Williams, R.L. Leyshon. 1996. Closed rupture of the common peroneal nerve: an unusual sporting injury. *Injury* 27(9):668-669.

Hyslop, G.H. 1941. Injuries to the deep and superficial peroneal nerves complicating ankle sprain. *American Journal of Surgery* 11(2):436-438.

Jackson, D.L. and B. Haglund. 1991. Tarsal tunnel syndrome in athletes: case reports and literature review. *American Journal of Sports Medicine* 19(1):61-65.

Jackson, D.L. and B.L. Haglund. 1992. Tarsal tunnel syndrome in runners. *Sports Medicine* 13(2):146-149.

Jenkins, David B. 1991. *Hollinshead's functional anatomy of the limbs and back,* 6th edition. Philidelphia: Saunders.

Jones, B. and M. Ward. 1980. Myositis ossificans in the biceps femoris muscles causing sciatic nerve palsy. *Journal of Bone and Joint Surgery (British)* 62-B:506-507.

Kanbe, K., H. Kubota, K. Shirakura, A. Hasegawa, E. Udagawa. 1995. Entrapment neuropathy of the deep peroneal nerve associated with the extensor hallucis brevis. *Journal of Foot and Ankle Surgery* 34(6):560-562.

Kashani, S.R., A.H. Moon, W.D. Gaunt. 1985. Tibial nerve entrapment by a Baker Cyst: case report. *Archives of Physical Medicine and Rehabilitation* 66:49-51.

Katirji, M.B. and A.J. Wilbourn. 1988. Common peroneal mononeuropathy: a clinical and electrophysiologic study of 116 lesions. *Neurology* 38:1723-1728.

Krivickas, L.S. and A.J. Wilbourn. 1998. Sports and peripheral nerve injuries: report of 190 injuries evaluated in a single electromyography laboratory. *Muscle and Nerve* 21:1092-1094.

Krivickas, L.S. and A.J. Wilbourn. 2000. Peripheral nerve injuries in athletes: a case series of over 200 injuries. *Seminars in Neurology* 20(2):225-232.

Kuntzer, T., G.V. Melle, F. Regli. 1997. Clinical and prognostic features in unilateral femoral neuropathies. *Muscle and Nerve* 20:205-211.

Langenhove, M.V., A. Pollefliet, G. Vanderstraeten. 1989. A retrospective electrodiagnostic evaluation of footdrop in 303 patients. *Electromyography and Clinical Neurophysiology* 29:145-152.

Leach, R.E., M.B. Purnell, A. Saito. 1989. Peroneal nerve entrapment in runners. *American Journal of Sports Medicine* 17(2):287-291.

Lindenbaum, B.L. 1978. Six boot compression syndrome. *Clinical Orthopaedics and Related Research* 140:109-110.

Lipscomb, A.B. and A.A. Ibrahim. 1977. Acute peroneal compartment syndrome in a well conditioned athlete: report of a case. *American Journal of Sports Medicine* 5(4):154-157.

Logue, E.J. and D. Drez. 1996. Dermatitis complicating saphenous nerve injury after arthroscopic debridement of a medial meniscal cyst. *Arthroscopy* 12(2):228-231.

Lorei, M. and E. Hershman. 1993. Peripheral nerve injuries in athletes: treatment and prevention. *Sports Medicine* 16(2):130-147.

Macgregor, J. 1977. Meralgia paresthetica—a sports lesion in girl gymnasts. *British Journal of Rheumatology* 11(1):16-19.

Malizos, K.N., T. Xenakis, A.N. Mavrodontidis, A. Xanthis, A.B. Korobilias, P.N. Soucacos. 1997. Knee dislocations and their management. *Acta Orthopaedica Scandinavia* 68:80-83.

Mann, R. 1995. Entrapment neuropathies of the foot. In J. DeLee and D. Drez, eds.: *Orthopaedic Sports Medicine*, 1831-1841. Philadelphia: Saunders.

Marinacci, A. 1968. The neuropathies of the nerves of the foot (painful foot). *Applied Electromyography*, 191-198. Philadelphia: Lea & Febiger.

McGeorge, D., M. Sturzenegger, V. Buchler. 1992. Tibial nerve mistakenly used as a tendon graft. *The Journal of Bone and Joint Surgery* 74-B(3):365-366.

McMahon, M.S. and S.M. Craig. 1994. Interfascicular reconstruction of the peroneal nerve after knee ligament injury. *Annals of Plastic Surgery* 32:642-644.

Meals, R.A. 1977. Peroneal-nerve palsy complicating ankle sprain. *Journal of Bone and Joint Surgery (American)* 59-A(7):966-968.

Miller, D.B. 1988. Arthroscopic meniscus repair. *American Journal of Sports Medicine* 16(4):315-320.

Miller, E.H. and F.E. Benedict. 1985. Stretch of the femoral nerve in a dancer. *Journal of Bone and Joint Surgery (American)* 67-A(2):315-317.

Moeller, J.L., J. Monroe, D.B. McKeag. 1997. Cryotherapy induced common peroneal nerve palsy. *Clinical Journal of Sports Medicine* 7:212-216.

Moller, B.N. and S. Kadin. 1987. Entrapment of the common peroneal nerve. *American Journal of Sports Medicine* 15(1):90-91.

Montgomery, T.J., F.H. Savoie, J.L. White, T.S. Roberts, J.L. Hughes. 1995. Orthopedic management of knee dislocations. *American Journal of Knee Surgery* 8(3):97-103.

Murphy, P.C. and D.E. Baxter. 1985. Nerve entrapment of the foot and ankle in runners. *Clinics in Sports Medicine* 4(4):753-763.

Myles, S.T., N.G.H. Mohtadi, J. Schnittker. 1992. Injuries to the nervous system and spine in downhill skiing. *Canadian Journal of Surgery* 35(6):643-660.

Nakano, K. 1978. Entrapment neuropathy from Baker's cyst. *Journal of American Medical Association* 239(2):135.

Nakano, K. 1987. Sciatic nerve entrapment: the piriformis syndrome. *Journal of Musculoskeletal Medicine* 4:33-37.

Nitz, A.J., J.J. Dobner, D. Kersey. 1985. Nerve injury and grades II and III ankle sprains. *American Journal of Sports Medicine* 13(3):177-182.

Nobel, W. 1966. Peroneal palsy due to hematoma in the common peroneal nerve sheath after distal torsional fractures and inversion ankle sprains. *Journal of Bone and Joint Surgery (American)* 48-A(8):1484-1495.

Oh, S.J., H.S. Kim, B.K. Ahmad. 1984. Electrophysiological diagnosis of interdigital neuropathy of the foot. *Muscle and Nerve* 7:218-225.

O'Sullivan, M., T. O'Sullivan, J. Colville. 1992. Tarsal tunnel syndrome following an ankle fracture. *The British Journal of Accident Surgery* 23(3):198-199.

Peicha, G., A. Pascher, F. Schwarzl, G. Pierer, M. Fellinger, J.M. Passler. 1998. Transsection of the peroneal nerve complicating arthroscopy: case report and cadaver study. *Arthroscopy* 14(2):221-223.

Peri, G. 1991. The critical zones of entrapment of the nerves of the lower limb. *Surgical and Radiologic Anatomy* 13(2):139-143.

Phillips, L.H. and R. Morgan. 1993. Anomalous origin of the sural nerve in a patient with tibial-common peroneal nerve anastamosis. *Muscle & Nerve* 16:414-417.

Pla, M.E., T.R. Dillingham, N.T. Spellman, E. Colon, B. Jabbari. 1996. Painful legs and moving toes associated with tarsal tunnel syndrome and accessory soleus muscle. *Movement Disorders* 11(1):82-86.

Putukian, M., D.B. McKeag, S. Nogle. 1995. Noncontact knee dislocation in a female basketball player: a case report. *Clinical Journal of Sports Medicine* 5:258-261.

Rask, M.R. 1978. Medial plantar neurapraxia (Jogger's foot). *Clinical Orthopaedics and Related Research* 134:193-195.

Sammarco, G.J. and M. Stephens. 1990. Tarsal tunnel syndrome caused by the flexor digitorum accessorius longus. *Journal of Bone and Joint Surgery (American)* 72-A(3):453-454.

Sammarco, G.J. and M.M. Stephens. 1991. Neurapraxia of the femoral nerve in a modern dancer. *American Journal of Sports Medicine* 19(4):413-414.

Schon, L.C. 1994. Nerve entrapment neuropathy, and nerve dysfunction in athletes. *Foot and Ankle Injuries in Sports* 25(1):47-59.

Seckler, M.M. and V. DiStefano. 1996. Peroneal nerve palsy in the athlete: a result of indirect trauma. *Orthopedics* 19(4):345-348.

Solomon, S. and K.G. Cappa. 1987. Impotence and bicycling: a seldom-reported connection. *Postgraduate Medicine* 81(1):99.

Spindler, K. and J. Pappas. 1995. Neurovascular problems. In J. Nicholas and E. Hershman, eds.: *The lower extremity and spine in sports medicine,* 1345-1358. St. Louis: Mosby.

Stefko, C.R.M., M.W.C. Lauerman, J.D. Heckman. 1994. Tarsal tunnel syndrome caused by an unrecognized fracture of the posterior process of the talus (Cedell fracture). *Journal of Bone and Joint Surgery (American)* 76-A(1):116-118.

Stein, J. and C. Warfield. 1983. Two entrapment neuropathies. *Hospital Practitioner* 18:100A-100P.

Stewart, J.D. 2000. *Focal peripheral neuropathies,* 580. Baltimore: Lippincott, Williams & Wilkins.

Streib, E.W. 1983. Traction injury of the peroneal nerve caused by minor athletic trauma. *Archives of Neurology* 40:62-63.

Streib, E.W., S.F. Sun, R.F. Pfeiffer. 1982. Toe extensor weakness resulting from trivial athletic trauma: report of three unusual cases. *American Journal of Sports Medicine* 10(5):311-313.

Styf, J. 1989. Entrapment of the superficial peroneal nerve: diagnosis and results of decompression. *Journal of Bone and Joint Surgery (American)* 71-B(1):131-135.

Torre, P.R., G.G. Williams, T. Blackwell, C.P. Davis. 1993. Bungee jumper's foot drop: peroneal nerve palsy caused by bungee cord jumping. *Annals of Emergency Medicine* 22(11):143-144.

Vanderford, L. and M. Meyers. 1995. Injuries and bungee jumping. *Sports Medicine* 20(6):369-374.

Vogel, C.M., R. Albin, J.W. Albers. 1991. Lotus footdrop: sciatic neuropathy in the thigh. *Neurology* 41:605-606.

Wascher, D.C., P.C. Dvirnak, T.A. DeCoster. 1997. Knee dislocation: initial assessment and implications for treatment. *Journal of Orthopedic Trauma* 11(7):525-529.

Weiss, B.D. 1985. Nontraumatic injuries in amateur long distance bicyclists. *American Journal of Sports Medicine* 13(3):187-192.

Wilbourn, A.J. 1986. AAEE case report #12: common peroneal mononeuropathy at the fibular head. *Muscle and Nerve* 9:825-836.

Wilbourn, A.J. 1992. The anterior tarsal tunnel revisited. *Muscle and Nerve* 15:1175.

Worth, R.M., D.B. Kettelkamp, R.J. DeFalque, K.U. Duane. 1984. Saphenous nerve entrapment: a cause of medial knee pain. *American Journal of Sports Medicine* 12(1):80-81.

Wu, K.K. 1996. Morton's interdigital neuroma: a clinical review of its etiology, treatment, and results. *The Journal of Foot and Ankle Surgery* 35(2):112-119.

Yamamoto, S., Y. Tominaga, S. Yura, H.Tada. 1995. Tarsal tunnel syndrome with double causes (ganglion, tarsal coalition) evoked by ski boots. *Journal of Sports Medicine and Physical Fitness* 35(2):143-145.

Yuen, E.C., R.K. Olney, Y.T. So. 1994. Sciatic neuropathy: clinical and prognostic features in 73 patients. *Neurology* 44:1669-1674.

Prevention
and Rehabilitation

7

General Principles of Peripheral Nerve Injury Rehabilitation

Brian A. Davis, MD, FACSM, FABPMR

$\mathbf{T}$he incidence of peripheral nerve injuries in sports is unknown (Clarke and Jordan 1998), but however often they occur, such injuries may lead to significant morbidity for the athlete.

It is essential for the care provider to establish an early and thorough diagnosis to prevent further injury, where possible, and to initiate rehabilitative measures that can reduce the associated impairments. Rehabilitation of nerve injuries is based not only upon which nerve or nerves have been affected but also on the cause of the injury. For example, in overuse-related nerve trauma, underlying abnormalities exist prior to the injury and contribute to it—suggesting that treatment must address not only the deficits from the nerve trauma but also will have to correct the predating abnormalities that induced the changes. Even though an acute traumatic event may cause a nerve injury, a clinician must try to identify preexisting biomechanical abnormalities that may have predisposed the athlete to the injury. Thus, health care providers for athletes must be exceptionally skilled in evaluating the neuromusculoskeletal system, so they not only can detect subtle nerve deficits but also can diagnose causes that are not readily apparent. This is most important in cases where overuse has directly induced the damage, but can also hold true for acute injuries where predisposing factors may be present.

In all athletic injuries, the clinician must rule out the possibility of nerve damage, whether or not it is suspected. Nerve injuries can be very subtle and must be recognized as early as possible to prevent further injury.

Early rehabilitation, taping, and bracing can provide athletes with faster return of strength and of cardiovascular and proprioceptive functions. Regardless of the injury, all athletes must be evaluated for deficits specifically affecting them, and programs should be individualized to meet their needs. This chapter discusses rehabilitation goals, treatment modalities, and rehabilitation following both complete and incomplete nerve injuries. For discussions of injury classification and electrodiagnostic testing, see chapter 1.

REHABILITATION GOALS

Care providers must be aware of the sports in which athletes participate, and whether an injury will affect that participation. The same injury may produce very different deficits for different athletes. For example, a median neuropathy can have very different effects on an athlete who primarily uses the upper extremities for sport versus one who primarily uses the lower extremities. But regardless of differences, all rehabilitation programs should address pain control, improve range of motion and strength, restore proprioception, and retrain for sport-specific activity. Programs should advance the athlete from less difficult to more difficult tasks and should be modified if they cause significant discomfort or undesirable compensation patterns. It is our belief that any athlete with nerve injury resulting in even minor deficits should receive therapeutic intervention. This program should be directed by a physician, certified athletic trainer, therapist, or other licensed professional knowledgeable in biomechanics, anatomy, therapeutic modalities, pain control, and sports conditioning.

Pain Control

Pain control is essential for allowing athletes to begin and maintain a rehabilitation program. Pain should be considered a guide as to what is safe and what is excessive. In addition to being caused by acute trauma and tissue damage, pain can arise from release of inflammatory mediators, muscle hyperactivity, *deafferentation (neuropathic pain)*, or instability and overuse. Determining the type of pain and its cause, and then applying the appropriate treatment(s) via medications, modalities, or other therapy techniques, can ultimately achieve relief.

deafferentation—The removal of afferent (incoming) nerve supply.

Drugs

Nonsteroidal anti-inflammatory drugs (NSAIDs) can be used to simultaneously treat both inflammation and pain. High doses of these medications should be used cautiously and probably only for short periods of time (probably for a maximum of two to three weeks), as there is significant potential for development of gastropathy, impaired hemostasis, or nephrotoxicity (Zuckerman and Ferrante 1998). Other idiosyncratic adverse effects such as hepatic, dermatologic, or central nervous system reactions can also occur (Zuckerman and Ferrante 1998). Some report that NSAIDs can reduce bone-healing rates (Altman 1995, Giannoudis et al. 2000, Martin et al. 1999). If the health practitioner has any question about using these agents after a fracture, he should consult a physician with experience in this area.

Compounds containing acetaminophen can be used safely for pain control, with doses up to 4,000 mg per 24-hour period (Zuckerman and Ferrante 1998). Acetaminophen compounds and NSAIDs may be used simultaneously. Use of *opiate/opioid* agents in association with nerve injury is controversial. Short-term use is acceptable and safe when other agents cannot control pain; but as soon as possible, the dose and frequency of opiates/opioids should be reduced and replaced with less potent compounds. Practitioners should closely monitor athletes for signs of abuse and quickly taper the medication if abuse is suspected.

Some practitioners have used oral corticosteroid medications after nerve injury to help reduce pain and inflammation. Steroid compounds, however, are banned by some athletic organizations such as the United States Olympic Committee (USOC) and the International Olympic Committee (IOC) and cannot be prescribed to many athletes (Fuentes and Rosenberg 1999). Epidural and selective nerve root injections are not banned by these organizations and may be helpful for radicular pain (Weinstein et al. 1995); review chapter 5 for an extensive discussion of these injections. Oral steroid use appears to be associated with a dose-dependent risk of avascular necrosis of the hip (Felson and Anderson 1987). In the low doses used for radiculopathies, the risks are probably quite small but need to be outweighed by the potential benefits. The decision to use oral steroids should be thoroughly discussed with the athlete.

Deafferentation (neuropathic pain) is common after neurologic injury and can be very difficult to treat (Lipman 1998). Pain is secondary to injury-induced biomechanical abnormalities of the affected nerves. A number of medications are available for treatment of these abnormalities and can be prescribed separately or in combinations. Some examples include tricyclic compounds (amitriptyline, nortriptyline, and desipramine), anticonvulsants (valproic acid, phenytoin, carbamazepine, gabapentin, lamotrigine, and zonisamide), alpha-2 agonists (clonidine or tizanidine), or anti-arrhythmic compounds (mexilitene). Medications with purported muscle relaxation properties (baclofen, carisoprodol, cyclobenzaprine, methocarbamol, metaxalone, orphenadrine, and zanaflex) may reduce neuropathic pain via several different mechanisms. Caution should be used when combining opiate/opioid and muscle relaxant medications, as significant potentiation may occur. Additionally, when carisoprodol is combined with opiates/opioids, the potential for abuse is often increased due to euphoric side effects. Use of epidural, selective nerve root, or caudal blocks is controversial in the management of acute radiculopathies but probably does have some role (Weinstein et al. 1995). These injections appear to be most successful when pain is referred to the extremity. See chapter 5 for a discussion of epidural corticosteroid injections.

Nonpharmaceutical Pain Relief

Many practitioners use *ultrasound* in the acute or subacute stages of musculoskeletal or nerve injuries. The author discourages the use of ultrasound in the acute phases of inflammation, regardless of the cause. A number of researchers report that inflammation and edema can be increased by the use of ultrasound, and nonthermal effects such as cavitation or acoustic streaming can cause tissue damage or chemical abnormalities (Abramson et al. 1960, Bickford and Duff 1953, Child et al. 1990, Rivenburgh 1992, Tarantal and Canfield 1994). Ultrasound may help decrease muscle spasm and associated muscle pain, however, but should only be used in areas away from sites of presumed acute inflammation. One controlled study suggested that ultrasound may help with tissue repair of surgically tenotomized animals (Enwemeka 1989) and suggested that this modality may be helpful under certain controlled surgical situations. Pulsed ultrasound has recently gained greater popularity in the treatment of musculoskeletal injuries, due to belief that the mechanical benefits of ultrasound can be achieved without the thermal effects of continuous ultrasound. Pulsed ultrasound reduces thermal effects by utilizing on-off cycles. It is unclear whether pulsed ultrasound has any effect on muscle spasm or on pain. It is recommended that ultrasound be used only after inflammation has subsided, and only when necessary for reducing muscle hyperactivity. Because denervated muscles have reduced blood supply (Sunderland 1978), ultrasound should not be used in areas of denervation.

High-voltage galvanic electrical stimulation (150-300 V, < 100 Hz) and transcutaneous electrical stimulation (TENS, variable intensities and frequencies) have been theorized to reduce pain by blocking afferent input from small A-delta and C pain fibers. This practice is based on a theory by Melzack and Wall (1965) that afferent input from larger A-beta fibers can block or "gate" information from incoming smaller fibers. A large body of literature describes the use of these modalities for pain control, and the full discussion is beyond the scope of this text, but the results are rather mixed with respect to efficacy. At the very least, electrical stimulation to control pain does not harm a patient and may be tried to obtain relief. Later in this chapter I discuss the potential risks and benefits of electrical stimulation for denervated muscles.

Electricity should never be used over the heart, carotid sinus, or demand pacemakers. High-voltage electrical stimulation probably should not be used on patients with vasculopathy, pregnancy, or seizure disorders (Nelson and Currier 1987).

Areas affected by dysesthesia can be treated by desensitization techniques. Desensitization is used to provide a higher tolerance for tactile stimulation or temperature changes or both (Fairchild et al. 1986). A number of techniques are available to desensitize the sensory systems (Schutt and Bengtson 1998, Umphred and McCormack 1990) and include tapping, massage (deep, light, or with ice), transcutaneous electrical stimulation, contrast baths, and whirlpool baths to name just a few. Efficacy studies on the benefit of desensitization are lacking, but this author has identified significant improvement in patients suffering from deafferentation pain who have been treated with desensitization techniques.

Pain can result from joint instability or overuse from abnormal substitution patterns. Therapy programs directed toward recovery of both strength and proprioception can help reduce pain that results from these problems. The chapters on rehabilitation will discuss the treatment of these issues in greater detail.

Flexibility/Range of Motion

A large body of evidence suggests a relationship between flexibility, performance, and injury rates (Carter 1994, Corbin 1984, Krivickas and Feinberg 1996, Marey et al. 1991, Smith et al. 1991). Rehabilitation programs need to restore flexibility and range of motion (ROM), which can be seriously affected following a nerve injury. In this situation, the weakened or paralyzed muscles leave the antagonist muscles unopposed—creating the risk of antagonistic muscle shortening and possibly frank contracture. The degree of imbalance between agonist and antagonist depends on the severity of weakness of the agonist and the relative strength of the antagonist. To prevent loss of ROM and maintain flexibility, different types of stretching exercises are available to the clinician and athlete. This author recommends static stretches. These are performed by slowly advancing the muscle to its limit of stretch (to a mild stretching discomfort but not pain) and holding it at this maximal point. A recent study by Bandy et al. (1998) demonstrated that static stretching significantly improved hamstring flexibility when compared to dynamic (ballistic) stretching. Slow, prolonged stretches should provide ample time for the gamma motor system to reset, thereby reducing associated muscle tone; they also should overcome the muscles' tendency to contract due to the stretch reflex (Bandy et al. 1998, Corbin 1984, Irrgang 1994). Several studies recommend holding the stretch for at least 30 seconds once daily (Bandy and Irion 1994, Bandy et al. 1997).

Other stretching techniques, such as *proprioceptive neuromuscular facilitation (PNF)* (Sady et al. 1982, Wallin 1985), may provide similar or greater improvements in flexibility, but static stretching is the author's preferred method as it is easily learned and is easily reproducible. The risk for harm with static and PNF stretches is also minimal compared to ballistic stretches, which may tear the muscle or tendon units (Bandy et al. 1998, Corbin 1984). Herbison et al. (1983b) caution that overstretching partially denervated muscles may cause further damage and weakness.

> **proprioceptive neuromuscular facilitation (PNF)—** Exercise programs designed to facilitate recovery using neuromuscular patterns and sensory receptors to either enhance or inhibit movement.

Clinicians sometimes forget that peripheral nerves contain connective tissue that can become contracted and can also be stretched. *Nerve gliding* within the surrounding connective tissue is imperative for normal nerve function. Neuropathic pain *(neuritis)* may develop if nerve motion is restricted or if connective tissue constriction is present. Stretching peripheral nerves should probably be performed with a slow, steady movement (Byron 1995) that does not exceed the nerve's allowable stretch limits—typically around 20%. Excessive stretch may lead to intraneural tearing, with associated axonal and fascicle disruption and hemorrhage (Smith 1995) that can result in increased pain as well as neurologic injury.

> **nerve gliding—**A nerve has flexibility within its connective tissue that allows it to glide.

> **neuritis—**Nerve inflammation or irritation.

Strengthening

Strengthening after a nerve injury is critical to maintain function in those muscles unaffected by the injury, to prevent atrophy to muscle innervated by the damaged nerve, to maintain muscle perfusion, and to minimize scarring.

Resistance Training

Muscle strengthening regimens vary among practitioners. In the past, it was thought that endurance and strength were diametrically opposed and that separate regimens were required to obtain one or the other (DeLorme 1945, 1946). This dichotomy may be true for the extremes, but for most athletes, programs can easily be designed that simultaneously generate both muscle power and endurance (DeLateur et al. 1968). We recommend that athletes perform exercises with a 10-15 repetition maximum—that is, the weight can be lifted only 10-15 times before complete fatigue. One should look for maladaptive substitution patterns and correct them. Free weights are the desired strengthening modality: Since athletes must perform their own three-dimensional stabilization of the weight, they improve proprioception while strengthening. Therabands™ can similarly be used for strengthening. Band resistance can be increased to result in fatigue after 10-15 repetitions. Two to three sets of the 10-15 repetition maximum routine should be performed at least once daily. In sports where endurance is required, a greater number of repetitions (up to 50 or 100) should probably be performed using light weights.

Strengthening programs should advance from those that require the least tension to those requiring the most (Joynt et al. 1993). We often start our athletes with concentric (shortening muscular activation) routines, as they subject the injured noncontractile elements to less strain. We then advance the athlete to either isometric (stable muscle length with activation) or eccentric (lengthening muscular activation) programs. We do not recommend isometric programs for some athletes because of the possible risk that they will overload the musculotendinous unit, and individuals with hypertension should not perform isometrics because these exercises can have a hypertensive effect (Mitchell and Wildenthal 1974). Isometric or co-contraction (simultaneous muscle activation of agonist and antagonist, often at stable muscle length) exercises can be of significant value when athletes must maintain strength but their joint has limited mobility or needs to be protected—for example, in postoperative situations, following proprioceptive losses, or during flare-ups of acute inflammatory arthropathy. Isometrics may also be useful for athletes with diminished joint proprioception, since the exercises confer stability to hypermobile joints while protecting local soft tissue and neurologic structures. *Isokinetic exercises* (stable velocity during muscular activation) have become popular with new technology. However, there is significant debate concerning their applicability to strength training and retraining, due to the fact that isokinetic exercises do not activate muscles at uniform tensions.

isokinetic exercise—One in which the muscle moves at a constant angular velocity during activation.

Once athletes have advanced to near-normal strength, they can begin *plyometric* (prestretching) exercises when indicated. These exercises use a muscle's ability to contract with the greatest force and tension immediately after a stretch has been applied to it (Asmussen 1968, Lamb 1978); in theory, plyometric stretches use the normal neurophysiologic tendon stretch reflex arc to help muscle activation. An example is a soccer striker practicing a kick against resistance: As the hip extends to initiate the kick cycle, the rectus femoris and iliopsoas are stretched, followed by their explosive contraction to complete the strike. The athlete can practice the maneuver against resistance to the explosive phase using weights or a Theraband, or in a pool. Strengthening muscles in patterns that are used during play or competition can provide greater control and specificity for the required activity. For this reason, sport-specific training should be initiated as early as possible during rehabilitation. Whatever method the practitioner uses for enhancing muscle strength, it is important to monitor the exercise program constantly to prevent overuse, excessive fatigue, or other form of injury due to incorrect performance. Severely denervated muscles should not be overworked (Challenor 1998, Lieberman et al. 1981), as this may increase muscle enzyme losses and ultimately reduce recovery and strength (Herbison, Jaweed, et al. 1973).

plyometric exercise—One in which the muscle is stretched and then activated to achieve a very forceful muscular response.

Electrical Stimulation

Electrical stimulation has been used for many years in attempts to maintain muscle bulk or increase muscle strength after nerve injury. There is a massive amount of literature regarding electrical stimulation and denervation. In order to understand the recommendations made in this section concerning electrical stimulation, one must be familiar with some of the literature concerning this subject.

Documented positive effects of electrical stimulation after denervation include reduction of muscle enzyme losses (Nemeth 1982), muscle atrophy (Fischer 1939, Guttman and Guttman 1944, Herbison, Teng, and Gordon 1973, Herbison et al. 1983a), connective tissue infiltration (Guttman and Guttman 1944), and fibrillation potentials (Herbison 1983a). Fischer (1939) demonstrated that electrical stimulation can maintain muscular excitability, but at the expense of increased oxygen consumption. Abdel-Moty et al. (1994) studied individuals with lower-extremity postradiculopathy weakness. Using a crossover design with individuals acting as their own controls, they found that stimulated muscles improved more than muscles not having stimulation and that electrical stimulation improved strength more than exercise alone did. Because muscle strength was tested only after completion of each treatment, however, it is unclear whether the strength gains remained after the electrical stimulation was discontinued. Note that the patients in this study were not completely denervated at the time—they had "weakness" due to previously documented radiculopathy, but there was no evidence that they were "denervated" during the time of the study. Therefore, it cannot be claimed that the electrical stimulation paradigm employed was beneficial for denervated muscle. Indeed, the stimulus parameters reported were not those for stimulating denervated muscles; see Spielholz (1999) for review of these requirements.

Several studies have demonstrated a positive effect of electrical stimulation on nerve growth and muscle recovery after nerve transection. Politis et al. (1988) applied direct current across severed nerves in rats and found that nerve regeneration was improved in the treatment group. Al-Amood and colleagues (1991) evaluated electrical stimulation on rats with extensor digitorum longus and soleus muscle denervation caused by sciatic nerve transection. Directly stimulated muscles were significantly stronger than the unstimulated group. However, the strength generated by the treatment group reached only 4-5% of normal, innervated muscles. These studies suggest that electrical stimulation may be able to improve distal nerve growth and maintain muscle strength after denervation, but whether functional outcome will be improved in humans through the use of electrical stimulation is questionable (Spielholz 1999).

Other studies have demonstrated no effect with electrical stimulation. Doupe et al. (1943) and Boonstra et al. (1987) observed no clinical or statistical difference in outcome variables of atrophy or muscle recovery after application of electrical stimulation. However, the authors of both studies identified no negative effects. It should be noted that Boonstra and colleagues demonstrated a greater amount of denervation potentials in the control group at 14 weeks after denervation (Boonstra et al. 1987). While the significance of this observation is unclear, one must consider the possibility that electrical stimulation may adversely affect nerve regeneration by inhibiting the release of nerve growth factors.

Some question exists about whether the stimulation variables were properly evaluated in early studies on electrical stimulation (Spielholz 1999). Chor and colleagues (1939) experimentally transected and repaired sciatic nerves in rhesus monkeys. They then compared treatment groups that received either electrical stimulation, passive range of motion combined with massage, or limb immobilization. The group with the best muscular recovery was the range of motion/massage group, with the electrical stimulation group displaying the next best improvement. Girlanda et al. (1982) performed crush experiments on the sciatic nerve of rabbits. They then stimulated the denervated soleus and extensor digitorum longus muscles of one group and used another as a control. Although the group receiving electrical stimulation had less type 2b fiber atrophy than the control group, the amount of type 1 fiber atrophy was greater in the treatment group. There was no difference in the time required for reinnervation.

There is some concern that electrical stimulation may harm denervated muscles. Studies by Brown and Ironton (1977) and Ironton et al. (1978) suggest that electrical stimulation can inhibit terminal sprouting of nerves in denervated muscles—possibly due to decreased hypersensitivity to acetylcholine of the denervated muscle fibers or to decreased production of "guidance" factors by the denervated-stimulated muscles. In other words, signals emitted by denervated muscle fibers may be reduced by electrical stimulation, resulting in decreased nerve regeneration and sprouting. Other theories suggest that electrical stimulation may retard the release of trophic factors produced and released by denervated muscles (for review see Spielholz 1999).

Electrical stimulation has also been evaluated for strength gains in individuals with intact peripheral nerves (i.e., with innervated muscles). Currier and Mann (1983) evaluated quadriceps strength changes in four groups of such individuals (three treatment groups and one control group). Subjects received either electrical stimulation alone, electrical stimulation with isometric strengthening, isometric strengthening alone, or neither intervention. No training group demonstrated greater strength improvement than any other, but clear improvement was noted in all individuals receiving treatment as compared to the control group.

In summary, despite the large volume of literature on electrical stimulation after denervation, there is sufficient controversy to question its use. Most importantly, no controlled human studies have suggested that electrical stimulation is beneficial to denervated muscles awaiting reinnervation (Ogard and Stockert 1990). As for partially denervated muscles, electrical stimulation may inhibit the release of trophic factors and the nerve sprouting they induce. In light of the available literature, it is probably wise to withhold electrical stimulation solely for the purpose of maintaining strength of partially or completely denervated muscles until more human research can further evaluate this modality. Basford (1990) has also recommended not using electrical stimulation for lower motor neuron disorders.

Proprioception

Proprioception is defined as the individual's conscious and subconscious awareness of position and movement (Barr and Kiernan 1988). Proprioception contributes to the motor planning for neuromuscular control required for precision movements; it also contributes to muscle reflexes, providing dynamic joint stability (Lephart et al. 1997). Proprioception affects the ability to correctly detect joint angular velocity (and associated vectors), muscle and joint capsule tension, and muscle length. This sensory pathway also allows for awareness of object recognition based upon size, weight, and movement of body segments on one another. Proprioceptive information is carried by sensory fibers originating from afferent receptors in skin, muscles, ligaments, and joint capsules (Clark and Burgess 1975, Horch et al. 1975, Kennedy et al. 1982, Miyatsu et al. 1993, Schultz et al. 1984); it travels through the dorsal column pathways and is relayed primarily to centers within the sensory cortex and the cerebellum. Modulation of motor control through sensory information occurs mainly at the level of the cerebellum and to a lesser extent at the level of the spinal cord (Joynt et al. 1993). Abnormalities in any one of these capacities may significantly affect athletic performance (Harrelson 1991, Jewell 1990).

Importance of Proprioceptive Training

When proprioception is impaired by advancing age (Skinner et al. 1984), joint effusion (Kennedy et al. 1982), fatigue (Yaggie et al. 1999), or local anesthesia, an athlete must attempt to improve feedback to central centers by increasing information from other joints and structures within the same limb or in areas nearby the injury. When muscles, tendons, ligaments, and joint capsule structures are damaged, injury may also occur to the afferent neural structures that play a vital role in proprioception (Forkin et al. 1996, Freeman et al. 1965). Kennedy and colleagues (1982) suggested a similar theory—that nociceptive sensory nerve injury from direct trauma to knee structures can cause prolonged knee pain. If this is the case, then injuries such as muscle strains or contusions may cause proprioceptive as well as nociceptive deficits. Similarly, ligament injuries have been associated with impaired proprioception (Barrett 1991, Beard et al. 1994, Forkin et al. 1996, Tropp et al. 1984). This loss may be caused by damaged neural structures residing within the ligament. Brand (1986) theorized that injured structures once responsible for afferent input, such as ligaments or joint capsules, might become reinnervated with healing. For these reasons, proprioceptive retraining should be provided for almost all injuries involving soft tissue. This may be more important for trained athletes than for the average individual, since trained athletes consistently demonstrate greater levels of whole-body coordination, dynamic and static balance (Golomer et al. 1997, Kioumourtzoglou et al. 1997), and knee proprioception (in the form of joint kinesthesia) than do untrained persons (Barrack et al. 1984, Lephart et al. 1996). It is likely that this trend also exists for other joints required for sport activity by athletes: If an athlete suffers a nerve injury, then the proprioceptive losses will probably be more functionally significant than for an untrained individual. Proprioceptive retraining should be performed as early as possible to attempt to recover the lost function.

With respect to gender, Golomer et al. (1997) found that trained female adolescent athletes displayed better dynamic equilibrium control than did male athletes. However, Barrack and colleagues (1984) found no difference in joint kinesthesia between the sexes.

Techniques of Proprioceptive Training

Proprioceptive exercises should include sudden alterations in joint position, velocity, and speed, as well as balance and postural activities, with and without visual input (Beard et al. 1994, Lephart et al. 1997). Proprioceptive exercises may be *open-chain* (limb is not fixed to either the wall or ground) or *closed-chain* (limb is fixed to the wall or ground). Common upper-extremity proprioceptive open-chain techniques include exercises using Therabands, free weights, Body Blades, plyometric balls, and medicine balls. Common lower-extremity open-chain programs include the use of Therabands or free weights. Upper-extremity closed-chain proprioceptive exercises may include push-ups or pull-ups. Lower-extremity closed-chain exercises often incorporate a leg press machine, single-limb squats, minitrampoline, or ankle disk. Figures 7.1 through 7.14 demonstrate several examples of upper- and lower-extremity proprioception exercises. Reeducation of sensory awareness should include training toward recovering awareness of shape, weight, and texture and perception of position in space (Challenor 1998). A study by Sheth et al. (1997) evaluated the effect of a training program using an ankle disk on the muscle reaction times of healthy individuals' anterior and posterior tibialis, peroneus longus, and flexor digitorum longus muscles. Monitored with fine-wire intramuscular electromyogram (EMG) electrodes to detect muscle responses, individuals were subjected to sudden ankle varus via *trap-door experiments.* One group used the ankle disk daily for eight weeks, while the other group acted as the control. A second set of trap-door experiments was conducted, and all muscle onset latencies were compared between groups and to pretreatment groups. The treatment group had slower anterior and posterior tibialis reaction times as compared to the other muscles, compared to the control group, and compared to pretreatment values. The authors proposed that slowed contraction of the invertors allowed the evertors to work more efficiently at controlling the ankle varus caused by the trap door— and proprioception exercises may help prevent ankle sprains through a similar mechanism.

open-chain exercise—One in which the limb is not fixed to either the wall or the ground.

closed-chain exercise—One in which the limb is fixed to either the wall or the ground.

trap-door experiment—Research design where ankle is suddenly forced into new position by dropping out a trapdoor. The most commonly used design is forced inversion (ankle varus).

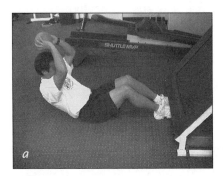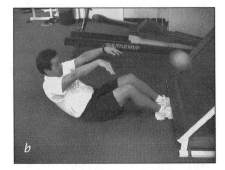

Figure 7.1 Upper-extremity open-chain trampoline exercises. *(a-b)* Athlete stabilizes lower body and trunk and throws a medicine ball at a trampoline. This exercise strengthens all extremities and simultaneously improves trunk mechanics. The lower extremities are acting in a closed-chain environment, while the uppers are working in an open-chain environment.

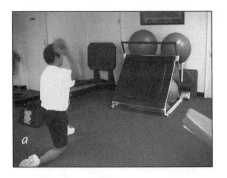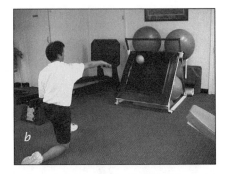

Figure 7.2 Upper-extremity open-chain trampoline exercises. *(a-b)* Athlete is positioned on one knee and throws the medicine ball at the trampoline. This exercise focuses on upper-extremity and trunk control, with the upper extremity working in an open-chain environment. The lower extremity is working in a closed chain.

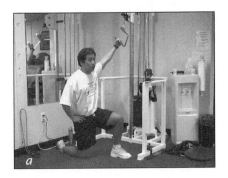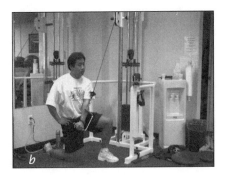

Figure 7.3 Upper-extremity open-chain stack weight exercises. *(a-b)* Athlete is positioned on one knee and performs strengthening exercises on a stack weight machine. Here, the athlete is performing exercises that work on specific patterns of recovery for the upper extremity in an open-chain environment, while the lower extremity works in a closed-chain environment.

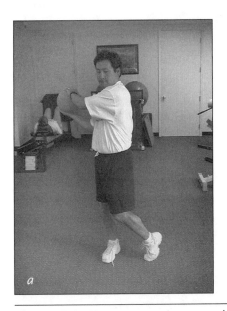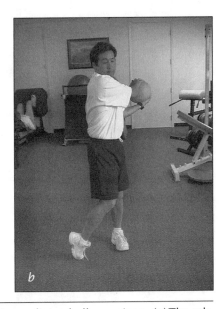

Figure 7.4 Upper-extremity open-chain medicine ball exercises. *(a)* The athlete starts with the trunk rotated to the right side. *(b)* The athlete rotates the limb and trunk all the way to the left. This exercise allows for one limb to work off of the strength and guidance of the second. Again, the lower extremity is acting in a closed chain.

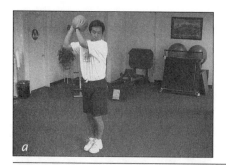 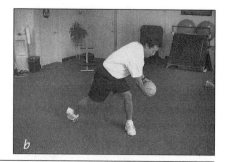

Figure 7.5 Upper-extremity open-chain medicine ball exercises. *(a)* The athlete starts with the limbs and trunk in line with one another. *(b)* The athlete then throws the medicine ball in patterns that assist with upper-extremity (open-chain) and lower-extremity (closed-chain) recovery.

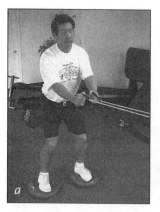 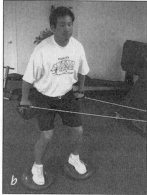

Figure 7.6 Advanced upper- and lower-extremity proprioception exercises. *(a-b)* Athlete uses ankle disks (closed-chain) to challenge the lower extremities while simultaneously challenging the upper extremities and trunk with elastic cords (open-chain). Athletes advance to this level of exercises after mastering less challenging exercises.

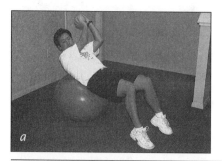 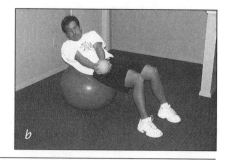

Figure 7.7 Advanced upper- and lower-extremity proprioception exercises. *(a-b)* Athlete uses a plyometric ball to challenge the entire body for balance. The athlete uses the medicine ball in recovery patterns (open-chain), while the lower extremities are fixed to the floor. This exercise can be made even more challenging by elevating one of the legs, forcing even greater trunk and four-limb control.

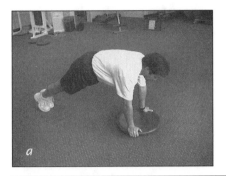 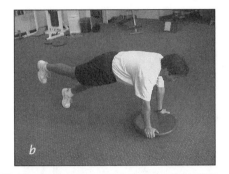

Figure 7.8 Open-chain lower-extremity exercise with closed-chain upper-extremity exercises. *(a)* Athlete uses an ankle disk to stabilize the upper extremities in a closed chain. *(b)* The athlete then alternates lifting his legs off the ground to force four-limb and trunk control. The athlete can add ankle weights, elastic cords, Therabands, or stack weights to make the exercise more challenging.

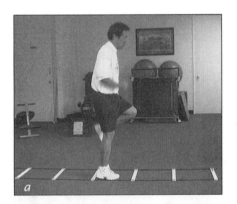 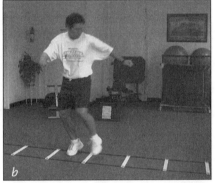

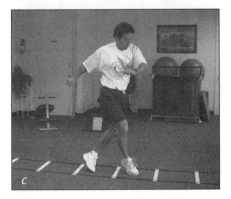

Figure 7.9 Lower-extremity open-chain ladder exercises. Athlete runs along a ladder laid out along the ground. *(a)* The athlete runs in a straight line. *(b-c)* The athlete performs a carioca along the ladder. (A carioca is an exercise that requires rotation of the trunk and lower extremities while the body is in motion.) These exercises challenge the athlete to control limb velocity and placement, as well as coordination with the other limb and with the trunk. Although the limb does touch the ground at some points during the exercise, the majority of the activity requires the limbs to be off the ground and should be classified as an open-chain activity.

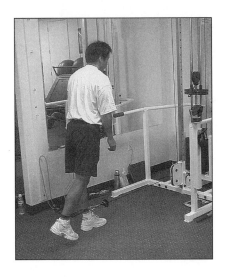

Figure 7.10 Lower-extremity stack weight exercises. Athlete is forcing the right limb to work in an open chain, while the left works in a closed-chain environment.

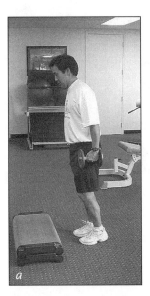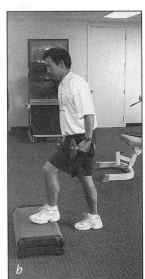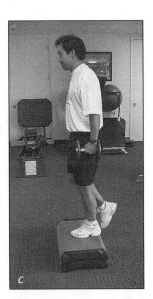

Figure 7.11 Lower-extremity closed-chain stair exercises. *(a-c)* Athlete performs step-up and step-down repetitively. He is forced to stabilize the trunk on the limb that is in stance phase; he needs to have full awareness that the limb is being moved and placed appropriately either on the step or on the ground. The activity is made more difficult by adding weight either to the upper or lower extremities.

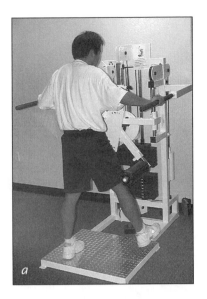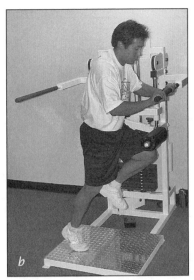

Figure 7.12 Lower-extremity closed-chain hip machine exercises. Athlete performs hip strengthening exercises with the hip machine. *(a)* Strengthening the right hip abductor, while simultaneously forcing the left limb to balance the trunk in a closed-chain environment. *(b)* Strengthening the left hip flexor, while simultaneously forcing the right limb to balance the trunk in a closed-chain environment.

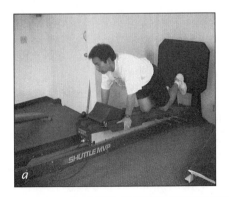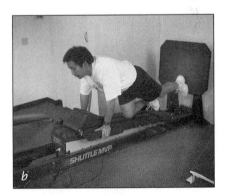

Figure 7.13 Lower-extremity closed-chain shuttle exercises. *(a)* Athlete is in a quadruped position, with the left limb on the base of the shuttle. *(b)* He then extends and flexes the left leg and must stabilize the trunk and upper extremities in a closed-chain environment.

161

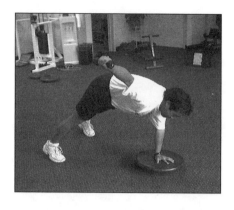

Figure 7.14 Advanced upper-extremity open-chain exercises with free-weights and closed-chain lower-extremity proprioception exercises. Athlete is demonstrating a more advanced form of proprioception exercise that requires four-limb and trunk stabilization. This type of exercise, and ones similar to it, are reserved for the last stages of rehabilitation since they require the greatest functional demands on the injured and uninjured extremities.

PNF exercises use a series of facilitation and synergy patterns to obtain strengthening. The muscles are reeducated and strengthened by using stronger muscles to support weaker ones (Ogard and Stockert 1990). PNF can also improve motion by maximally stretching and shortening the muscle of interest (Andrews et al. 1995). *Tai chi quan* has also been evaluated as an exercise to improve proprioception for older people. Wolf and colleagues compared tai chi quan to a computerized balance training program for efficacy in decreasing fall rates and improving balance and postural stability. Tai chi quan reduced fall rates (Wolf et al. 1996) but was less effective in improving balance (Wolf et al. 1997). Since tai chi quan can be easily learned and requires no formal equipment, it can be useful in retraining older athletes who have suffered nerve injuries.

tai chi quan—An exercise program that involves changes in posture in linked movements. It focuses on balance, coordination, concentration, and stress relief.

Elastic bandages or taping techniques can enhance proprioception by improving cutaneous sensory feedback; they also appear to help both uninjured (Perlau et al. 1995) as well as injured joints (Karlsson and Andreasson 1992). Even though tape can lose its structural support within a fairly short period of time (Greene and Hillman 1990, Manfroy et al. 1997), it may continue to enhance proprioception.

Proprioceptive exercises should be instituted as early as possible to have the best functional outcome (Lephart et al. 1997). The exercises should first target the most proximal stabilizing structures: This allows for proximal stabilization, upon which the more distal structures can be strengthened. Visual input also appears to be important in task acquisition and balance (Robertson and Elliot 1996). The athlete should be trained to use these visual cues as much as possible to determine position, quality, and quantity of movement. Similarly, biofeedback may help athletes with diminished proprioception by providing external cues to impaired internal awareness of muscle activation and by discouraging undesirable compensatory strategies (Challenor 1998).

Sport-Specific Retraining

Optimum athletic function requires complex pattern *(engram)* formation (Crossman 1959) in the extrapyramidal system. Practicing the required skill over and over during development and skill acquisition forms these engrams. Engram modulation and coordination requires input from other centers within the cerebrum, basal ganglia, brainstem, and spinal cord (Hasan et al. 1985). Because the pyramidal system can influence the engram pattern, early return to the desired activity can help re-form selected patterns or help develop new, compensatory ones (Kottke 1990). The reformation of appropriate patterns required for activities of daily living, work, musical performance, or sports activity is crucial to maximizing return to participation.

> **engram**—Patterns of movement, including velocity, vector, position, and multiple other variables, that are stored in central and peripheral centers for subsequent use.

Additionally, as motor skills improve, so does the efficiency of performing that skill. Therefore, more work can be accomplished with less energy expenditure. Unfortunately, this component of rehabilitation is often the last to be addressed. Yet sport-specific retraining should begin as early as athletes are able to tolerate the basic movements and strength requirements of their sports (Challenor 1998).

TREATMENT MODALITIES

Many passive or semipassive treatments are available to help speed recovery by reducing pain and inflammation, facilitating proprioception, providing support to injured structures, and limiting unwanted compensation patterns. Clinicians should understand the benefits and limitations of these modalities—and it is important that they use them only as adjuncts for treating athletes with nerve injuries, not as the primary mode of treatment.

Cryotherapy

Cryotherapy is the application of cold for the treatment of injury and is used widely in sports medicine. Cold can be applied via ice packs, ice baths/slushes, ice towels, ice massage, gel packs, and vapocoolant sprays (Rivenburgh 1992, Swenson et al. 1996). Cooling produces an initial period of vasoconstriction (Basford 1998, Lemons and Downey 1994), which may or may not be followed by a reactive vasodilation (the latter is thought to occur as a result of cold-induced paralysis of the vascular smooth muscle). Some researchers suggest that changes in skin color associated with vasodilation may be caused by diminished tissue metabolism and oxygen utilization (Nadler 2001). Blood flow in arteries, soft tissue, and bone is reduced as exposure time to cold increases (Ho et al. 1994, 1995). Cold reduces edema (McMaster et al. 1978, Rivenburgh 1992) through its vasoconstrictive effects and through its decrease of enzymatic activity and production of inflammatory mediators. Ice application also appears to decrease metabolic activity and muscle tone (Eldred et al. 1960, Lehman and DeLateur 1990). The following discussion centers on ice application, which is the most common form of applying cold in sports medicine; ice also cools tissues more rapidly than gel or refrigerant cooling agents (McMaster et al. 1978) and is the best cooling option available to the clinician.

Cryotherapy has long been used as an analgesic acutely after injury, as well as during the chronic stages (Basford 1998, Bierman 1955, Grant 1964, Rivenburgh 1992, Starkey 1976, Swenson et al. 1996). Cold application can also be very helpful for pain and edema control in athletes with nerve injury. Pain control via cryotherapy is not completely understood. One possibility is that nerve conduction is either blocked, causing transient neurapraxia, or the number of nociceptive afferent volleys is significantly diminished once the area is numbed by cold. Another possibility is that the reduction in muscle tone, or "spasm," through cooling may be responsible for pain control (Rivenburgh 1992), via two different mechanisms. First, decreased muscular contraction should reduce local metabolite production and associated pain. Second, if increased muscle tone triggers nociceptive afferent volleys, then decrease in tone should decrease the associated pain. Perhaps these mechanisms contribute to the rapid pain reduction experienced with ice application. However, cryotherapy is known to cause both immediate and long-lasting pain control. Reduced enzymatic activity and inflammatory mediator production are more likely to result in the analgesia seen well after the cold has been removed.

Ice packs, compression wraps, and ice slushes can reduce temperatures very quickly. Treatments should be applied for only 20-30 minutes at a time, as further application can induce frostbite or other tissue injuries. Ice massage consists of rubbing a block of ice over the area of injury. Although analgesic levels are achieved after around 7-10 minutes of use (Basford 1998), treatments usually last 10-15 minutes until the skin has become numb. Ice massage appears to decrease tissue temperatures faster than ice packs, probably due to the presence of continuous contact of the cold environment to the skin (Zemke et al. 1998). Whirlpools can also cool very quickly and are often used for 20-30 minutes. Whirlpool and ice pack cooling rates are similar, but rewarming has been found to be faster for ice packs. This is not entirely understood. One would want to keep skin/ muscle temperatures as low as possible for as long a period of time as possible. There have been numerous studies that have evaluated rewarming just for this reason.

Absolute contraindications to the use of cryotherapy include Raynaud's phenomenon, cryoglobulinemia, paroxysmal cold hemoglobinuria, and cold urticaria. Note also that areas affected by severe peripheral vascular disease should not be exposed to cold, which will increase the already unhealthy level of vasoconstriction characteristic of such regions. Ice should also be avoided in asensate regions due to the risk of frostbite. Ice or other cold application should be used cautiously on areas with reduced sensation or vascular supply.

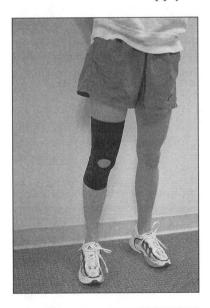

Figure 7.15 Neoprene knee orthosis for improving proprioception. This device would aid in improving cutaneous feedback from the knee region, especially in cases of patellofemoral abnormalities.

Orthoses and Taping

Orthoses and taping may be helpful after a peripheral nerve injury, because they provide mechanical support and enhance afferent neurologic input. They provide functional stability to a weak segment and can prevent overstretching of weak muscles by the unaffected antagonists (Berger and Schaumburg 1988). Nerve injuries can impair cutaneous nociceptive and local proprioceptive sensory input. Orthoses and taping may be able to restore some of this lost input (figures 7.15 and 7.16). Although it is unclear how orthoses and tape improve proprioception, one potential explanation is the following: With an injury to the superficial peroneal nerve, sensation on the dorsum of the foot would likely be affected, and to some degree the proprioceptive information from the same region would also be affected. Tape could be applied to the

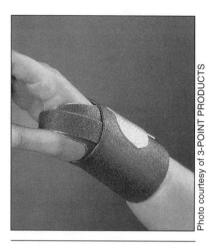

Photo courtesy of 3-POINT PRODUCTS

Figure 7.16 Flexible wrist orthosis for improving proprioception. Many commercial devices are available for the upper and lower extremities to enhance proprioception.

entire ankle region to cover both areas of decreased or absent sensation, as well as sensate areas such as those supplied by the sural or saphenous nerves. Ankle motion will generate tension through the tape to the skin. The referred information can be converted into proprioceptive information and relayed to central centers for processing. One concern is that taping or bracing, by providing artificial support, may lead to a loss of the normal physiologic proprioceptive protective mechanisms.

Although this author believes that orthoses and taping can help improve proprioceptive responses, literature in this area has demonstrated mixed results. Perlau et al. (1995) showed that knee proprioception can be improved via elastic bandages used in athletes with uninjured joints. His group found that elastic bandage application improved proprioception most in athletes with the poorest initial ability to detect changes in joint angle. This effect remained after light activity. Wojtys et al. (1996) studied what they termed "spinal cord reflex" (short-latency), "intermediate response" (intermediate-latency), and "voluntary" (long-latency) reaction times of the quadriceps and hamstring muscles of patients with anterior cruciate ligament (ACL) deficiency. An anterior translation force was applied to the tibia, and these superficial electromyographic responses were recorded. The degree of anterior translation was also measured. They found that anterior tibial translation was most significantly reduced with bracing and simultaneous muscular contraction. Spinal reflex reaction times of the quadriceps and lateral hamstring also improved with bracing, whereas the medial hamstring muscle responses were variably affected (percent changes not specified). The intermediate response reaction times were variable for all muscles tested. Bracing slowed voluntary quadriceps and hamstring reaction times. These results suggest that bracing can reduce some reaction times but may increase others. The overall significance of these results is unclear, as these reflexes and responses are not well characterized, and whether they are functionally important in athletic performance also remains in question (Wojtys et al. 1996).

Brodersen and Symanowski (1993) studied the effect of prophylactic bracing on the incidence of knee injuries in collegiate athletes. The number and severity of knee injuries decreased with bracing, but no analysis was presented on the reported increase in meniscal and ankle injuries in those who were braced. Burks et al. (1991) found that, in healthy athletes, several different ankle supports impaired performance on tasks such as vertical jumps or shuttle runs, but the researchers did not directly evaluate proprioceptive performance. Other studies have shown that taping can help prevent ankle sprains, especially in those with previous ankle sprains (Garrick and Requa 1973, Tropp et al. 1985). Tropp and colleagues (1985) showed that ankle orthoses might help prevent recurrence of sprains in athletes, but no more effectively than rehabilitative exercises. As there remains no clear consensus on the ability of bracing or taping to assist with lost proprioception, it is recommended that they be used only in conjunction with standard rehabilitation techniques. I also recommend that only foot orthoses be used prophylactically unless there is some compelling reason to institute other forms of prophylactic devices.

Football players frequently tape their fingers and wrists. Many report that the finger taping improves hand strength and that the wrist taping improves wrist/forearm strength and reduces undesirable wrist extension during play. Rettig et al. (1997) compared dominant and nondominant grip strength before taping to wrist-taped nondominant hands, finger-taped dominant hands, and finger- and wrist-taped dominant hands. Finger- and wrist-taped dominant hands exhibited significantly lower grip strength than untaped dominant hands ($p = 0.02$). The authors state that although grip strength did not improve in their study, players taping their fingers or wrists may perceive a benefit from a "kinesthetic sensory feedback phenomenon" similar to that of a neoprene brace. The authors further theorized that the pressure from the taping, especially over the pulley system of the finger flexors, may "enhance a perception of increased pressure during a grasp," but they did not pursue this theory in their study, nor did they investigate the degree to which wrist taping prevented wrist extension. The authors admitted that the dominant-hand finger- and wrist-taping trial was the last of six trials and that fatigue may have affected the results, but they did not statistically evaluate this possibility. They also reported an unspecified amount of variability between the two grip strength trials of each test, which may have also affected the results. Regardless of the flaws reported, there is probably no significant clinical benefit—and there may even be drawbacks—to prophylactic use of finger or wrist taping to improve grip strength. Further studies are needed to evaluate the role of taping on strength and proprioception in both the upper and lower extremities.

Biofeedback

The term biofeedback applies to any process whereby instrumentation converts a covert physiologic process into a detectable and quantifiable one (Wolf 1991). Biofeedback typically utilizes EMG signals, pressure gauges, position sensors, or other measuring devices and converts the information received from muscles into auditory or visual data for the individual to view. Although other forms of feedback are available, the most commonly used forms are audio and visual. Individuals are trained to modify the feedback by altering their activity, and with practice, they learn to control muscular activation through the feedback system. Biofeedback can be used to strengthen muscles, coordinate skilled movement (Basmajian 1998), modify maladaptive substitution patterns, and assist with reintegration of sensory information. Through biofeedback, athletes can be trained to contract weakened muscles or utilize muscles on command more effectively and accurately. This section focuses on EMG biofeedback, as it is one of the most widely used in rehabilitation medicine, and a great deal of literature has addressed its effectiveness.

In EMG biofeedback training, athletes are instructed how to increase or decrease the intensity of EMG signals in order to reach a desired effect (Mirabelli 1990). EMG biofeedback has been more widely used in stroke rehabilitation than elsewhere (Basmajian 1998); its effectiveness as a therapy after sports-related nerve injury has not been well studied. Wolf (1994) noted that research has probably been limited by belief that the benefits of biofeedback are already clear and therefore warrant no further study. Literature regarding other sports-related injuries and postoperative scenarios suggests favorable outcomes with EMG biofeedback, and although this literature is not directly related to nerve injuries in athletes, some of the findings may be useful in training athletes who have suffered a nerve injury.

Draper (1990) evaluated the effect of biofeedback (11 patients) versus a control group (11 patients) on quadriceps isometric peak force after ACL reconstruction. Patients were randomized and matched for age, gender, and surgical repair. Each group received identical instruction, with the exception of the introduction of biofeedback to the treatment group. It appears that all subjects received electrical stimulation for the first two weeks of treatment. Quadriceps strength of the 22 patients was tested at 45, 60, and 90 degrees of knee extension at 1 and 12 weeks after surgery. The biofeedback group made statistically significant gains compared to the control group at all angles. A similar study by Draper and Ballard (1991) compared electrical stimulation to EMG biofeedback of the quadriceps muscles in 30 athletes recovering from ACL reconstruction. Both groups performed voluntary isometric strengthening exercises three times per week, using either biofeedback or electrical stimulation. Electrical stimulation was applied at 35 pulses per second, with a hold time of 10 seconds and an off time of 20 seconds. Stimulation intensity was increased from 15 mA to 40 mA during the course of the six-week treatment program. The biofeedback group developed greater quadriceps isometric peak torque (46.4% peak torque of unaffected limb) than the electrical stimulation group (37.9% peak torque, $p = 0.044$). It is unclear, however, how clinically significant this difference in peak torque is after just six weeks. Levitt and colleagues (1995) evaluated the role of EMG biofeedback (three times daily with five-second isometric contractions; number of repetitions was not identified) on recovery of quadriceps strength after arthroscopic knee surgery. Surgery was performed for synovitis, loose bodies, patellar chondromalacia, or a combination of these conditions. At two weeks after surgery, the authors found a statistically significant improvement in the quadriceps extensor torque and recruitment patterns of patients who received both exercises and feedback, compared to those who received only exercises. Finally, Maitland and colleagues (1999) reported one case where EMG biofeedback made significant improvement of gait and muscle activity in an individual with an unstable knee after ACL repair.

Biofeedback has been reported to be helpful in nerve injury. May et al. (1989) evaluated the efficacy of EMG biofeedback, surgery, and botulinum toxin on patients suffering from Bell's palsy. A total of 86 patients were studied, but only 13 received EMG biofeedback. Patients had facial paralysis ranging from 5-60 months, with the average length of paralysis being 12 months. Patients underwent EMG biofeedback to balance the smile (10 patients), improve separation of mouth and eye movements (7 patients), reduce hyperkinetic spasm (4 patients), or increase oral competence and overall facial motion (2 patients). Eight of the 13 EMG patients received one training session, and the other five received two sessions. Duration and frequency of treatment was not provided. Improvement was based upon a patient's subjective appearance and the physician's assessment of improvement based upon photographs and videos taken prior to initiation of treatment. Twelve of the 13 biofeedback patients reportedly improved. This paper had a number of shortcomings: There was no blinding, nor were the specific results identified for each patient (although the authors did address the difficulty of presenting such diversified data). The authors stated that the EMG biofeedback appeared to be helpful only for highly motivated patients and should probably be used prior to the full development of synkinesis and hyperkinesis. This study suggests that individuals suffering even from long-standing partial facial nerve injuries can benefit from EMG biofeedback.

LeVeau and Rogers (1980) studied the effects of a three-week (five days per week for one-half hour) EMG biofeedback training program on vastus medialis and vastus lateralis contractions in 10 healthy individuals. Following this training, subjects were able to increase the EMG output of the vastus medialis over baseline and also succeeded in increasing the vastus medialis to vastus lateralis output ratio.

Biofeedback of foot pressure during standing has been used with individuals suffering from balance disorders secondary to any form of neuromuscular dysfunction. Individuals can be trained on devices that detect sway from a central point and provide auditory and/or visual cues to help the patient correct position. This apparatus can also be used to present a target to the patient, who tries to pinpoint it by shifting weight.

Based upon all the above data, it appears that biofeedback should have a role in the recovery of athletes who have suffered a nerve injury. Available literature, however, has not adequately evaluated the long-term efficacy of biofeedback in these situations. It is probably safe to assume that athletic recovery will not be hindered by its use, and biofeedback is probably a reasonable adjunctive modality. If biofeedback is used, it probably should be initiated as early after the injury as possible. EMG biofeedback may be used as soon as muscle activity is identified (muscle strength 1/5 or greater). It may also be helpful when muscle strength is reduced (3-4/5), to retrain athletes to recruit the desired muscles instead of using substitution patterns.

TREATMENT OF ACUTE, COMPLETE, INCOMPLETE, AND CHRONIC INJURIES

As stated previously in this chapter, the mechanism (acute, chronic, overuse), degree of injury (complete, incomplete), and identity of affected nerves all dictate the appropriate treatment and rehabilitation program. This section discusses issues of treatment and rehabilitation from acute to chronic injury. The clinician addressing such injuries should not assume that the injury is a static one, but rather should change strategies as the deficits change and the injury "matures."

Acute Traumatic Nerve Injuries

Immediately after an athlete sustains a nerve injury, the affected region should be protected to prevent further nerve injury and secondary muscle injury (Perlmutter and Apruzzese 1998). Denervated muscles are especially prone to scarring and contracture, due to their impaired blood supply (Sunderland 1978) and decreased metabolic activity. Management of these athletes within the first week should reduce bleeding, risk of infection, local swelling, and overstretch of the affected nerve or muscles (Denny-Brown 1951, Sunderland 1978). Edema and swelling ultimately affect wound healing and tissue tensile strength (Ethicon 1988) and should be controlled as early as possible after an injury. The use of NSAIDs, cold, and electrical stimulation during this period has already been described. Compression via stockings or elastic bandages can also reduce swelling and keep it to a minimum but should not exceed capillary closing pressures, as this may lead to further blood pooling and worsen limb blood flow. Care should also be taken when blood flow is reduced in the extremity, since even minimal compression may overcome arterial pressures and lead to an ischemic limb. Limb elevation to a level above that of the heart also reduces swelling and should be employed where possible.

Local hematomas and edema can result in further neurologic compromise and should be treated aggressively. Treatment may include hematoma evacuation, drain placement, or fasciotomy if neurovascular compromise is present. Obviously, medical personnel skilled in this area should perform these procedures. Smaller hematomas can also be treated with local compression, ice, and elevation. After any athletic injury, and in particular after an acute nerve injury, pain may limit the athlete's ability to initiate and maintain a rehabilitation program. Pain control is therefore a very important part of an overall program. Many treatments aimed at reducing swelling will also reduce pain. Medications designed for reducing deafferentation pain may have side effects that limit their usefulness— typically, larger evening or bedtime doses of these medications can provide relief of nocturnal symptoms; lower doses during the day will reduce daytime sleepiness. In cases where there is significant inflammation in the region of the nerve injury, such as with nerve compression secondary to a disc herniation, corticosteroids can be delivered locally by injection (Weinstein et al. 1995). Chapter 5 (pages 91 to 95) thoroughly discusses use of corticosteroids in pain control and rehabilitation of lumbar radiculopathies and should be read carefully prior to any decision to inject corticosteroids.

Protective orthoses should be used as early as possible to prevent secondary injury to skin that may result from direct contact (especially if the limb has decreased or absent sensation, or healing wounds), or if weakened muscles result in poorly controlled motion of a joint. Some cases of joint instability may require surgical stabilization, and physicians with knowledge in this area should be consulted as needed.

Nerve trauma caused by or directly in association with a fracture should be addressed by setting the fracture appropriately. These patients should be referred to medical specialists in the treatment of such cases as soon as possible in the hopes of reducing vascular or neurologic compression. Because movement of the fracture can lead to further compression of the vascular or neurologic structures, setting the fracture reduces the risk of further nerve injury. Penetrating trauma resulting in neurovascular injury should be referred to medical specialists in the treatment of such cases as soon as possible. These wounds should be explored and determination made as to whether primary repair is indicated. A special situation results when a nerve injury occurs in association with a spine injury. Appropriate protection is required for the spinal cord and the surrounding nerve roots. If a spine injury is suspected, spinal precautions should be maintained and the athlete transported via collar and/or backboard to an appropriate medical center. Radiographic evaluation (computed tomography scanning, magnetic resonance imaging, or standard radiography) should be obtained as necessary to evaluate the skeletal and/or soft-tissue structures. Orthoses or surgical stabilization is required for an unstable spine or when further neurologic damage is feared and should be instituted immediately in the management of these disorders. If a spine injury is suspected or detected, a physician specializing in the area of spine surgery should be immediately consulted. Fortunately, most cervical spine injuries result only in neurapraxic root injury (Torg 1987)—only rarely do athletes suffer complete nerve transection without penetrating or extreme deceleration trauma.

Rehabilitation Following Complete Nerve Injuries (Axonotmesis/Neurotmesis)

After appropriate local management of the wound has been applied, swelling has been controlled, and orthoses used to prevent contractures, the athlete can begin the rehabilitative phase of her injury. Rehabilitation strategies ultimately depend on the expected chances of recovery. Since the full prognosis may not be known until many months after the injury, the initial approach to care should assume that there will be recovery until proven otherwise. It is important to remember that significantly denervated muscle has diminished blood flow and is more susceptible to injury from extreme temperatures (e.g., ice packs or hot packs) and local trauma from overstretching and the like (Sunderland 1978). The initial program for all patients should include range-of-motion exercises to each affected joint's end range. Overstretch should not be applied to any weakened muscles, as it may cause local muscle damage and scarring, which may affect muscle strength if reinnervation occurs in the future. Overstretching also has the potential to damage the epineurium or other connective tissue structures that act as a framework for the regenerating nerve (chapter 1, pages 4-5). If the scaffolding for the nerve is disrupted, nerve regeneration may be faulty, with the nerve missing its intended target. Use of electrical stimulation directly to the affected muscles should probably be avoided, as previously discussed.

Athletes should begin strength training as soon as possible after injury but should avoid excessive stress to the weakened muscles. This is especially important when the weakened muscles are required to protect nerves, as further nerve damage could occur if they are overworked. Strength of muscles unaffected by the nerve injury should at least be maintained via lightweight, high-repetition exercises. The athlete should avoid fatiguing the unopposed muscles, as this will lead to strengthening of unaffected muscles and may lead to contracture formation due to the unopposed action of these muscles. Regular stretching of the muscle being strengthened may also prevent muscle shortening. The clinician needs to consider each region separately, because continued strength training does not always lead to muscle imbalances. As an example, consider a musculocutaneous nerve injury that results in weakness of the biceps, coracobrachialis, and to a lesser extent, the brachialis (the brachialis has dual innervation from both the musculocutaneous and radial nerves). Maintenance of triceps strength will not necessarily lead to a muscular imbalance at the elbow, since the brachialis may be functional. Additionally, these muscles act as primary shoulder and elbow flexors, and presumably, one would not want to strengthen the shoulder or elbow extensors. However, because the biceps also acts as a glenohumeral *coaptor* (holds together the glenohumeral joint), strengthening the extensor components of the deltoid and triceps may help reduce clinically significant shoulder subluxation when present. At this early stage, development of substitution patterns may emerge to compensate for lost muscular and sensory functions. This is most likely to occur when only one or two muscles have become denervated and other local musculature can attempt to compensate for lost strength. It is important to prevent the formation of substitution patterns that may lead to further dysfunction. Some would argue that substitution patterns not be allowed to form at all, in the belief that if eventual reinnervation occurs, these patterns will ultimately be detrimental to performance.

coaptor—A muscle or other structure that assists with joint stability by bringing joint surfaces together.

Nerves regenerate at the rate of approximately one-half inch to two inches per month (Buchthal and Kuhl 1979, Sunderland 1978. See also chapter 1, pages 8-9) Therefore, one can estimate the time necessary for recovery based upon the distance of regrowth required.

Proprioception exercises should also be instituted at this stage of recovery. These exercises may reduce the risk of forming maladaptive substitution patterns through reeducation. Clearly, care must be taken when performing proprioception exercises with moderately to severely weakened structures (i.e., 3/5) (Einarsson and Grimby 1987, Feldman and Soskolne 1987). Exercises should be nonfatiguing to avoid structural damage. These exercises should be maintained until evidence of muscle return is detected. The practitioner should be cautious about assuming that muscle function has returned in a previously denervated muscle solely based upon joint motion. This author has identified several cases (unpublished) where motion has returned, but electromyographic needle examination revealed persistent absence of innervation. The motion was probably the result of substitution patterns. Biofeedback may be used early in treatment to prevent undesirable substitution patterns but is probably not necessary after an athlete has reached reliable voluntary activation of desirable muscle tension levels (Challenor 1998). Once innervation has been identified, the clinician can treat athletes as if they have an incomplete nerve injury, as discussed in the following section.

Incomplete Nerve Injuries and Reinnervation

Nerve regeneration after axonal degeneration is heralded electromyographically by the return of motor unit potentials within a previously denervated muscle. As chapter 1 discussed, these "nascent" or "rebirth" potentials are typically very small in size (usually less than 300 µV), polyphasic (i.e., contain more than four phases), and of short duration, often being less than 5-10 milliseconds. In the early stages of recovery, only one or two motor units may be found, but as reinnervation continues, muscle strength improves and the polyphasic units become larger in amplitude and duration (mature polyphasic unit). Abnormal spontaneous activity may continue to be present. Nerves incompletely injured from the outset of an event display a third type of polyphasic unit when attempting to recover function: They are normal-appearing motor units containing satellite potentials (time-locked, very small, negative deflections) that represent terminal collateral sprouting from nearby functional units to denervated muscle fibers. As the nerve recovery progresses, all the polyphasic potentials mature and take on larger amplitude with normal to increased duration.

Strength and Proprioceptive Training

Strength maintenance may begin early in the course of muscular recovery but should be performed cautiously when muscle strength is 3/5 (Einarsson and Grimby 1987, Feldman and Soskolne 1987) or in the presence of immature polyphasic potentials, which indicate reinnervation and probable susceptibility to reinjury. In either of these cases, athletes should avoid overfatiguing a muscle in order to avoid paradoxical weakening. When muscles reach greater than 3/5 strength, strengthening exercises can probably approach fatigue without concern for causing damage. Exercises should advance from those that require the least force (concentric) to those that require the most (plyometric). One should begin by reestablishing proximal stability and proprioception; once that has been accomplished, the more distal structures can be strengthened and undergo proprioceptive training.

Proprioceptive exercises should also be performed at a very early stage to restore central awareness to the area. As with strengthening, proprioceptive exercises should also target proximal structures before being applied to the more distal ones. Before beginning the next phase of rehabilitation—sport-specific retraining—the practitioner should make certain that the athlete's proprioceptive capacity is at or near normal levels. For this reason, practitioners need to establish protocols for testing proprioception for each limb and spine region. Proprioception can be formally tested, but is not usually necessary. If the athlete has an unimpaired extremity, proprioception may simply be compared to that side. The upper extremity is more likely to reveal better proprioception on the dominant side, and this should be accounted for. Each clinician will need to decide what form of testing is required before advancing an athlete to a higher level of training or return to play.

Muscle strength can also be formally evaluated if needed. Testing equipment is more readily available for muscle strength testing than for proprioception and may be an attractive option in helping staff decide whether to allow an athlete to advance to the next level of training or return to play. More simply, if the contralateral limb is unaffected, the examiner may compare the sides for symmetry. The nondominant upper extremity should be no weaker than 90% of the strength of the dominant limb. It is important to recognize that neither full strength nor proprioception alone allow for optimal athletic performance; these two factors need to be simultaneously maximized.

Substitution Patterns

Substitution patterns are counterproductive for athletes who have the potential for complete recovery. As long as a chance remains for complete recovery, emerging substitution patterns should be corrected or prevented. A physician, trainer, coach, therapist, or similar professional knowledgeable in athletic biomechanics should closely monitor performance to correct patterns that are detrimental to the athlete and to prevent further injury. This is particularly important in the rehabilitation of incomplete injuries, which have much greater potential for full recovery than do complete injuries.

Although substitution patterns can be maladaptive for the athlete who eventually recovers full muscle strength and control, those athletes who do not regain full capacity may need to use substitution patterns for athletic participation and for some daily activities. The degree of residual dysfunction and the need to use substitution patterns for participation will determine whether an athlete can compete in able-bodied events or at the disabled level. Thus, once clinicians have determined that no further recovery will occur, they should encourage substitution patterns. Establishing the completion of recovery can be difficult but can be suggested by needle study of the recovering muscle. If the polyphasic potentials present within a muscle do not display any satellite potentials, regeneration polyphasic potentials are no longer identified, and a reasonable time needed for recovery has elapsed, this would suggest that no further significant nerve recovery is taking place.

Chronic/Overuse Injuries

A chronic injury is any that has persisted for at least six months or more, regardless of the cause. These can arise out of acute injuries that have been only partially treated or simply have not improved, or when an injury is not recognized and the damage is cumulative—typical of acute-on-chronic nerve injuries often seen with overuse musculoskeletal injuries. Acute nerve injuries have not had sufficient time to develop compensation patterns, whereas chronic ones (either from acute or overuse injury) typically have. The clinician's role in chronic nerve injuries is to determine the following: (1) What is the cause of the chronic injury (i.e., acute versus overuse)? (2) What neurologic and muscular structures have been affected? (3) What compensation patterns have developed? (4) Is full neurologic recovery expected? (5) Can the athlete be restored to baseline capacity or greater, and how? (6) If full neurologic recovery is not expected, which compensation patterns should be facilitated to allow for elite or adapted competition?

Acute injuries that have merely become chronic due to lack of treatment or lack of response to treatment are caused by a one-time event. Treatment is geared toward protecting the nerve from further damage and facilitating recovery through strengthening and sport-specific return. Nerve injuries that have resulted from musculoskeletal overuse are due to failure of the structures surrounding the nerve and have accumulated over a period of time. The clinician must first determine the cause of the overuse that led to the nerve injury. A common overuse nerve injury is seen in baseball pitchers who have poor mechanics that lead to ulnar collateral ligament failure and subsequent ulnar neuropathy. The practitioner must first recognize that there is not only ligament but also nerve damage. Treatment immediately consists of preventing further ligament and nerve injury, followed by appropriate strengthening and mechanical analysis and retraining.

Typically, injuries to the neurovascular structures from overuse are secondary to demyelination (neurapraxia); or if axon damage occurs, it is an incomplete lesion. These injuries usually occur insidiously, and athletes may complain of pain, numbness, tingling, or decreased strength during sports activity. Athletes may not even be aware of these symptoms of nerve damage and may complain only of decreasing performance. The history of dysfunction should be carefully questioned, with specific attention paid to when the symptoms occur and how performance is affected. Because certain sports are known to be associated with distinct nerve injuries, the examiner should attempt to elicit history specific to these injuries. Examples include asking about shoulder dysfunction and associated suprascapular neuropathy in volleyball players or ulnar neuropathy associated with medial collateral ligament laxity at the elbow in overhead athletes. The physical examination should also focus on these possibilities, even if athletes do not spontaneously offer history to suggest such disorders.

An electrodiagnostic study can help determine whether or not the dysfunction is, in fact, due to an overuse or an acute injury. If the nerve has been acutely damaged, the denervation changes will all be of an age correlating to that injury. After the muscle has been denervated, the muscles will begin to display large fibrillation potentials (Kraft 1990) and positive sharp waves. As time passes, these potentials diminish in size (Kraft 1990). Several polyphasic motor unit potential characteristics can also suggest the acuity of a nerve injury. Intact axons sprout to supply local denervated muscles. Initially, these sprouts are very small, lack mature myelin, and innervate a small number of muscle fibers. Often, these newly innervated fibers fire in a time-locked orientation to the native muscle fibers, giving rise to the satellite potential. As the nerve sprouts mature, the resultant motor unit potential increases in amplitude and become less polyphasic. Overuse injuries typically cause acute-on-chronic damage to the affected nerve. A needle electromyogram may display large and small fibrillation potentials and positive sharp waves, along with polyphasic potentials of varying size and shape, characteristic of this acute-on-chronic damage.

Once the degree and location of the nerve injury are determined, it is up to the practitioner to discover the nature of the overuse injury and the mechanics or training errors that produced the nerve damage. If there remains question as to the underlying cause of the injury, it would be advisable for a physician, coach, trainer, therapist, or similar practitioner knowledgeable in athlete biomechanics to observe the athlete during performance. This observation will provide information about what structures need strengthening and what mechanical errors need to be addressed—factors that clearly must be determined prior to returning the athlete to sport.

Edema is not likely to be a problem in this set of athletes, but ice application can help with pain control. Inflammation typically is minimal, as the process has been present for an extended period of time. However, acute episodes of inflammation may coexist with chronic changes and may improve with NSAID use. Pain is typically less severe with chronic nerve injuries than with acute cases, thereby negating the need for opioid analgesics in most athletes. Oral steroid use in chronic disease is usually not recommended, unless concomitant significant acute nerve injury is also felt to be present. Steroid injection for radiculopathy is unlikely to provide significant benefit after 3-6 months of disease (Brown 1977, Green et al. 1980). Orthoses may be needed in the early stages of injury to prevent excessive forces from being applied across the affected nerve. These devices are most needed when an athlete is incapable of preventing abnormal joint motion that may result in further nerve damage. For example, if an athlete suffers a severe tear of the ulnar collateral ligament, the ulnar nerve is unprotected from valgus forces at the elbow. A valgus-controlling device will protect the ulnar nerve from further injury and should be initiated as soon as possible for treatment. These devices should not be ordered routinely; they are expensive and may not be necessary under all circumstances. They should be ordered and instructions provided only by practitioners knowledgeable about the products and their actual use. If possible, the orthosis should be capable of assisting during both the rehabilitation and the functional phases of return to sports activity.

Strength training is essentially the same for chronic as for acute injuries. Strengthening not only should target muscles weakened by the nerve injury but also should focus on muscles throughout the kinetic chain responsible for the injury. As with acute injuries, any loss of proximal control needs to be targeted first to prevent further neurovascular injury from proximal instability. Sport-specific retraining should be performed once the athlete displays an acceptable level of strength and stability.

The Kinetic Chain

The kinetic chain refers to the order and control of movement that occur at all levels of the body associated with activity. There is a typical pattern of events that requires proper sequence and adequate strength to achieve smooth, coordinated movement (Freidhoff et al. 1998). The most important practical concepts regarding the kinetic chain that the rehabilitation specialist must keep in mind are the following:

- The more proximal structures control more motion than the more distal ones.
- The entire limb and torso must act as a unit to activate and control motion.
- Therefore, any weak proximal muscles must be strengthened and provided appropriate proprioceptive awareness before the more distal muscles are treated.
- If the above principles are not taken into account, a weakened muscle within the kinetic chain may not be capable of properly controlling the motion, and this lack of control may lead to substitution muscle firing of other muscles that are not weak or inhibited. Such altered firing patterns can be quite difficult to normalize.

Thus, if the kinetic chain is ignored during rehabilitation, the patient may acquire new and rather intractable problems as a result of a poorly conceived and monitored course of treatment.

Management of incomplete injuries secondary to overuse is quite similar to management for neurapraxic injuries. The major difference in treatment is that the resultant strength and proprioceptive deficits may take longer to return, if there is complete return at all. Neurapraxia-related nerve injury usually resolves within 4-6 weeks once the offending cause is removed. The return of function should be nearly complete unless axonal damage has occurred. Once axonal damage has taken place, there is potential for incomplete recovery. Under these circumstances, the athlete may develop abnormal substitution patterns from both the weakness and proprioceptive changes. Additionally, abnormal patterns responsible for the overuse injury may reemerge. The athlete must be watched very closely during this period to prevent these substitution patterns. If full nerve recovery is not expected, then substitution patterns may be allowed, but the practitioners working with the athlete must be certain that the athlete will not induce further injury from the new pattern.

CONCLUSION

Peripheral nerve injuries can be very mild and may even go unnoticed by the athlete. When the injury is due to overuse, the athlete will probably present with symptoms not directly associated with the nerve injury. It is at this point that treatment is most successful and will prevent further injury. When an acute injury occurs, it is important to prevent secondary injury through early recognition and treatment by health professionals specializing in such disorders. Electrodiagnostic studies can help determine how complete an injury is and can assist in determining the athlete's prognosis. These studies can also be used during treatment to determine if and when recovery is occurring. This information can help direct proper strength, proprioception, and sport-specific retraining and provide the athlete with the best possible outcome.

REFERENCES

Abdel-Moty E, Fishbain DA, Goldberg M, Cutler R, Zaki AM, Khalil TM, Peppard T, Rosomoff RS, and Rosomoff HL. Functional electrical stimulation treatment of postradiculopathy associated muscle weakness. *Arch Phys Med Rehabil* 1994; 75(6):680-686.

Abramson DI, Burnett C, Bell Y, Tuck S, Rejal H, and Fleischer CJ. Changes in blood flow, oxygen uptake and tissue temperatures produced by therapeutic physical agents: I. Effect of ultrasound. *Am J Phys Med* 1960; 39:51-62.

Al-Amood WS, Lewis DM, and Schmalbruch H. Effects of chronic electrical stimulation on contractile properties of long-term denervated rat skeletal muscle. *J Physiol* 1991; 441:243-256.

Altman RD, Latta LL, Keer R, Renfree K, Hornicek FJ, and Banovac K. Effect of nonsteroidal antiinflammatory drugs on fracture healing: a laboratory study in rats. *J Orthop Trauma* 1995; 9(5):392-400.

Andrews JR, Schemmel SP, Whiteside JA, and Timmerman LA. Evaluation, treatment, and prevention of elbow injuries in throwing athletes. In: Nicholas JA and Hershman EB (eds.), *The upper extremity in sports medicine*, 2nd edition. St. Louis: Mosby, 1995:749-788.

Asmussen E. The neuromuscular system and exercise. In: Falls HB (ed.), *Exercise physiology*. New York: Academic Press, 1968:3-42.

Bandy W and Irion J. The effect of time on static stretch on the flexibility of the hamstring muscles. *Phys Ther* 1994; 74(9):845-850.

Bandy W, Irion J, and Briggler M. The effect of time and frequency of static stretch on flexibility of the hamstring muscles. *Phys Ther* 1997; 77(10):1090-1096.

Bandy WD, Irion JM, and Briggler M. The effect of static stretch and dynamic range of motion training on the flexibility of the hamstring muscles. *J Orthop Sports Phys Ther* 1998; 27(4):295-300.

Barr ML and Kiernan JA. General sensory systems. In: Barr ML and Kiernan JA (eds.), *The human nervous system: an anatomical viewpoint*, 5th edition. Philadelphia: Lippincott, 1988: 277-295.

Barrack R, Skinner H, Brunet M, and Cook S. Joint kinesthesia in the highly trained knee. *J Sports Med* 1984; 24(1):18-20.

Barrett DS. Proprioception and function after anterior cruciate reconstruction. *J Bone Joint Surg [Br]* 1991; 73(5):833-837.

Basford JR. Electrical therapy. In: Kottke FJ and Lehmann JF (eds.), *Krusen's handbook of physical medicine and rehabilitation*, 4th edition. Philadelphia: Saunders, 1990:375-401.

Basford JR. Physical agents. In: DeLisa JA and Gans BM (eds.), *Rehabilitation medicine: principles and practice*, 3rd edition. Philadelphia: Lippincott-Raven, 1998:483-503.

Basmajian JV. Biofeedback in physical medicine and rehabilitation. In: DeLisa JA and Gans BM (eds.), *Rehabilitation medicine: principles and practice*, 3rd edition. Philadelphia: Lippincott-Raven, 1998:505-520.

Beard DJ, Dodd CAF, Trundle HR, and Simpson AHRW. Proprioceptive enhancement for anterior cruciate ligament deficiency. *J Bone Joint Surg [Br]* 1994; 76(4):654-659.

Berger AR and Schaumburg HH. Rehabilitation of focal nerve injuries. *J Neuro Rehab* 1988; 2(2):65-91.

Bickford RH and Duff RS. Influences of ultrasonic radiation of temperature and blood flow in the human skeletal muscle. *Circ Res* 1953; 1:534-538.

Bierman W. Therapeutic use of cold. *JAMA* 1955; 157:1189-1192.

Boonstra AM, van Weerden TW, Eisma WH, Pahlplatz VB, and Oosterhvis HJ. The effect of low-frequency electrical stimulation on denervation atrophy in man. *Scand J Rehab Med* 1987; 19:127-134.

Brand RA. Knee ligaments: a new view. *Trans ASME* 1986; 108:106-110.

Brodersen MP and Symanowski JT. Use of double upright knee orthosis prophylactically to decrease severity of knee injuries in football players. *Clin J Sports Med* 1993; 3(1):31-35.

Brown FW. Management of diskogenic pain using epidural and intrathecal steroids. *Clin Orthop* 1977; 129:72-78.

Brown MC and Ironton R. Suppression of motor nerve terminal sprouting in partially denervated mouse muscles. *J Physiol* 1977; 272:70P-71P.

Buchthal F and Kuhl V. Nerve conduction, tactile sensibility, and the electromyogram after suture or compression of peripheral nerve: a longitudinal study in man. *J Neurol Neurosurg Psych* 1979; 42:436-451.

Burks RT, Bean BG, Marcus R, and Barker HB. Analysis of athletic performance with prophylactic ankle devices. *Am J Sports Med* 1991; 19(2):104-106.

Byron PM. Upper extremity nerve gliding: programs used at the Philadelphia Hand Center. In: Hunter JM, Mackin EJ, and Callahan AD (eds.), *Rehabilitation of the hand: surgery and therapy*. Philadelphia: Mosby, Inc., 1995:951-956.

Carter RL. Competitive diving. In: Fu FH and Stone DA (eds.), *Sports injuries, mechanisms, prevention, treatment*. Philadelphia: Williams & Wilkins, 1994:261-281.

Challenor YB. Rehabilitation of the neurologically impaired athlete. In: Jordan BD, Tsairis P, and Warren RF (eds.), *Sports neurology*, 2nd edition. Philadelphia: Lippincott-Raven, 1998:125-134.

Child SZ, Hartman CL, Schery LA, and Carstensen EL. Lung damage from exposure to pulsed ultrasound. *Ultrasound Med Biol* 1990; 16:817-825.

Chor H, Cleveland D, Davenport HA, Dolkart RE, and Beard G. Atrophy and regeneration of the gastrocnemius-soleus muscles: effects of physical therapy in the monkey following section and suture of sciatic nerve. *JAMA* 1939; 113(11):1029-1033.

Clark FJ and Burgess PR. Slowly adapting receptors in the cat knee joint: can they signal joint angle? *J Neurophysiol* 1975; 38(6)1448-1463.

Clarke KS and Jordan BD. Sports neuroepidemiology. In: Jordan BD, Tsairis P, and Warren RF (eds.), *Sports neurology*, 2nd edition, Philadelphia: Lippincott-Raven, 1998:3-13.

Corbin CB. Flexibility. *Clin Sports Med* 1984; 3(1):101-117.

Crossman ERFW. A theory of acquisition of speed-skill. *Ergonomics* 1959; 2:153-166.

Currier DP and Mann R. Muscular strength development by electrical stimulation in healthy individuals. *Phys Ther* 1983; 63(6):915-921.

Daube JR. AAEM minimonograph #11: needle examination in clinical electromyography. *Muscle Nerve* 1991; 14:685-700.

DeLateur BJ, Lehman JF, and Fordyce WE. A test of the DeLorme axiom. *Arch Phys Med Rehabil* 1968; 49(5):245-248.

DeLorme TL. Restoration of muscle power by heavy resistance exercises. *J Bone Joint Surg* 1945; 27(4):645-667.

DeLorme TL. Heavy resistance exercises. *Arch Phys Med Rehabil* 1946; 27:607-630.

Denny-Brown D. The influence of tension and innervation on the regeneration of skeletal muscle. *J Neuropath Exp Neurol* 1951; 10:94-96.

Doupe J, Barnes R, and Kerr AS. The effect of electrical stimulation on the circulation and recovery of denervated muscle. *J Neurol Psychiat* 1943; 6:136-140.

Draper V. Electromyographic biofeedback and recovery of quadriceps femoris muscle function following anterior cruciate ligament reconstruction. *Phys Ther* 1990; 70(1):11-17.

Draper V and Ballard L. Electrical stimulation versus electromyographic biofeedback in the recovery of quadriceps femoris muscle function following anterior cruciate ligament surgery. *Phys Ther* 1991; 71(6):455-461.

Einarsson G and Grimby G. Strengthening exercise program in post-polio subjects. In: Halstead LS and Weichers DO (eds.), *Research and clinical aspects of the late effects of poliomyelitis*. White Plains, NY: March of Dimes Birth Defects Foundation, 1987:275-283.

Eldred E, Lindsley DE, and Buchwald JS. The effect of cooling on mammalian muscle spindles. *Exp Neurol* 1960; 2:144-157.

El-Khoury GY, Ehara S, Weinstein JN, Montgomery WJ, and Kathol MH. Epidural steroid injection: a procedure ideally performed with fluoroscopic control. *Radiology* 1988; 168:554-557.

Enwemeka CS. The effects of therapeutic ultrasound on tendon healing: a biomechanical study. *Am J Phys Med* 1989; 68(6):283-287.

Ethicon, Inc. Wound healing. In: *Wound closure manual.* Ethicon, Inc., Johnson & Johnson Company, 1988:3-14.

Fairchild VM, Salerno LM, Wedding SL, and Weinberg E. Physical therapy. In: Raj PP (ed.), *Practical management of pain.* Chicago: Yearbook Medical Publishers, 1986:839-852.

Feldman RM and Soskolne CL. The use of non-fatiguing strengthening exercises in post-polio syndrome. In: Halstead LS and Weichers DO (eds.), *Research and clinical aspects of the late effects of poliomyelitis.* White Plains, NY: March of Dimes Birth Defects Foundation, 1987:335-341.

Felson DT and Anderson JJ. Across-study evaluation of association between steroid dose and bolus steroids and avascular necrosis of bone. *Lancet* 1987 Apr 18;1(8538):902-6.

Fischer E. The effect of faradic and galvanic stimulation upon the course of atrophy in denervated skeletal muscles. *Am J Physiol* 1939; 127(4):605-619.

Forkin DM, Koczur C, Battle R, and Newton RA. Evaluation of kinesthetic deficits indicative of balance control in gymnasts with unilateral chronic ankle sprains. *J Orthop Sports Phys Ther* 1996; 23(4):245-250.

Freeman MAR, Dean MAR, and Hanham IWF. The etiology and prevention of functional instability of the foot. *J Bone Joint Surg [Br]* 1965; 47:678-685.

Freidhoff G, Davies G, and Malone T. Rehabilitation: Chain links: rehabilitation program should balance open and closed kinetic chain activities. *Biomechanics* 1998; 5(3).

Fuentes RJ and Rosenberg JM. Anabolic steroids and the athlete. In: Fuentes RJ and Rosenberg JM (eds.), *Athletic drug reference '99.* Durham, NC: Clean Data, Inc./Glaxo-Wellcome, 1999:131-160.

Garrick J and Requa R. Role of external ankle support in the prevention of ankle sprains. *Med Sci Sports Exerc* 1973; 5(3):200-203.

Giannoudis PV, MacDonald DA, Matthews SJ, Smith RM, Furlong AJ, and DeBoer P. Nonunion of the femoral diaphysis. The influence of reaming and non-steroidal anti-inflammatory drugs. *J Bone Joint Surg [Br]* 2000; 82-B(5): 655-658.

Girlanda P, Dattola R, Vita G, Oteri G, LoPresti F, and Messina C. Effect of electrotherapy on denervated muscles in rabbits: an electrophysiological and morphological study. *Exp Neurol* 1982; 77:483-491.

Golomer E, Dupui P, and Monod H. Sex-linked differences in equilibrium reactions among adolescents performing complex sensorimotor tasks. *J Physiol (Paris)* 1997; 91(2):49-55.

Grant AE. Massage with ice (cryokinetics) in the treatment of painful conditions of the musculoskeletal system. *Arch Phys Med Rehabil* 1964; 45:233-237.

Green PWB, Burke AJ, Weiss CA, and Langan P. The role of epidural cortisone injection in the treatment of diskogenic low back pain. *Clin Orthop* 1980; 153:121-125.

Greene TA and Hillman SK. Comparison of support provided by a semirigid orthosis and adhesive ankle taping before, during and after exercise. *Am J Sports Med* 1990; 18:498-506.

Guttman E and Guttman L. The effect of galvanic exercise on denervated and re-innervated muscles in the rabbit. *J Neurol Neurosurg Psychiat* 1944; 7:7-17.

Harrelson GL. Introduction to rehabilitation. In: Andrews JR and Harrelson GL (eds.), *Physical rehabilitation of the injured athlete*. Philadelphia: Saunders, 1991:165-195.

Hasan Z, Enoka RM, and Stuart DG. The interface between biomechanics and neurophysiology in the study of movement: some recent approaches. *Exerc Sport Sci Rev* 1985; 13:169-234.

Herbison GJ, Jaweed M, and Ditunno JF. Acetylcholine sensitivity and fibrillation potentials in electrically stimulated crush-denervated rat skeletal muscle. *Arch Phys Med Rehabil* 1983a; 64(5):217-220.

Herbison GJ, Jaweed M, and Ditunno JF. Exercise therapies in peripheral neuropathies. *Arch Phys Med Rehabil* 1983b; 64(5):201-205.

Herbison GJ, Jaweed MM, Ditunno JF, and Scott CM. Effect of overwork during reinnervation of rat muscle. *Exp Neurol* 1973; 41:1-14.

Herbison GJ, Teng C, and Gordon EE. Electrical stimulation of reinnervating rat muscle. *Arch Phys Med Rehabil* 1973; 54(4):156-160.

Ho SS, Coel MN, Kagawa R, and Richardson AB. The effects of ice on blood flow and bone metabolism in knees. *Am J Sports Med* 1994; 22(4):537-540.

Ho SSW, Illgen RL, Meyer RW, Torok PJ, Cooper MD, and Reider B. Comparison of various icing times in decreasing bone metabolism and blood flow in the knee. *Am J Sports Med* 1995; 23:74-76.

Horch KW, Clark FJ, and Burgess PR. Awareness of knee joint angle under static conditions *J Neurophysiol* 1975; 38(6):1436-1447.

Ironton R, Brown RC, and Holland RL. Stimuli to intramuscular nerve growth. *Brain Res* 1978; 156:351-354.

Irrgang JJ. Rehabilitation: evaluation, training and special concerns. In: Fu FH and Stone DA (eds.), *Sports injuries: mechanisms, prevention and treatment*. Philadelphia: Williams & Wilkins, 1994:81-95.

Jewell MJ. Overview of the structure and function of the central nervous system. In: Umphred DA (ed.), *Neurological rehabilitation*, 2nd edition. St. Louis: Mosby, 1990:27-41.

Jones AC. Clinical observations in the use of ultrasound. *Am J Phys Med* 1954; 33:47-53.

Joynt RL, Findley TW, Boda W, and Daum MC. Therapeutic exercise. In: DeLisa JA and Gans BM (eds.), *Rehabilitation medicine: principles and practice*, 2nd edition. Philadelphia: Lippincott, 1993:526-554.

Karlsson J and Andreasson GO. The effect of external ankle support in chronic lateral ankle joint instability. *Am J Sports Med* 1992; 20(3):257-260

Kennedy JC, Alexander IJ, and Hayes KC. Nerve supply of the human knee and its functional importance. *Am J Sports Med* 1982; 10(6):329-335.

Kimura J. Anatomy and physiology of the peripheral nerve. In: Kimura J (ed.), *Electrodiagnosis in diseases of nerve and muscle: principles and practice*, 2nd edition. Philadelphia: Davis, 1989:55-77.

Kioumourtzoglou E, Derri V, Mertzanidou O, and Tzetzis G. Experience with perceptual and motor skills in rhythmic gymnastics. *Percep Motor Skill* 1997; 84(3 pt 2):1363-1372.

Kottke FJ. The neurophysiology of motor function. In: Kottke FJ and Lehman JF (eds.), *Krusen's handbook of physical medicine and rehabilitation*, 4th edition. Philadelphia: Saunders, 1990:234-269.

Kraft GH. Fibrillation potential amplitude and muscle atrophy following peripheral nerve injury. *Muscle Nerve* 1990; 13(9):814-21.

Kraft GH. Fibrillation potentials and positive sharp waves: are they the same? *Electroenceph Clin Neurophysiol* 1991; 81:163-166.

Kraft GH. Are fibrillation potentials and positive sharp waves the same? No. *Muscle Nerve* 1996; 19(2):216-220.

Krivickas LS and Feinberg JH. Lower extremity injuries in college athletes: relation between ligamentous laxity and lower extremity muscle tightness. *Arch Phys Med Rehabil* 1996; 77(11):1139-1143.

Lamb DR. The physiological basis of muscular strength. In: Lamb DR (ed.), *Physiology of exercise: responses and adaptations*. New York: Macmillan, 1978.

Lehman JF and DeLateur BJ. Diathermy, and superficial heat, laser, and cold therapy. In: Kottke FJ and Lehmann JF (eds.), *Krusen's handbook of physical medicine and rehabilitation*, 4th edition. Philadelphia: Saunders, 1990:283-367.

Lemons DE and Downey JA. Control of the circulation in the limbs. In: Downey JA, Myers SJ, Gonzalez EG and Lieberman JS (eds.), *The physiologic basis of rehabilitation medicine*, 2nd edition. Boston: Butterworth-Heinemann, 1994:365-391.

Lephart SM, Giraldo JL, Borsa PA, and Fu FH. Knee joint proprioception: a comparison between female intercollegiate gymnasts and controls. *Knee Surg Traumatol Arthroscopy* 1996; 4(2):121-124

Lephart SM, Pincivero DM, Giraldo JL, and Fu F. The role of proprioception in the management and rehabilitation of athletic injuries. *Am J Sports Med* 1997; 25(1):130-137.

Levitt R, Deisinger JA, Remondet Wall J, Ford L, and Cassisi JE. EMG feedback-assisted postoperative rehabilitation of minor arthroscopic knee surgeries. *J Sports Med Phys Fitness* 1995; 35:218-223.

LeVeau BF and Rogers C. Selective training of the vastus medialis muscle using EMG biofeedback. *Phys Ther* 1980; 60(11):1410-1415.

Lieberman JS, Taylor RG, and Fowler WM. Fatiguing muscle weakness: an overlooked phenomenon in patients with neurogenic dysfunction. *Arch Phys Med Rehabil* 1981; 62:515.

Lipman AG. Pharmacological approaches to pain management: nontraditional analgesics and analgesic adjuvants. In: Ashburn MA and Rice LJ (eds.), *The management of pain*. New York: Churchill Livingstone, 1998:111-140.

Maitland ME, Ajemian SV, and Suter E. Quadriceps femoris and hamstring muscle function in a person with an unstable knee. *Phys Ther* 1999; 79(1):66-75.

Manfroy PP, Ashton-Miller JA, and Wojtys EM. The effect of exercise, prewrap, and athletic tape on the maximal active and passive ankle resistance to ankle inversion. *Am J Sports Med* 1997; 25(2):156-163.

Marey S, Boleach LW, Mayhew JL, and McDole S. Determination of player potential in volleyball: coaches' rating versus game performance. *J Sports Med Phys Fitness* 1991; 31:161-164.

Martin GJ, Boden SD, and Titus L. Recombinant human bone morphogenetic protein-2 overcomes the inhibitory effect of ketorolac, a nonsteroidal anti-inflammatory drug (NSAID), on posterolateral lumbar intertransverse process spine fusion. *Spine* 1999; 24(21):2188-2193.

May M, Croxson GR, and Klein SR. Bell's palsy: management of sequelae using EMG rehabilitation, botulinum toxin, and surgery. *Am J Otology* 1989; 10(3):220-229.

McMaster WC, Liddle S, and Waugh TR. Laboratory evaluation of various cold therapy modalities. *Am J Sports Med* 1978; 6:291-294.

Mehta M and Salmon N. Extradural block. Confirmation of the injection site by x-ray monitoring. *Anaesthesia* 1985; 40:1009-1012.

Melzack R and Wall PD. Pain mechanisms: a new theory. *Science* 1965; 150:971-979.

Mitchell JH and Wildenthal K. Static (isometric) exercise and the heart: physiological and clinical considerations. *Ann Rev Med* 1974; 25:369-381.

Mirabelli L. Pain management. In: Umphred DA (ed.), *Neurological rehabilitation*, 2nd edition. St. Louis: Mosby, 1990:755-771.

Miyatsu M, Atsuta Y, and Watakabe M. The physiology of mechanoreceptors in the anterior cruciate ligament: an experimental study in decerebrate-spinalised animals. *J Bone Joint Surg [Br]* 1993; 75(4):653-657.

Nadler SF, Weingand KW, Stitik TP, and Kruse RJ. Pain relief runs hot and cold. *Biomechanics* 2001; 8(1):83-90.

Nelson MN and Currier DP. In: Nelson MN and Currier DP (eds.), *Clinical electrotherapy 1987*. Norwalk, CT: Appleton & Lange, 1987.

Nemeth PM. Electrical stimulation of denervated muscle prevents decreases in oxidative enzymes. *Muscle Nerve* 1982; 5(2):134-139.

Ogard WK and Stockert BW. Peripheral neuropathies. In: Umphred DA (ed.), *Neurological rehabilitation*, 2nd edition. St. Louis: Mosby, 1990:333-345.

Perlau R, Frank C, and Fick G. The effect of elastic bandages on human knee proprioception in the uninjured population. *Am J Sports Med* 1995; 23(2):251-255.

Perlmutter GS and Apruzzese W. Axillary nerve injuries in contact sports: recommendations for treatment and rehabilitation. *Sports Med* 1998; 26(5): 351-361.

Politis MJ, Zanakis MF. and Albala BJ. Facilitated regeneration in the rat peripheral nervous system using applied electric fields. *J Trauma* 1988; 28(9):1375-1381.

Renfrew DL, Moore TE, Kathol MH, El-Khoury GY, Lemke JH, and Walker CW. Correct placement of epidural steroid injections: fluoroscopic guidance and contrast administration. *AJNR* 1991; 12:1003-1007.

Rettig AC, Stube KS, and Shelbourne KD. Effects of finger and wrist taping on grip strength. *Am J Sports Med* 1997; 25(1):96-98.

Rivenburgh DW. Physical modalities in the treatment of tendon injuries. *Clin Sports Med* 1992; 11(3):645-658.

Robertson S and Elliot D. Specificity of learning and dynamic balance. *Research Quarterly for Exercise and Sport* 1996; 67(1):69-75.

Sady SS, Wortman M, and Blanke D. Flexibility training: ballistic, static or proprioceptive neuromuscular facilitation? *Arch Phys Med Rehabil* 1982; 63:261-263.

Schultz RA, Miller DC, Kerr CS, and Michelli L. Mechanoreceptors in human cruciate ligaments. *J Bone Joint Surg [Am]* 1984; 66:1072-1076.

Schutt AH and Bengtson KA. Hand rehabilitation. In: DeLisa JA and Gans BM (eds.), *Rehabilitation medicine: principles and practice*, 3rd edition. Philadelphia: Lippincott-Raven, 1998:1717-1732.

Seddon HJ. Three types of nerve injury. *Brain* 1943; 66:237-288.

Sheth P, Yu B, Laskowski ER, and An KN. Ankle disk training influences reaction times of selected muscle in a simulated ankle sprain. *Am J Sports Med* 1997; 25(4):538-543.

Shiflett SC, Schoenberger NE, Diamond BJ, Nayak S, and Cotter AC. In: DeLisa JA and Gans BM (eds.), *Rehabilitation medicine: principles and practice*, 3rd edition. Philadelphia: Lippincott-Raven, 1998:873-885.

Skinner HB, Barrack RL, and Cook SD. Age-related decline in proprioception. *Clin Orthop* 1984; 184(Apr):208-211.

Smith AD, Stroud L, and McQueen C. Flexibility and anterior knee pain in adolescent elite figure skaters. *J Ped Orth* 1991; 11:77-82.

Smith KL. Nerve response to injury and repair. In: Hunter JM, Mackin EJ, and Callahan AD (eds.), *Rehabilitation of the hand: surgery and therapy.* Philadelphia: Mosby, Inc., 1995:609-626.

Spielholz NI. Electrical stimulation of denervated muscle. In: Nelson RM, Hayes KW and Currier DP (eds), *Clinical electrotherapy,* 3rd edition. Norwalk, CT: Appleton & Lange, 1999:411-446.

Starkey JA. Treatment of ankle sprains by simultaneous use of intermittent compression and ice packs. *Am J Sports Med* 1976; 4:142-144.

Sunderland S. Treatment. General considerations. In: Sunderland S (ed.), *Nerves and nerve injuries,* 2nd edition. Edinburgh: Churchill Livingstone, 1978.

Swenson C, Swärd L, and Karlsson J. Cryotherapy in sports medicine. *Scand J Med Sci Sports* 1996; 6:193-200.

Tarantal AF and Canfield DR. Ultrasound induced lung hemorrhage in the monkey. *Ultrasound Med Biol* 1994; 20:65-72.

Torg JS. Management guidelines for athletic injuries to the cervical spine. *Clin Sports Med* 1987; 6(1):53-60.

Trojaberg W. Early electrophysiologic changes in conduction block. *Muscle Nerve* 1978; 1:400-403.

Tropp H, Askling C, and Gillquist J. Prevention of ankle sprains. *Am J Sports Med* 1985; 13(4):259-262.

Tropp H, Ekstrand J, and Gillquist J. Stabilometry in functional instability of the ankle and its value in predicting injury. *Med Sci Sports Exer* 1984; 16(1):64-66.

Tsairis P. Electromyography: clinical applications. In: Jordan BD, Tsairis P and Warren RF (eds.), *Sports neurology,* 2nd edition. Philadelphia: Lippincott-Raven, 1998:3-13.

Umphred DA and McCormack GL. Classification of common facilitatory and inhibitory treatment techniques. In: Umphred DA (ed.), *Neurological rehabilitation,* 2nd edition. St. Louis: Mosby, 1990:111-161.

Wallin D, Ekblom B, Grahn R, and Nordenborg T. Improvement of muscle flexibility: a comparison between two techniques. *Am J Sports Med* 1985; 13(4):263-268.

Weinstein SW, Herring SA, and Derby R. Contemporary concepts in spine care: epidural steroid injections. *Spine* 1995; 20:1842-1846.

Wojtys EM, Kothari SU, and Huston LJ. Anterior cruciate ligament functional brace use in sports. *Am J Sports Med* 1996; 24(4):539-546.

Wolf SL. Electromyographic biofeedback: an overview. In: Nelson RM and Currier DP (eds.), *Clinical electromyography,* 2nd edition. Norwalk, CT: Appleton & Lange, 1991:361-384.

Wolf SL. Biofeedback. In: Downey JA, Myers SJ, Gonzalez EG, and Lieberman JS (eds.), *The physiologic basis of rehabilitation medicine,* 2nd edition. Boston: Butterworth-Heinemann, 1994: 563-572.

Wolf SL, Barnhart HX, Ellison GL, Coogler CE, and Atlanta FICSIT Group. The effect of tai chi quan and computerized balance training on postural stability in older subjects. Atlanta FICSIT Group. Frailty and Injuries: Cooperative Studies on Intervention Technique. *Phys Ther* 1997; 77(4):371-381.

Wolf SL, Barnhart HX, Kutner NG, McNeely E, Coogler C, Xu T, and Atlanta FICSIT Group. Reducing frailty and falls in older persons: an investigation of tai chi and computerized balance training. *J Am Geriatr Soc* 1996; 44:489-497.

Yaggie JA, McGregor S, and Armstrong CW. The effects of isokinetic fatigue on balance and the ranges of postural control. *Med Sci Sports Exerc* 1999; 31(5S):S284.

Zemke JE, Andersen JC, Guion WK, McMillan J, and Joyner AB. Intramuscular temperature responses in the human leg to two forms of cryotherapy: ice massage and ice bag. *J Orthop Sports Phys Ther* 1998; 27(4):301-307.

Zuckerman LA and Ferrante FM. Nonopioid and opioid analgesics. In: Ashburn MA and Rice LJ (eds.), *The management of pain*. New York: Churchill Livingstone, 1998:111-140.

8

Rehabilitation of Upper-Extremity Nerve Injuries

Gerard A. Malanga, MD
Robert Savarese, DO

The rehabilitation of upper-extremity nerve injuries can be quite challenging. Pathologies encountered range from mild compressive *neuropathies* to complex postoperative complications of peripheral nerve trauma. Injuries can occur from traction, compression, ischemia, or laceration. In order to incorporate biomechanical modifications into the rehabilitation process, clinicians need to understand the mechanisms of injuries.

> **neuropathy**—A functional disturbance or pathologic change in the peripheral nervous system.

The first rule following any injury is to prevent further injury of the involved nerve, either through positioning, splinting, or casting. Any activity that would cause compression or excess traction is also prohibited. After an appropriate period of relative rest and sometimes immobilization, restoration of motion is essential. The fact that peripheral nerves contain connective tissue, which can become contracted and can also be stretched, is often forgotten. Adherence of the nerve to local soft-tissue or bony structures may limit *nerve glide*, leading to excessive traction or compression. To help address this problem, peripheral nerve stretching should be performed with a short-duration, repetitive type of stretch because it is probable that prolonged stretch causes ischemia of the nerve vasculature, resulting in pain and injury to the nerve.

nerve glide—Normal physiologic movement of a nerve within connective tissue as a response to bodily movements.

Following restoration of normal range of motion, a progressive strengthening program of the muscles supplied by that nerve should be started when there is enough muscle strength to overcome gravity (3/5):

1. Muscles significantly weakened from denervation are initially strengthened by *isometric* co-contractions when the arc of motion needs to be limited.

2. *Isotonic* lightweight (with high repetition) *concentric* strengthening follows this. Lightweight concentrics can be initiated early and may even be preferable to isometrics when an arc of motion is permitted and when there has been injury to the noncontractile musculotendinous structures.

3. Although muscles are often strengthened initially in isolation, this can potentially overload them and lead to maladaptive patterns. Thus, a more functional strengthening program that requires the synergistic activation of multiple muscle groups should be initiated as soon as an individual can begin them. This approach not only prevents overload to the involved muscle but also helps to reestablish proper motor engrams.

4. The final phase of rehabilitation involves training the affected area in work-specific or sport-specific activities. This allows for the reestablishment of engrams and proprioception, which can be crucial for activities of daily living, work, musical performance, and sports.

isometric contraction—Muscle contraction that increases tension without a shortening or lengthening of the muscle.

isotonic contraction—Muscle contraction that results in a shortening of the muscle without a change in its tension.

concentric contraction—Muscle contraction that results in the approximation of the muscle's origin and insertion.

Denervated or minimally innervated muscles may respond to electrical stimulation. Although recent literature supports the use of electrical stimulation to preserve muscle mass following nerve injuries (Politis et al. 1988), its functional benefit has not been demonstrated. Electric stimulation has been extensively discussed on pages 151-153 in chapter 7. Certainly, once the patient is able to volitionally activate a muscle, active strengthening is preferred over electrical stimulation. Moreover, strengthening of contralateral extremities can result in strength gains through central effects.

For detailed discussions of the general principles of nerve injury management, consult chapter 7.

MEDIAN NERVE INJURIES

As noted in chapter 4, the median nerve may be injured or compressed at several sites along its course in the upper extremity, including at the ligament of Struthers and between the two heads of the pronator teres. A thickening of a fascial band between the biceps tendon and the flexor carpi radialis has also been described as a source of median nerve constriction (Spinner 1970). The pronator syndrome and injury to the anterior interosseous nerve can also occur. For a full discussion of anatomy and diagnosis, see pages 61-67 in chapter 4.

Proximal Median Neuropathies

Nonoperative treatment of these more proximal median neuropathies begins with a period of relative rest, which limits repetitive or forceful elbow flexion and forearm pronation for a four- to six-week period. During this time, muscle lengthening is achieved with a passive, prolonged stretch of greater than thirty seconds that is repeated four to six times. Such stretching should be done three to five times a day. A warm-up exercise, such as on an upper-extremity bike (figure 8.1), will enhance the therapeutic benefit of stretching.

Following this period of relative rest, a gradual progressive strengthening program may begin, with every strengthening session followed by stretching. Isometrics are the type of muscle contractions least stressful to the nerve and are started initially. Light weights with a high number of repetitions (18-20), including both concentric and *eccentric* strengthening, should begin as soon as the acute, painful symptoms have resolved. The proper weight is identified by having the last two repetitions be completed with maximal effort. Examples include wall push-ups,

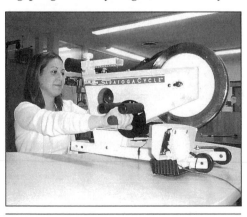

Figure 8.1 Upper-extremity bike.

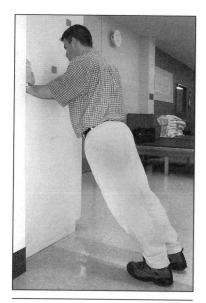

Figure 8.2 Wall push-ups.

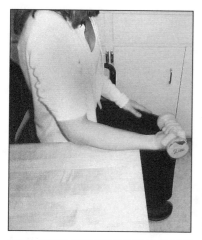

Figure 8.3 Biceps curls.

biceps curls, forearm curls, and pronation strengthening with Therabands (figures 8.2 through 8.4). It is generally recommended that two to three sets be performed three times a week. Once symmetric strength to the opposite limb is achieved, a more functional strengthening program can begin. At this stage, athletes can use medicine balls or resistive rubber tubing or bands in motions that mimic various sport activities such as tennis strokes or a baseball pitch (figures 8.5 through 8.7). Throwing and catching a medicine ball against a minitrampoline is a functional exercise that also allows the athlete to focus on proper body mechanics (figure 8.8). The rehab specialist must remain aware of the interactions of the elements of the kinetic chain involved, being careful to insure that the more proximal elements are functioning well before proceeding to the more distal elements and watching for dysfunctional substitution muscle firing patterns. Patients unresponsive to this nonoperative approach may need to consider operative treatment.

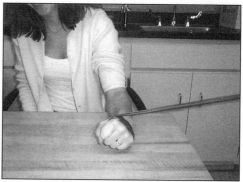

Figure 8.4 Pronation strengthening with a Theraband.

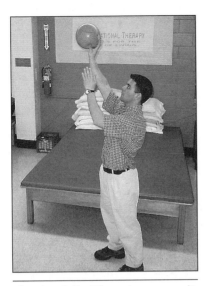

Figure 8.5 Throwing a medicine ball like a basketball.

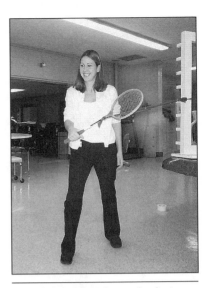

Figure 8.6 Using a badminton racquet attached to a Theraband—forward stroke.

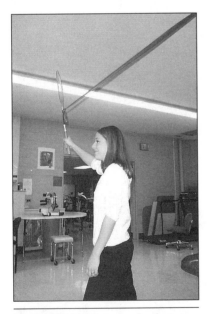

Figure 8.7 Using a badminton racquet attached to a Theraband—overhead stroke.

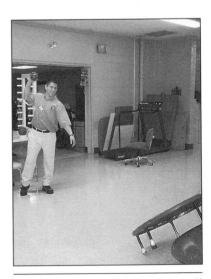

Figure 8.8 Throwing a small medicine ball like a baseball at a minitrampoline.

eccentric contraction—Muscle contraction that results in a lengthening of the muscle's origin and insertion.

Carpal Tunnel Syndrome

The most common median neuropathy occurs at the carpal tunnel. Although the carpal tunnel is rarely injured by trauma, it can become symptomatic from overly repetitive flexion and extension at the wrist as well as via ulnar and radial wrist movements. It is well accepted that wrist flexion and extension result in increased pressure within the carpal tunnel (Gelberman et al. 1981). Such movements can occur in activities such as volleyball, baseball, and racquet sports. Direct pressure for prolonged or repetitive periods can also result in median nerve irritation, as can vibration (such as cyclists experience). The irritation likely stems from intraneural ischemia.

Knowing the causes of median neuropathy at the carpal tunnel can help a clinician devise appropriate treatment. Obviously, positions that increase symptoms and pressure within the carpal tunnel should be avoided. Inflammation within the carpal tunnel should also be addressed in the early phase of treatment. This is done with local icing, splinting the wrist in a neutral position, and a short course of nonsteroidal anti-inflammatory medications. If the symptoms are mild, splinting can be limited to nighttime use; for severe or recurrent symptoms, daytime use should be considered for three to four weeks. This can be effective in up to two-thirds of all patients (Kruger 1991).

Local steroid injection can help patients who do not respond to less invasive measures. Proper placement is imperative. The exact dosage has not been clearly delineated in the literature. Depomedrol can be used along with a short-acting anesthetic with a total volume of 1-2 ml. Giannini et al. (1991) found that steroid injection was effective in over 90% of patients treated with the injection. Gelberman and colleagues (1981), however, found that only 40% of patients were successfully treated with injection into the carpal tunnel. Green (1990) noted a significant recurrence rate after injection, with only 11% having no recurrences up to 45 months— note, however, that only 46% of the patients with recurrent symptoms ultimately required surgical treatment.

Kaplan et al. (1984) defined five factors that were predictive of a poor outcome in nonoperative treatment of carpal tunnel syndrome. These factors included age greater than 50 years, more than 10 months of symptoms prior to treatment, constant paresthesias, stenosing *tenosynovitis*, and a positive Phalen's test in less than 30 seconds. Kaplan and colleagues (1984) treated 331 patients with splinting and nonsteroidal anti-inflammatory medication. Sixteen percent also received intracarpal steroid injection. Patients were considered "cured" if they reported no symptoms after six months. Of the patients who had none of the factors listed above, two-thirds had a successful nonoperative treatment outcome and were considered cured. Nonoperative treatment failed in 93% of the patients who had three or more of the above factors.

tenosynovitis—Inflammation of the tendon sheath.

In addition to NSAIDs, splinting, and steroid injection, other techniques can benefit patients with carpal tunnel syndrome. *Iontophoresis* of corticosteroid was found to be comparable to injection in a study by Banta (1994)—58% of patients were successfully treated with iontophoresis using dexamethasone, along with splinting and NSAIDs.

iontophoresis—A physical modality in which soluble salts (most commonly steroids) are introduced into the body through the skin via an electrical current.

Finally, there are myofascial stretching techniques of the soft tissue about the wrist, including the transverse carpal ligament, that can be quite helpful in conjunction with the other treatments previously discussed. Patients can be instructed to do these stretches at home. The athlete places her palm on a wall as figure 8.9 illustrates and sustains the stretch for 15-30 seconds; she should advance her arm up the wall four to six times as tolerated. The usefulness of vitamin B-6 supplements is unclear, but certainly is not harmful in doses less than 200 mg/day. The role of acupuncture treatment is unclear, although it has been helpful in other painful conditions.

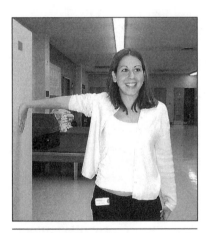

Figure 8.9 Myofascial stretching of the wrist to treat carpal tunnel syndrome.

It is important to make all possible biomechanical modifications to limit excess flexion, extension, and radial and ulnar deviation. In general, the biomechanics of most sports do not require extremes of flexion or extension. Cyclists should avoid prolonged periods in upright positions where the wrists are resting directly against the handlebars. They should work on strengthening their trunk and upper back muscles (e.g., the latissimus dorsi). Such strengthening reduces the need to rest on the wrists, which increases pressure within the carpal tunnel. Finally, properly padding the handlebars and using well-padded cycling gloves can help decrease vibrational irritation and pressure on the median nerve.

ULNAR NERVE INJURIES

Ulnar nerve injury and compression are relatively common in athletes who perform repetitive overhead activities—for example, baseball pitchers and javelin throwers. In these athletes the ulnar nerve is subject to both compressive and distractive forces at the elbow, particularly as it passes through the cubital tunnel (see pages 67-68 for a complete discussion and illustration of the anatomy). This area decreases as the elbow flexes. The arcuate ligament tightens at approximately 45 degrees of elbow flexion, and at 90 degrees of flexion the flexor carpi ulnaris also tightens (Vanderpool et al. 1968). Elbow flexion also causes the ulnar collateral ligament to relax and bulge into the tunnel, sometimes causing further encroachment. Macnicol (1982) measured increased pressures as the elbow was flexed and the shoulder abducted. This position corresponds to the cocking position in throwing and to other overhead sports movements. Osteophytes can also cause compression on the ulnar nerve, typically while the elbow goes into extension during the follow-through phase of throwing. Traction effects on the nerve also occur during elbow flexion. Finally, shoulder abduction with elbow flexion—a common position of the arm during sleep—can exacerbate an already irritated ulnar nerve. Proximal nerve compression or lack of proper nerve glide in the shoulder region can result in distal nerve irritation as an athlete changes the shoulder position, especially if the athlete increases stress on the elbow by leading with the elbow instead of the shoulder and trunk.

In addition to these biomechanical causes for ulnar nerve compression at the elbow, anatomic changes can further narrow the cubital tunnel and increase the compressive force on the ulnar nerve. These include thickening and fibrosis of the arcuate ligament and osteophyte formation at the elbow joint. These changes are common in older athletes who have been involved in repetitive overload activities. The combination of the normal biomechanical changes within the cubital tunnel and the pathoanatomic changes from repetitive overload of the tissues of the elbow result in compression that may cause neural ischemia and swelling.

Ulnar Neuropathies at the Elbow

The causes of ulnar nerve injuries at the elbow provide insight into appropriate treatment and rehabilitation of this condition. Treatment begins by attempting to reduce pain and inflammation through NSAIDs, icing, and relative rest. Splinting can play an important role in minimizing further compression on the nerve. By limiting elbow flexion, a splint can decrease the compressive forces on the ulnar nerve. Elbow flexion should be limited to less than 45 degrees in order to decrease the tightening of the arcuate ligament and reduce buckling of the ulnar collateral ligament. This should help decrease compressive forces and ischemia to the nerve. The splint can initially be worn only at bedtime. If symptoms persist in spite of nighttime splint use or in cases of severe symptoms, both day and night splinting should be considered. Serror (1993) used night splinting in 22 patients and found that it improved symptoms in all of them, including three for whom surgical treatment had failed. Instruction on modifying sleep position to avoid shoulder abduction and elbow flexion may assist in decreasing traction on the nerve. A night splint can help prevent some of these positions. Injection of corticosteroids into the cubital tunnel has been performed, although there is no scientific evidence to support its use. Theoretically, it may have some benefit in reducing perineural edema, which can cause pain and sensory complaints. We recommend that injections be used cautiously and sparingly in cases that are refractory to other forms of treatment.

Once the sensory and pain complaints have improved, restoration of normal upper-extremity range of motion is important. Pectoral stretching, cervical spine stretching, and specifically ulnar nerve gliding techniques (figure 8.10) can help restore upper-extremity range of motion—including the shoulder, wrist, and hand as well as the cervical spine, trunk, and lower extremities. The entire kinetic chain is involved in generating forces in the throwing motion, and alterations in any of the links can have effects further down the chain. This is especially true for anything that would increase elbow flexion, such as weakness of the triceps. Altered elbow biomechanics caused by repetitive throwing can lead to hypertrophic changes, osteophytes around the elbow joint, and soft-tissue contractures—all of which can result in loss of full elbow extension. Athletes who have experienced such a loss begin their motion with some degree of elbow flexion, which increases as they accelerate their arms.

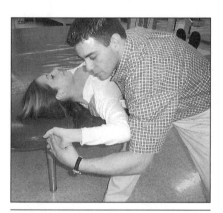

Figure 8.10 Ulnar nerve gliding technique. With the patient supine, the therapist depresses the shoulder while externally rotating the upper extremity and extending the wrist and fingers. The therapist should hold this position for 15 to 30 seconds for four to six repetitions.

Strengthening the muscles about the elbow can help to protect its static structures by limiting the compressive and distractive forces to which it is subjected. The entire kinetic chain should be addressed, with emphasis on the shoulder girdle muscles including the scapular stabilizers and rotator cuff muscles. Stretching the pectoralis muscles may reduce compression of the medial cord proximally, which, if tight, may make the ulnar nerve more susceptible to traction at the elbow. Elbow and forearm muscles

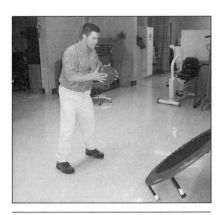

Figure 8.11 Throwing/catching a medicine ball, using a mini-trampoline.

should be strengthened with both concentric and eccentric exercises. Eccentric overload to the triceps occurs in the cocking phase of the throwing motion. Eccentric overload to the biceps and distraction of the joint capsule occur in the follow-through phase. Inadequate deceleration at the elbow can result in distracting forces to the joint and nerve. Low-weight, high-repetition strengthening is recommended initially, with gradual increase in weight and progression to functional strengthening exercises. Exercises including narrow-based push-ups and throwing and catching a large medicine ball against a minitrampoline will help strengthen the triceps and help decrease the amount of elbow flexion (figure 8.11).

Finally, a knowledgeable coach or certified athletic trainer should examine the athlete's throwing mechanics in order to correct any biomechanical flaws that increase stress to the elbow joint. Examples: lack of lumbar extension, diminished hip rotation, or abdominal weakness—which, by decreasing the force generated proximal to the arm, requires greater force generation at the shoulder and elbow. Athletes with this flaw tend to "lead with the elbow" in throwing and racquet sports, thereby increasing stress across the elbow joint.

Ulnar Neuropathies at the Wrist

Injuries usually occur from compression of the distal ulnar nerve within Guyon's canal (see chapter 4, pages 67-68). Cyclists often experience this injury from compression on the handlebars. Treatment initially is similar to ulnar nerve injuries at the elbow (NSAIDs, icing, and relative rest). To control the forces through the tunnel, cyclists should limit the amount of time spent in the "drop" position and frequently change positions. Increasing the padding in the gloves and the handlebars can also limit the compressive and vibrational forces to the hand. Riding on smoother surfaces can also reduce vibrational forces. The seat height and position are also of significant importance, since improper position can result in the upper body's assuming a forward position—which increases the weight borne by the wrists and hands. Cyclists also tend to rest on the handlebars if they have weak muscles in the upper trunk and shoulder girdle—again, increasing pressure through the wrists and hands and on the ulnar nerves in the hands. Therefore, a strengthening program of the scapular stabilizers and the upper trunk is an important part of the rehabilitation and can help prevent ulnar nerve compression at the wrist.

This sort of wrist injury is also common in tennis. The problem can often be solved by using tennis rackets made of more flexible materials that dampen vibration. If preventive measures are not helpful (whether for cyclists, tennis players, or anyone else), it may be necessary to temporarily end participation in the sport that is causing the symptoms. A gradual return to the activity is then recommended, with the hope that the symptoms do not return or that they can be controlled.

RADIAL NERVE INJURIES

The posterior interosseous nerve traverses through the radial tunnel to enter the forearm from the volar to the dorsal compartments, supplying the wrist and finger extensors. The nerve can be compressed by a fibrous band, a sharp edge of the extensor carpi radialis brevis, or within the arcade of Frohse, which is formed by the fibrous edge of the superficial head of the supinator. Clinically, patients present with weakness and achiness without sensory loss. Chapter 4 discusses radial nerve anatomy and etiology of injury at length (see pages 70-72).

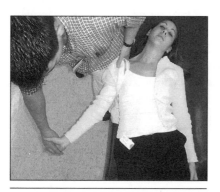

Figure 8.12 Radial nerve gliding technique. With the patient supine and cervical spine laterally flexed to the contralateral side, the therapist depresses the shoulder while extending the upper extremity. The patient's forearm should be fully supinated and the wrist extended. The therapist should hold this position for 15 to 30 seconds for four to six repetitions.

Successful nonoperative treatment includes the use of relative rest and splinting to control supination and pronation and hands-on treatment by a hand therapist to perform myofascial release. A deep heating modality such as ultrasound occasionally is required to facilitate mobilization of the soft tissues. Alternatively, active upper-extremity exercise on an upper-body ergometer may increase blood flow into the upper extremity and help raise the temperature in the soft-tissue structures. Nerve gliding techniques can also be of significant benefit (figure 8.12).

Although there is no strong scientific evidence to support their use, injections are sometimes tried—including trigger-point injections of the supinator and other forearm muscles, which are generally performed to control pain and in hopes of reducing muscle irritability and relaxing spasm. This approach is recommended only if more conventional therapy fails. Return of extensor carpi ulnaris function is usually the earliest sign of recovery in severe injuries with wrist drop (Bateman 1967). Proper positioning of the wrist and hand is important to allow for improved function of the finger flexors and to avoid further stretch and injury to the nerve.

Entrapment of the superficial radial nerve between the extensor carpi radialis longus and the brachioradialis can occur from local trauma or from repetitive use of pronation/supination (Dellon and Mackinnon 1996). These injuries are usually best treated by removing the source of compression, by protecting the nerve with padding, and by avoiding repetitive pronation and supination. Neuritic symptoms can be managed with low-dose tricyclic medications such as amitriptyline or nortriptyline. Full recovery generally occurs.

MUSCULOCUTANEOUS NERVE INJURIES

Injury to the motor portion of the musculocutaneous nerve is rare in isolation, but the nerve can be compressed as it passes through a hypertrophied coracobrachialis, as has been reported in weightlifters (Braddom 1978). Chapter 3 discusses anatomy and injury of the nerve at length (page 53). Relaxation of muscle tone may be accomplished with soft-tissue mobilization and electrical stimulation. Nerve glide techniques may also relieve neural tension.

Injuries to the lateral antebrachial cutaneous nerve are uncommon but have been reported in baseball pitchers, racquetball players, and swimmers doing the backhand stroke (Basset and Nunley 1982, Felsenthal et al. 1984). Injury to the nerve is usually secondary to a forceful pronation with the elbow extended (Weinstein and Herring 1992). Compression occurs between the biceps tendon and the brachial fascia. Recall that the symptoms of aching pain must be distinguished from epicondylitis (page 53). Nonsurgical treatment consists of rest, a trial of iontophoresis, and gentle stretching of the area. It is important also to address the possible biomechanical cause for the nerve injury by avoiding forceful pronation as the elbow extends. Athletes may need to modify their throwing or racquet swing motion by working with a high-level coach. If symptoms persist, splinting with an extension block of 20-40 degrees may be helpful (Weinstein and Herring 1992). Topical creams can be tried as well. Combinations with ketoprofen, lidocaine, and many other medications can be mixed and topically applied to the area for symptom control. With rest, protection, and time these injuries should resolve. If symptoms persist, surgical release should be considered.

AXILLARY NERVE INJURIES

The axillary nerve is most commonly injured as a result of shoulder dislocation. This occurs in 9-18% of all anterior shoulder dislocations (Blom and Dahlback 1970, Mendoza and Main 1990). The axillary nerve can also be compressed or entrapped without trauma. Cahill and Palmer (1983) described entrapment within the quadrilateral space, coining the term "quadrilateral space syndrome" whereby the axillary nerve is compressed along with the posterior circumflex artery. Bennett (1941) described chronic irritation of the axillary nerve in professional baseball pitchers from osteophytes at the posterior, inferior aspect of the glenoid.

Although the axillary nerve supplies both the deltoid and teres minor, the most clinically and functionally significant problems involve the loss of deltoid muscle function. In severe injuries, there is obvious weakness of shoulder flexion and abduction, and over time atrophy becomes evident. EMG studies can be very helpful in determining prognosis and in guiding treatment. If no motor units can be activated on EMG, the prognosis is poor and electrical stimulation on a daily basis should be considered. The scientific basis for and against electrical stimulation of denervated muscle is reviewed elsewhere in this textbook (see pages 151-153). The shoulder should be protected and splinted in approximately 30 degrees of abduction to reduce any "wringing out" effect on the rotator cuff and to place the limb in a good functional position for most daily activities (Bateman 1967). Gentle passive and active assisted range-of-motion exercises should be done at least twice a day to prevent contractures. If no motor unit activity develops after two to four months, surgical exploration and possible nerve grafting should be considered (Mendoza and Main 1990).

For less severe injuries, the shoulder should be protected, although splinting is probably not necessary. Forceful overhead activity and contact sports should be avoided. Stretching should be performed twice daily with 5-10 repetitions. Strengthening should begin slowly and carefully to avoid overactivation of immature nerve sprouts and collaterals. Initially, isometric strengthening should be employed at multiple angles of abduction and forward flexion. Closed kinetic upper-extremity strengthening can also be very beneficial, as it activates several muscle groups in positions that are stable to the shoulder joint. Lightweight isotonic strengthening should begin after the athlete has full active range of motion. Progressive resistance can then be gradually started. Ultimately, strengthening should be progressed to functional activities that replicate the sport of the athlete. These activities should not be started until the muscle can fire appropriately; beginning too early will result in a substitution pattern of muscle activation. Functional strengthening can be done, using resistive rubber tubing or bands in various planes of motion, to replicate a particular task such as a tennis stroke or baseball pitch. Plyometric exercise and eccentric strengthening are important activities to prepare the athlete for the muscular demands necessary for most overhead sports. Plyometric exercise can include the use of medicine balls that are thrown and caught in various planes.

LONG THORACIC NERVE INJURIES

The serratus anterior is essential for the stabilization of the scapula and for normal shoulder girdle function. Chapter 3 discusses the anatomy of the nerve on pages 42-43. Injury to the long thoracic nerve has been reported in various sports including tennis, racquet sports, football, hockey, weightlifting, wrestling, and basketball (Mendoza and Main 1990). The long thoracic nerve is commonly involved in acute brachial neuritis and should be suspected in athletes without any acute or repetitive type injury. Fortunately, the prognosis is good in most individuals.

Injury to the long thoracic nerve results in weakness of the serratus anterior and medial winging of the scapula. Depending on the degree of scapular winging, normal shoulder motion is impaired. Complete loss of serratus anterior function usually leads to impairment of forward flexion and abduction beyond 90 degrees, resulting in significant functional loss (particularly in the overhead athlete). Some patients are able to compensate using the trapezius muscle in substitution. In addition, patients often complain of burning and aching pain about the shoulder, and secondary rotator cuff impingement often occurs.

Johnson and Kendall (1955) reported a good response to nonoperative treatment in 111 patients with long thoracic neuropathy. The goal of treatment is to prevent stretching of the serratus muscle and prevent contracture of other muscles, while facilitating neurologic recovery. Overstretching of the serratus results in an altered length-tension relationship, reducing the force that can be generated by an already weakened muscle. Proper positioning of the shoulder and arm is the key to preventing this problem. Various braces have been designed to maintain the scapula in proper position (Truong 1979). Manual stabilization, however, is probably the most reliable way of maintaining proper scapula positioning. Marin (1988) described a new brace for the management of scapular winging from long thoracic nerve injury. He felt that this brace provided proprioceptive feedback to remind patients to avoid active forward flexion, and that the brace

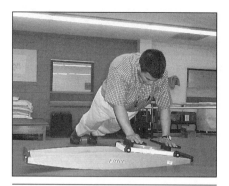

Figure 8.13 With the athlete's hands placed on the rolling track, he can move the sled from side to side. This provides dynamic scapula stabilization exercises in the transverse plane. This exercise can be modified to incorporate the vertical plane by turning the rolling track 90 degrees. This technique can be made easier by having the athlete perform the exercise while on his knees.

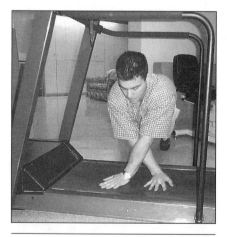

Figure 8.14 If a rolling track is not available, a treadmill can be used to provide dynamic scapula stabilization. The athlete can "walk" his hands along the treadmill belt. The belt can also be modified to a vertical plane, and the exercise can be made easier by having the athlete perform it while on his knees.

transferred contralateral shoulder protraction force to the affected scapula. Patients reported decreased pain and increased shoulder flexion strength with this brace. This brace may be helpful during the pain control and muscle reeducation phases of treatment. Results from using this brace have not been documented. Taping may also help provide cutaneous feedback and enhance proprioceptive training.

In addition to bracing and taping, treatment should include stretching of the rhomboids and pectoralis muscles that tend to tighten with this condition. The use of electrical muscle stimulation should be considered in severe cases. The athlete should be instructed to avoid activities of the involved shoulder until full shoulder motion is achieved and scapulothoracic motion has normalized. Isolated strengthening of the serratus should begin as normal motion is restored and scapula winging resolves. Serratus strengthening commonly requires some form of biofeedback, with either taping techniques or hands-on feedback from a physical therapist. The athlete must be reeducated to appropriately fire the serratus in various planes of shoulder motion. Once athletes have demonstrated appropriate activation of the serratus and the other scapulothoracic muscles at low loads, they can progress gradually to heavier upper-extremity resistive training. As always, the strengthening should include eccentric, plyometric, and functional training. Figures 8.13 and 8.14 illustrate some advanced scapula stabilization training techniques.

SUPRASCAPULAR NERVE INJURIES

The suprascapular nerve may be injured from acute trauma (such as after shoulder dislocation), from stretching in overuse injuries (such as volleyball players and baseball pitchers experience), and, at times, without any clear inciting etiology. Injuries can occur at the origin of the suprascapular nerve (from the upper trunk) following a fall and traction to the nerve. There can be entrapment and injury at the suprascapular notch, resulting in dysfunction of both the supraspinatus and infraspinatus, or there can be entrapment at the spinoglenoid notch that spares the supraspinatus. Chapter 3 discusses the anatomy and diagnosis of suprascapular neuropathy on pages 45-47.

Once the diagnosis of suprascapular neuropathy has been made and localized, the treatment will depend on the etiology of the nerve dysfunction. Cysts and other anatomic causes for compression should be surgically addressed before rehabilitation is instituted. For injuries from repetitive traction and compression, nonoperative treatment is highly successful. The mainstay of treatment begins with determining and correcting the biomechanical cause for traction on the nerve. Suprascapular nerve traction often occurs in overhead athletes with weakness of the scapular stabilizers, which can cause lateral and medial winging of the scapula. As this type of athlete cocks the shoulder back prior to the acceleration phase (e.g., in preparing for a volleyball serve), it has been theorized that there is excess tracking of the scapula, resulting in traction of the suprascapular nerve by the abnormal positioning of the scapula. Treatment therefore centers on strengthening the scapular stabilizers, which are key in maintaining a stable scapula for proper functioning of the rotator cuff and in limiting traction on the suprascapular nerve. The rotator cuff muscles, which weaken secondary to the nerve injury and from impingement from secondary instability, also need to be strengthened. The teres minor, which is innervated by the axillary nerve, assists the infraspinatus with external glenohumeral rotation and can be trained to compensate for loss of infraspinatus function. Stretching the pectoralis muscles and posterior shoulder capsule is important in restoring a balanced shoulder. Strengthening the shoulder should be gradual, beginning with isotonic and progressing to eccentric and plyometric activities. Overhead activities are avoided until there is no pain, full motion, normal scapulothoracic rhythm, and symmetric strength.

The biomechanics of overhead athletes must be critically examined. These athletes should generate a significant amount of force from their trunks and lower extremities. Weakness in these proximal muscles leads to great stress on the distal and smaller muscles of the shoulder girdle and arm. Many sports also require adequate rotation at the hip joint for proper force output. Restriction in motion results in altered motion at other joints along the kinetic chain, whereby the trunk rotates too early and causes the shoulder to lag behind the trunk. This causal chain is seen, for example, in a pitcher whose loss of hip rotation causes him to "open up too soon." It is imperative that a rehabilitation program addresses the entire kinetic chain from the ground up.

CONCLUSION

While the rehabilitation of upper-body peripheral nerve injuries can be challenging, a step-wise approach to treatment can maximize the outcome in patients with these injuries. Localizing the site of the injury is important, as is understanding what factors caused the injury in the first place. Reducing further compression or other trauma to the nerve is the first step in rehabilitation. Following this, modalities, splinting, and stretching and strengthening exercises can all be helpful in the rehabilitation process. The majority of these problems can be successfully treated without surgery.

REFERENCES

Banta CA. A prospective, nonrandomized study of iontophoresis, wrist splinting, and antiinflammatory medication in the treatment of early-mild carpal tunnel syndrome. J Occ Med 1994; 36(2): 166-168.

Basset FH, Nunley JA. Compression of the musculocutaneous nerve at the elbow. J Bone Joint Surg 1982; 64A: 1050-1052.

Bateman JE. Nerve injuries about the shoulder in sports. J Bone Joint Surg 1967; 49A: 785-792.

Bennett GE. Shoulder and elbow lesions of the professional baseball pitcher. JAMA 1941; 117: 510-514.

Blom S, Dahlback LO. Nerve injuries in dislocations of the shoulder joint and fractures of the neck of the humerus. Acta Chir Scand 1970; 136: 461-466.

Braddom R. Musculocutaneous nerve injury after heavy exercise. Arch Phys Med Rehabil 1978; 59: 290.

Cahill BR, Palmer RE. Quadrilateral space syndrome. J Hand Surg 1983; 8: 65-69.

Dellon AL, Mackinnon SE. Radial sensory nerve entrapment in the forearm. J Hand Surg 1996; 11A: 199-205.

Eversmann WW. Entrapment and compression neuropathies. In: Green DP (ed.) *Operative Hand Surgery*, 2nd edition. New York: Churchill Livingstone; 1988: 1430-1440.

Felsenthal G, Mondell DL, Reischer MA, Mack RH. Forearm pain secondary to compression syndrome of the lateral cutaneous nerve of the forearm. Arch Phys Med Rehab 1984; 65: 139-141.

Gelberman RH, Hergenroeder PT, Hargens AR, Lundborg GN, Akeson WH. The carpal tunnel syndrome: a study of carpal canal pressures. J Bone Joint Surg 1981; 36A: 380.

Gelberman RH, Aroson D ,Weismann MH. Carpal tunnel syndrome—results of a prospective trial of steroid injection and splinting. J Bone Joint Surg 1980; 62A: 1181-1184.

Giannini F, Passero S, Cioni R, Paradiso C, Battistini N, Giordano N, Vaccai D, Marcolongo R. Electrophysiologic evaluation of local steroid injection in carpal tunnel syndrome. Arch Phys Med Rehabil 1991; 72: 738-742.

Green DP. Diagnostic and therapeutic value of carpal tunnel injection. J Hand Surg 1990; 15B: 243-248.

Herbison GJ, Teng C, Gordon EE. Electrical stimulation of reinnervating rat muscle. Arch Phys Med Rehabil 1973; 54(4): 156-160.

Johnson JT, Kendall HO. Isolated paralysis of the serratus anterior muscle. J Bone Joint Surg 1955 ; 37A: 567-574.

Kaplan SJ, Glickel SZ, Eaton RG. Predictive factors in the nonsurgical treatment of carpal tunnel syndrome. J Hand Surg 1984; 9A: 850-854.

Kruger VL, Kraft GH, Deitz JC, Ameis A. Carpal tunnel syndrome: objective measure and splint use. Arch Phys Med Rehab 1991; 72: 517-520.

Macnicol MF. Extraneural pressures affecting the ulnar nerve at the elbow. Hand 1982; 14: 5-11.

Marin R. Scapula winger's brace: a case series on the management of long thoracic nerve palsy. Arch Phys Med Rehabil 1988; 79: 1226-1230.

Mendoza FX, Main K. Peripheral nerve injures of the shoulder in the athlete. Clin Sports Med 1990; 9(2): 331-342.

Politis MJ, Zanakis MF, Albala BJ. Facilitated regeneration in the rat peripheral nervous system using applied electric fields. J Trauma 1988; 28(9): 1375-1381.

Serror PJ. Treatment of ulnar nerve palsy at the elbow with a night splint. J Bone Joint Surg 1993; 75B(2): 322-327.

Slater RR, Bynum DK. Diagnosis and treatment of carpal tunnel syndrome. Orthopedic Review 1993; 22: 1095-1105.

Spinner M. The anterior interosseous nerve syndrome with special attention to its variation. J Bone Joint Surg 1970; 52A: 84-94.

Truong AB. Orthotic devices for serratus anterior palsy: some biochemical considerations. Arch Phys Med Rehabil 1979; 60: 66-69.

Vanderpool SW, Chalmers J, Lamb DW, Whiston TB. Peripheral compression lesions of the ulnar nerve. J Bone Joint Surg 1968; 50B: 792-803.

Weinstein SM, Herring SA. Nerve problems and compartment syndromes in the hand, wrist, and forearm. Clin Sports Med 1992; 11(1): 161-188.

9
Rehabilitation in Radiculopathies and Lower-Extremity Peripheral Nerve Injuries

Brian A. Davis, MD, FACSM, FABPMR

Peripheral nerve injury can be devastating to athletic performance, as there may be loss to muscle strength, proprioception, or cutaneous sensation. The principles of upper-extremity rehabilitation differ from those for the lower extremity, as lower limbs do not require the fine coordination skills of the upper. As a general rule, moreover, mild to moderate nociceptive perception impairment of the lower extremity is not as critical for athletic participation as it may be for the upper extremity. The lower extremity is the focus of balance for the trunk and acts as the ultimate platform upon which the upper extremity functions. This allows for greater focus on overall strength and limb awareness. This chapter discusses appropriate rehabilitation and use of orthoses in situations where joint proprioception is significantly impaired, the deficits caused by muscle denervation, the biomechanical abnormalities associated with specific lower-extremity nerve injuries, and the resultant strength expected after rehabilitation. Note that any of the lower-extremity nerve injuries described in this chapter may cause paresthesia, hypesthesia, or dysesthesia—conditions that can interfere with athletic function and that should be addressed using approaches described in chapter 7.

RADICULOPATHY

Radiculopathy affecting lumbar or sacral nerve roots accounts for the majority of lower-extremity peripheral nerve injuries among athletes. Although the causes of radiculopathies are similar for lumbar and sacral roots, approaches to rehabilitation can differ. Treatment can be markedly different for an L5 than for an S1 radiculopathy. Moreover, one athlete with an L5 radiculopathy may present very differently (in terms of muscles affected and degree of involvement) from the way another athlete presents with a radiculopathy at the same level. The rehabilitation programs and recommendations for compensatory techniques, taping, or bracing will also vary based upon the individual deficits.

Disc Herniation

Disc herniation is the most common cause of lumbar radiculopathies in young athletes. Recommended treatment varies for acute disc herniations and associated radiculopathies (Saal and Saal 1989, Saal et al. 1990, Weber 1983). Control of herniation-associated inflammation remains controversial, but many physicians treat athletes with anti-inflammatory doses of NSAIDs or with brief doses of steroids (e.g., methylprednisolone in a Medrol Dose Pack; or perhaps 60 mg prednisone for three days, with 10-mg taper daily for a total of eight days of treatment). As of 1999, corticosteroid preparations for medical treatment, taken by mouth, were banned by the United States Olympic Committee and the International Olympic Committee, but not by the National Collegiate Athletic Association (Fuentes and Rosenberg 1999). Epidural or selective nerve root steroid injections are playing a greater role in both acute and chronic management and should be considered in recalcitrant cases or when athletes cannot actively participate in a therapy program. For a discussion of selected spinal injection procedures, see chapter 5 (pages 91-95). Epidural and selective nerve root injections are not banned by the organizations named above.

Some authorities advocate three days of bed rest (Deyo et al. 1986), while others suggest active exercise programs with adequate pain control. R.A. McKenzie (1981) has developed a treatment technique known as *centralization*. Radiculopathy treatment by centralization attempts to reduce disc pressures and decrease radiation of symptoms into the buttock or extremity. Literature remains variable as to its success, but this author has found the program exceptionally useful in clinical practice. Determination of centralization appears to be reliable regardless of a clinician's level of training in physical therapy (Fritz et al. 2000). Evidence suggests that individuals who can centralize pain have a higher self-reported functional outcome (Sufka et al. 1998) than those who cannot; they also are less likely to require surgical intervention (Donelson et al. 1991, 1997) and are more likely to return to work (Karas et al. 1997). These data were not obtained in athletes, but one would expect a similar pattern in athletic populations. It has been this author's experience that those who can centralize pain are also more likely than others to respond positively to epidural steroid injections and discectomy when these are required. After athletes learn how to centralize pain, they can begin advancing to other exercises that reduce disc pressures and provide stabilization. To learn more about centralization, study McKenzie's 1981 publication (see *For Further Reading on . . .*, page 209).

> **centralization**—A treatment technique that the examiner uses to determine what lumbar positions reduce leg pain (i.e., "centralize" the pain to the lumbar or gluteal regions). Activities are initiated in this position of centralization to reduce disc pressures and nerve irritability.

Most patients with disc herniations and associated radiculopathies display flexion-biased pain and usually respond to extension-biased exercise programs (McKenzie 1981) that include prone-on-elbow and press-up (patient lies prone and performs trunk extension) exercises. Some athletes with disc herniations have pain upon extension and need to modify their programs to add flexion or more neutral-biased exercises before advancing to more advanced techniques. Postural exercises are of critical importance for athletes with disc-related disorders, as abnormal postures are known to increase disc pressures (Nachemson 1981).

Athletes often display tightness of muscle groups surrounding the hip region and lumbosacral junction. Muscles that may exhibit reduced flexibility include the iliopsoas, hamstrings, rectus femoris, gluteal/erector spinae muscles, and tensor fascia lata/iliotibial band. Although the etiology of the inflexibility is unclear, it is known that reduced flexibility and relative weakness lead to alteration of the lumbo-sacro-femoral angle and subsequent changes of the associated spine mechanics. As the lower extremity is in the stance phase, tight muscles inserting into the femur (or tibia) may act on the pelvis or lumbar region by a reversed origin-insertion (i.e., closed-chain) action. Moreover, if a muscle is tight, it is not at optimum length prior to contraction, making it functionally weaker. This weakness has the greatest impact during ballistic and plyometric muscle activation, since the relative or absolute decrease in muscle strength may lead to activation of other muscles not normally required for a task. Abnormal muscle substitution patterns can result, leading to further injury. Additionally, a muscle's inability to stretch to its fullest extent may lead to decreased joint range of motion and subsequent need for some other joint or area to account for the needed motion. In the case of the lumbar spine, increased motion may be transferred to the discs, *facet joints*, or other structural components of the spine, creating abnormally high stresses. These stresses can prevent healing of injured discs and lead to further injury at other disc levels.

Therapy programs for disc herniation eventually should be advanced to include *stabilization exercises* (McKenzie 1981), which help provide normal spine mechanics during all sports and required daily activities. It is important to remember how intimately the pelvis is associated with lumbar spine mechanics. Athletes cannot achieve proper spine stabilization without pelvic stabilization and proper lumbosacral pelvic rhythm. Techniques used to stabilize the spine include performing leg extension or arm elevation from a quadriped position, and later performing simultaneous arm elevation and contralateral leg extension (White et al. 1990). Other exercises include using a ball under the athlete's abdomen while performing the same or similar tasks.

> **stabilization exercise**—One that places the injured spine area into the most balanced position (usually neutral) while maintaining that position through the use of muscular contraction. These exercises are advanced from basic to advanced activities while maintaining the spine in a balanced, anatomic pain-free state.

For Further Reading on . . .

Disc Herniation

McKenzie RA. In: McKenzie RA (ed.), *The lumbar spine: mechanical diagnosis and therapy*. Waikanae, New Zealand: Spinal Publications, 1981.

Norris CM. *Back stability*. Champaign, IL: Human Kinetics, 2000.

White AH, McKenzie R, Paris SV, Stein D, Floman Y, and Mayer TG. Rehabilitation. In: Weinstein JN and Wiesel SW (eds.), *The lumbar spine*. Philadelphia: Saunders, 1990:772-779.

Stenosis and Apophyseal Lesions

As with most degenerative conditions, the risk of stenosis increases with age. Stenosis of the neuroforamen or the central canal can cause radiculopathy in older athletes, who almost universally exhibit lumbosacro-femoral inflexibility. The lack of flexibility forces individuals into abnormal postures (usually with the hips flexed) and subsequently into aberrant placement of the body's center of gravity during upright activities.

Compensatory lumbar spine extension can lead to overload and hypertrophy of facet joints, thus increasing compression on the exiting nerve root within the intervertebral foramen and leading to radiculopathy. Such people typically display almost rigid lumbar spines and usually present with significant limitations of extension. Flexibility exercises should target the iliopsoas, hamstrings, rectus femoris, and gluteal/erector spinae muscles, as well as the tensor fascia lata/iliotibial band. Stretching these muscles and the underlying soft-tissue structures can allow for greater motion within the spine and possibly increase the relative size of the neuroforamina. Once the athlete's flexibility is improved, stabilization exercises should help maintain the spine mechanics to prevent future compression episodes. Approaches to pain control should be chosen on an individual basis, as should consideration of epidural or selective nerve root steroid injections for recalcitrant cases.

Posterior limbus vertebrae (posterior lumbar apophyseal lesions) may also cause radiculopathy or cauda equina syndrome and may occur as a result of trauma or vigorous physical exercise. Baba and colleagues (1996) observed that these lesions were present mostly in younger gymnasts. The L4-L5 level was the most frequently involved by this lesion, with the L3-L4 level being the next most likely involved. Limbus vertebrae lesions at the L5-S1 level occurred in only 3 of 29 patients.

Specific Radiculopathies

The consequences and treatment of specific radiculopathies are discussed below. Treatment of lumbar radiculopathies needs to be individualized to each athlete depending upon the degree of involvement to major muscle groups and the witnessed dysfunction. This section will discuss the possible consequences of the lumbar radiculopathies and treatments geared toward these deficits.

L2 and L3 Radiculopathies

The L2 and L3 nerve roots form a portion of the femoral and obturator nerves and provide a share of the innervation for the spine/hip flexors, knee extensors, and adductors. Via the obturator, femoral, and accessory obturator nerves, the L2 and L3 nerve roots supply innervation to the hip joints (Crafts 1985, O'Rahilly 1986b, Wertheimer 1952); and via the femoral (Gardner 1948) and saphenous nerves, they supply the knee joints. The obturator nerve (Kennedy et al. 1982) may provide a variable degree of innervation to the knee with L3 fibers. The iliopsoas and rectus femoris appear to be quite active during the hip flexion component of early swing phase during running (Montgomery et al. 1994). Significant loss of strength of the hip flexors and adductors can lead to gait abnormalities throughout the gait cycle, especially with loss of adductor function (discussed later in this chapter, pages 225-226).

Hip and Quadriceps Strengthening Exercises

Hip flexor losses may lead to excessive lumbar flexion at initial contact during ambulation and running as compensation for this weakness. In most cases, athletes should be able to re-strengthen either the iliopsoas or adductor group sufficiently to compensate and ultimately provide normal or near-normal function. Focused strengthening of the hip flexors can be performed using Therabands or similar elastic strengthening devices. The athlete is seated with the knee flexed to 90 degrees and places the Theraband around the distal upper leg. The band is held under the opposite foot, while hip flexion is performed against resistance (figure 9.1). The iliopsoas may also be strengthened to a lesser degree through straight-leg raises with increasing weight as tolerated. While adductor group strengthening will occur simultaneously to some degree, more directed exercises are necessary. Adductor muscles can be strengthened by performing short-arc (end-range) squat exercises with a ball between the knees. Limiting the squat to the first 45-60 degrees of flexion (end range) usually reduces the potential for patellofemoral joint irritation. Adductor strengthening may also be achieved by performing leg adduction from a modified side-lying position against Theraband resistance, or by adding weights as tolerated (figure 9.2). Adduction strength training is also easily performed with progressive resistance equipment.

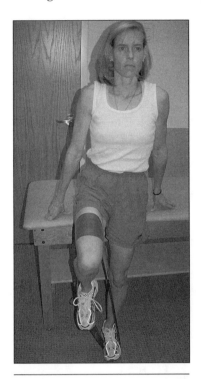

Figure 9.1 Strengthening hip flexors using a Theraband. The athlete holds the band under the opposite foot and flexes the hip against the resistance.

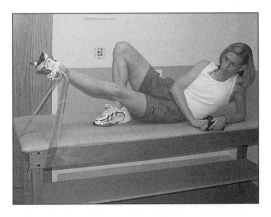

Figure 9.2 Strengthening hip adductors using a Theraband. The athlete lies on her side and adducts against the resistance.

The quadriceps group is quite active during the terminal swing phase and the initial contact and loading phase of stance during running (Montgomery et al. 1994) and ambulation. Quadriceps weakness may result in a gait deviation with *genu recurvatum*. When recurvatum is present, the individual increases knee extension during stance phase by maximally contracting the hamstring and gluteus maximus muscles against the femur/tibia complex. This can result in significant weakening of the posterior capsular structures and the medial collateral ligament if the individual uses external hip rotation to compensate for the weak stabilizers of knee extension. Quadriceps weakness also predisposes athletes to patellofemoral pain, and appropriate precautions should be instituted. Strengthening is accomplished with resistive straight-leg raises (figure 9.3) or by increasing weight as tolerated. Strengthening can also be performed via cycling exercises, leg press exercises, short-arc squats, and terminal end-range knee-extension exercises. Athletes with severe weakness or buckling of the knee are not likely to regain adequate knee stability and control through taping or the use of neoprene sleeves. Taping the knee or using a light neoprene sleeve may assist the athlete with mild strength deficits, however, by providing greater proprioceptive control. Braces capable of preventing hyperextension and buckling are available, but this degree of weakness usually prevents able-bodied competitive sports participation.

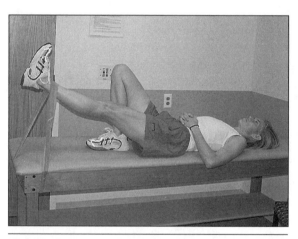

Figure 9.3 Strengthening quadriceps muscles with resistive straight-leg raises using a Theraband. The athlete lies supine and performs a straight-leg raise against the Theraband resistance.

Proprioceptive Enhancement Exercises

L2 or L3 injuries may result in decreased hip or knee joint proprioception. In the case of hip involvement, the athlete can enhance neurosensory input from the affected hip joint, the contralateral hip joint, and the ipsilateral foot, ankle, and knee joints and their associated muscles. Increasing sensory feedback from the ipsilateral hip, ankle, and foot joints could enhance knee joint proprioception. Athletes may begin proprioception training by standing on the contralateral leg, with toe-touch weightbearing of the affected leg. They gradually bear greater amounts of weight through

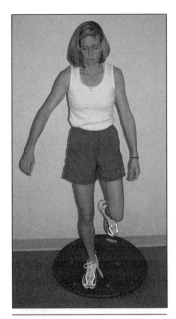

Figure 9.4 Using a BAPS board to enhance hip and knee joint proprioception. Difficulty is increased by changing the balance platform size, closing the eyes, or using the upper extremities.

the affected leg and remove weightbearing from the contralateral leg. Athletes also can use a movable platform—such as a biomechanical ankle platform system (BAPS board) or minitrampoline—with varying degrees of difficulty and changes of task, while trying to maintain balance (figure 9.4). A Pro-Fitter can also be used as a type of movable platform to increase proprioception for the entire lower extremity, either with one or both legs on the platform, by varying tasks while trying to maintain balance (figure 9.5, a-b). Once athletes master these tasks, they can begin hopping on a flat surface, then on a varied one. More advanced activities require the athletes to utilize only peripheral sensory perception and can be facilitated by having the athletes close their eyes and attempt to perform tasks similar to those just described. Caution should be taken not to advance athletes to more advanced proprioceptive exercises before they have mastered simpler tasks. Taping the hip joint to improve proprioception may help in some cases, but it is

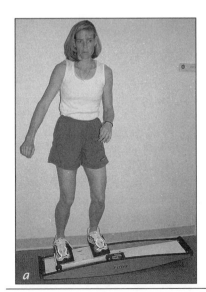

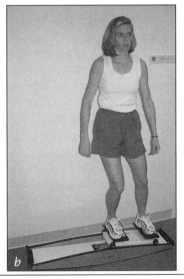

Figure 9.5 *(a-b)* Using a Pro-Fitter to enhance proprioception, stabilize muscles, mobilize joints, and increase strength in the lower extremities.

often too cumbersome and can limit performance. The knee, in contrast, is quite amenable to taping or bracing. Taping, elastic wraps, or neoprene sleeves may improve central awareness by substituting cutaneous feedback for the lost joint receptor input.

L4 Radiculopathy

L4 nerve root injuries occur slightly more often than those at the L2 or L3 levels, but are still uncommon (Borenstein et al. 1995, Spangfort 1972). Injury usually occurs in association with disc herniation or spinal stenosis. The L4 nerve root forms a portion of the femoral, obturator, superior gluteal, tibial, and common peroneal nerves. The L4 nerve root provides innervation for hip adduction, knee extension, and ankle dorsiflexion. Hip flexion, abduction, and external rotation, as well as long toe extension, receive a small degree of L4 nerve root supply. L4 nerve root fibers from either the femoral, superior gluteal, obturator, or accessory obturator nerves may supply the hip joint (Crafts 1985, O'Rahilly 1986b, Wertheimer 1952) and probably supply the knee joint via the femoral (Gardner 1948) and saphenous nerves. The obturator and common peroneal nerves may provide a variable degree of innervation to the knee joint (Kennedy et al. 1982, O'Rahilly 1986b).

The ankle joint may also receive L4 nerve supply through either the tibial, deep peroneal, or saphenous nerves (Champetier 1970, Gardner and Gray 1968). Feuerbach et al. (1994) conducted a study in which they anesthetized the anterior talofibular and calcaneofibular ligaments. They asked athletes to reproduce reference positions with and without anesthesia. Anesthetized athletes performed as well as controls, suggesting that sensory information from these ligaments is of little importance in providing ankle joint proprioception. Their study, however, used limited numbers of subjects, did not adequately demonstrate anesthesia of the ligaments, and did not account for the afferent information supplied by the remaining intact capsular and ligamentous structures (posterior talofibular ligament, anterior tibiofibular ligament, and posterior tibiofibular ligaments).

L4 nerve root injury may affect the strength and function of any of the muscle groups listed above. When dysfunction does occur, the strengthening program should be similar to those for an L2-L3 radiculopathy, but it also must address weakness in the tibialis anterior (see the following section).

L5 Radiculopathy

L5 nerve root injuries are quite common (Spangfort 1972). They are frequently a result of disc herniation at the L4-L5 level (Borenstein et al. 1995) or develop in association with spinal stenosis; they also have been commonly documented with pelvic fractures (Huittenen 1972, Huittinen and Slätis 1972). The L5 nerve root forms a portion of the superior gluteal, inferior gluteal, tibial, and common peroneal nerves; it also provides a significant share of innervation for hip abduction, hip extension, hip external rotation, knee flexion, ankle inversion, ankle eversion, toe flexion, and toe extension. The most significant clinical deficits, however, are seen in the ankle dorsiflexors. To a variable degree, the L5 root assists ankle plantarflexion and foot intrinsic musculature. Injuries to the L5 nerve root can significantly affect lower-extremity athletic function, with even moderate levels of muscular denervation preventing elite or subelite competition.

L5 nerve root fibers may supply the hip joint (Crafts 1985, O'Rahilly 1986b, Wertheimer 1952) and to a lesser extent the knee and ankle joint (Champetier 1970, Gardner and Gray 1968). L5 fibers may also provide information to the tarsal and metatarsal joints. Potential loss of proprioception of these joints should be addressed.

Anterior Tibialis Strengthening Exercises

The anterior tibialis has both L4 and L5 nerve root supply, but management of its weakness is discussed in this section because it is primarily an L5-innervated muscle. Results of damage to the L5 nerve root can range from mild weakness to a complete foot drop. Such damage mostly affects athletes during the stance phase at the time of initial foot contact, when the anterior tibialis is eccentrically activating to slow descent of the foot. Weakness of the anterior tibialis may lead to varying degrees of "foot slap," named for the sound made when the foot "slaps" the ground secondary to decreased eccentric control of the foot at initial contact. Athletes can easily learn and perform relevant Theraband strengthening exercises: The Theraband is wrapped around the dorsum of the weak foot, and the athlete dorsiflexes against the resistance of the band (figure 9.6). Initially, performing fatiguing exercises with a 10-15 repetition maximum will improve general strength. Increasing the number of repetitions (up to 30-50) with a lighter-strength band may also improve endurance of the anterior tibialis. The toe extensors can also be strengthened by performing toe dorsiflexion against the resistance of a very light Theraband.

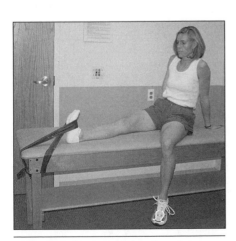

Figure 9.6 Strengthening the anterior tibialis by use of a Theraband. The athlete dorsiflexes against a band wrapped around the dorsum of the foot.

Mild ankle dorsiflexor weakness will usually be well controlled with a RocketSoc® or Swede-O® type of ankle-foot orthosis (AFO). These

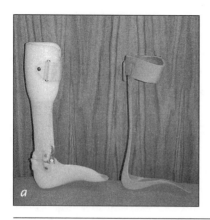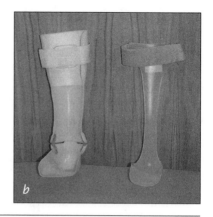

Figure 9.7 *(Left in a and b)* Hinged ankle-foot orthosis is used for more severe injuries than the *(right in a and b)* thinner posterior leaf spring orthosis.

devices are made from neoprene or canvas and are adjustable, but provide less dorsiflexion support than plastic or metal upright AFOs (figure 9.7, a-b). Athletes with adapted needs frequently use plastic or metal upright AFOs for recreational or competitive activities. Bracing and stretching should be initiated as early as possible to avoid overstretch of weak dorsiflexors by the more powerful plantarflexors (Berger and Schaumburg 1988). Taping may assist weak dorsiflexors, but the loss of support can occur within a fairly short period of time (Greene and Hillman 1990, Manfroy et al. 1997).

Semitendinosus and Semimembranosus Strengthening Exercises

The semitendinosus and semimembranosus muscles eccentrically activate during the initial contact of stance phase to prevent excessive hip/trunk flexion (Montgomery et al. 1994). Weakness in these muscles can lead to a gait characterized by excessive extension just prior to and inclusive of the initial contact. The gluteus maximus and biceps femoris muscles simultaneously resist hip flexion and may be able to compensate for significantly weakened semitendinosus and semimembranosus muscles. The hamstring muscles are also strong knee flexors and activate concentrically to flex the knee at lift-off. If knee flexion is affected by semitendinosus or semimembranosus weakness, gait may reveal a "hiking," that is, elevation of the hip to allow for limb clearance during the swing phase. Circumduction, or swinging the leg around to clear the limb, is another possible gait compensation seen with hamstring weakness.

The semitendinosus and semimembranosus are strengthened by targeting hip extension or knee flexion. Athletes strengthen hip extension muscles much as they do the hip abductors (see next section), except that

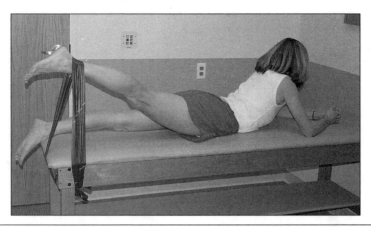

Figure 9.8 Strengthening hip extensors using a Theraband. The athlete lies prone and extends the hip against the resistance of the band and gravity.

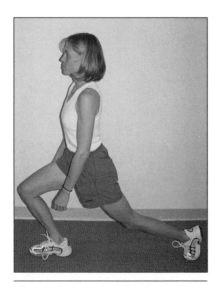

Figure 9.9 Using lunge exercise to strengthen hip extensor and knee flexor components of the hamstring muscles.

they lie prone and extend the hip against a Theraband or weight resistance and gravity (figure 9.8). Strengthening hip extensors using exercise machines while standing may require large weights to cause fatigue. Lunge exercises, with or without weights, can also strengthen both the hip extensor and knee flexor components of the hamstring muscles (figure 9.9). Hip extensor exercises also strengthen the gluteus maximus and biceps femoris muscles. "Stool walking" is a good exercise for strengthening the knee flexor component of the hamstrings. Here the athlete sits on a wheeled stool with the knees flexed to around 70-90 degrees. The athlete "walks" around, pulling her own weight (figure 9.10, a-b). Weight can be added onto a sled that the athlete pulls or can be held by the athlete during the exercise. Stool walking can also improve ankle and knee proprioception, which an L5 radiculopathy is likely to impair. The biceps femoris and gastrocnemius muscles can also be strengthened during knee flexion exercises and may be able to partially compensate for the weakened semimembranosus and semitendinosus muscles.

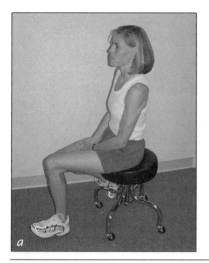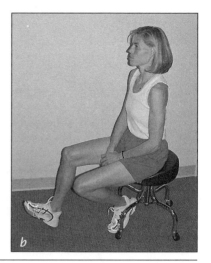

Figure 9.10 *(a-b)* "Stool walking" to strengthen the knee flexor component of the hamstring muscles.

Hip Abductor Strengthening Exercises

The major hip abductors (tensor fascia lata and gluteus maximus, medius, and minimus) control contralateral pelvic drop during the stance phase. This action is very important for reducing energy expenditures during gait by limiting motion of the body's center of gravity (Saunders et al. 1953). This reduction is achieved through the hip abductors' literally pulling the upper pelvis downward toward the lateral femur during stance phase. As the hip abductors have significant L5 root innervation, they are prone to neurologic dysfunction with L5 radiculopathies. Weakness leads to poor control of contralateral pelvis descent and stabilization during stance phase, leading to either a compensated or uncompensated *Trendelenburg gait* (a.k.a. "gluteus medius lurch" or "abductor lurch"). In an uncompensated Trendelenburg gait, the free limb sags while the weak side is in the stance phase. The individual's weight is thrust medial of the hip joint, and the athlete appears almost to fall to the opposite side and then suddenly appears to catch himself. In a compensated gait, the individual vaults the pelvis laterally over the hip joint in an attempt to reduce the need for hip abduction. If weakness is bilateral, there is a waddling gait due to the bilateral vaulting. Mild weakness frequently goes unnoticed until the strength of specific isolated abductor muscles is tested. Functional weakness may also be identified by asking the athlete to stand on one leg and to try to squat to 30-45 degrees of knee flexion. He should be able to perform this task without pelvic tilt and without allowing hip internal rotation. Abductor weakness is addressed most often through

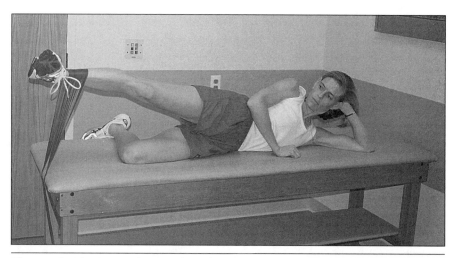

Figure 9.11 Strengthening hip abductors using a Theraband. The athlete lies on her side and abducts the hip against the resistance of the band and gravity.

Theraband or weight strengthening against resistance (figure 9.11). A hip machine (see figure 7.12 on page 161) is also frequently used for this purpose. Mild weakness may be tolerated by some athletes but can cause significant performance deficit in running athletes, pitchers (especially with *posting* leg weakness), and jumping athletes.

> **Trendelenburg gait**—Abnormal gait pattern that occurs when hip abduction weakness is present. The individual will either lean or vault to the side opposite hip weakness (uncompensated Trendelenburg gait) or to the side of hip weakness (compensated Trendelenburg gait).

> **posting**—Part of windup phase of pitching motion where the pitcher is stabilized on one limb.

Hip External Rotator Strengthening Exercises

The hip external rotators primarily receive L4, L5, and S1 innervation (gluteus minimus and medius) or L5, S1, and S2 innervation (gluteus maximus, piriformis, obturator externus, and the gemelli). Both of these groups are supplied mostly from the L5 and S1 roots, leaving the external rotators susceptible to weakness and dysfunction with L5 radiculopathies. Weakness of the hip rotators may go unnoticed by the clinician—but it may affect athletes during jumping or while posting (such as baseball pitchers require during a windup) and may cause a loss of force and control during any activity that requires hip stabilization. Athletes should strengthen the hip rotators by focusing on the extension, abduction, and rotation components of activation. Strengthening of hip extensors and abductors has already been discussed. Athletes can strengthen hip rotation by lying on their sides with knees and hips flexed to 90 degrees. They then externally rotate the hip against resistance with a Theraband or with an ankle weight. Strengthening can also be done by using a four-way hip machine, jumping on a miniature trampoline, or hopping.

Posterior Tibialis Strengthening Exercises

The posterior tibialis is a powerful invertor of the foot and also has weak plantarflexor capacity. It also acts eccentrically to slow calcaneal valgus (pronation/eversion) and foot pronation during the early and midstance phases of gait. During running, the posterior tibialis has strong muscle activity during midstance and is believed by some to be acting as an eccentric plantarflexor to slow dorsiflexion activity (Reber et al. 1993). The most important functional loss related to a weakened posterior tibialis is probably decreased foot arch control and subsequent excessive pronation. These failures can lead to excessive forces on the medial arch and osseous structures, resulting in stress fractures or lax spring (calcaneonavicular) ligaments. The decreased foot eversion strength can also lead to awkward mechanics and reduced efficiency during running activities.

Athletes can easily strengthen the posterior tibialis with Theraband exercises that focus on foot inversion (figure 9.12) and plantarflexion. Toe raises (figure 9.13) and cycling can strengthen the other plantarflexor and invertor muscles that have less reliance on L5 supply (gastrocnemius-soleus, flexor digitorum longus, and flexor hallucis longus). "Towel scrunches," in which the athlete slowly "scrunches up" a towel using the toe flexors, will also increase the strength and endurance of muscles with accessory inversion activity (figure 9.14, a-b). Picking up small weights with the toes may also improve short and long toe flexor strength. Medial arch control can be achieved through a full-length

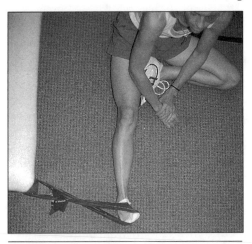

Figure 9.12 Strengthening the posterior tibialis through foot inversion exercises using a Theraband. The athlete inverts against the Theraband resistance.

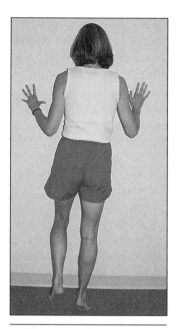

Figure 9.13 Using toe raises to strengthen the posterior tibialis and other plantar flexors.

semirigid orthosis posted in the forefoot to control excessive pronation; in less severe injuries, taping can support the arch. Severe invertor weakness may preclude activities that require running or walking.

Peronei Strengthening Exercises

The peronei are the primary foot evertors and have minimal plantarflexion (peroneus longus and brevis) or dorsiflexion (peroneus tertius) activity. Peroneus brevis, in particular, when measured by fine-wire electromyography, significantly increases its activity as running pace is quickened (Reber et al. 1993). The peronei act eccentrically to control calcaneal inversion (supination) during early stance phase, especially during the moments shortly after initial contact. Weakness of the peronei can cause excessive calcaneal varus and can lead to acute injury of either the anterior talofibular or calcaneofibular ligaments. Decreased eversion strength can also lead to an awkward gait that requires the athlete to compensate by increasing ankle valgus. This compensation leads to a dysfunctional gait for a running athlete and eventually to excessive lateral compressive forces on the fibula and ankle complex. The peronei

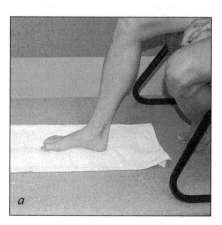 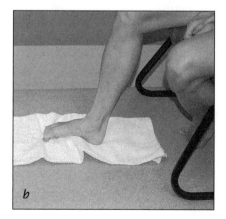

Figure 9.14 Using "towel scrunches" to strengthen accessory muscles used in inversion and arch control. *(a)* The athlete "scrunches" up a towel using her toes, *(b)* advancing along the length of the towel.

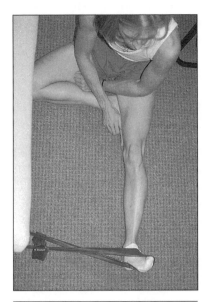

Figure 9.15 Strengthening foot evertors using a Theraband. The athlete everts the foot against the resistance of the Theraband.

can be strengthened by Theraband exercises that focus on eversion (figure 9.15). Strengthening plantarflexion will probably add little to peronei function, due to their weak activity as ankle plantarflexors. Taping or orthoses that place the ankle in a slightly everted position may be able to assist with mild weakness. Several commercial devices, such as the Swede-O or RocketSoc (figure 9.16, a-b) orthoses, can assist weak evertors with a piece of material on the lateral aspect that holds the lateral border of the foot more closely approximated to the lateral malleolus—that is, they increase calcaneal valgus. The Aircast® Airstir-up provides medial-lateral support for the ankle and may be able to prevent excessive eversion but does not increase calcaneal valgus to assist the peronei muscles. These

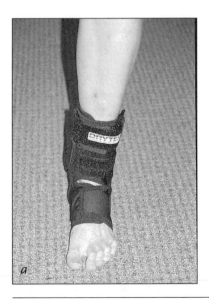

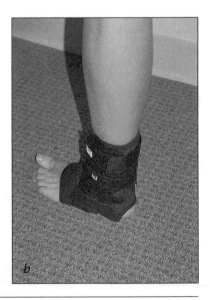

Figure 9.16 *(a-b)* A RocketSoc (ankle stabilizing orthosis) for assisting weak ankle evertors. Numerous devices are on the market to aid ankle evertor weakness. The RocketSoc aids the ankle evertors by utilizing eversion-assisting straps.

devices may also improve stability through proprioceptive actions. An orthosis incorporating a lateral flange into the rear foot may aid in proprioception and control in patients with lateral ligament injuries secondary to excessive calcaneal valgus. High-top basketball shoes do not appear to limit ankle inversion injuries in healthy athletes or in those with previous ankle sprains and are probably of no use to athletes with peronei weakness (Barrett et al. 1993).

S1 Radiculopathy

As with L5, injury to the S1 nerve root can cause significant disruption to athletic function if even moderate muscular weakness is present. The S1 nerve root provides innervation for all major muscle actions of the lower extremity and forms a portion of the superior gluteal, inferior gluteal, tibial, and common peroneal nerves. The S1 root may provide innervation to the hip via either the nerve to the quadratus femoris or the superior gluteal nerve (Crafts 1985, O'Rahilly 1986b, Wertheimer 1952). S1 fibers from either the tibial, sural, deep peroneal, or accessory deep peroneal nerves may supply the ankle joint (Champetier 1970, Gardner and Gray 1968). S1 fibers may also provide information to the tarsal and metatarsal joints through the medial plantar, lateral plantar, deep peroneal, or accessory deep peroneal nerves (Gardner and Gray 1968).

Of the muscles with S1 innervation, those most likely to be affected by an injury to the root include the semitendinosus, semimembranosus, peronei (longus, brevis, and tertius), posterior tibialis, gastrocnemius, soleus, and muscles of the foot (S1 and S2 innervation).

Weaknesses of the semitendinosus, semimembranosus, peronei, and posterior tibialis muscles have already been discussed. The gastrocnemius and soleus muscles are required primarily for the push-off that occurs in the late stance phase. They also provide most of the strength required for jumping and landing. During jumping, there is a concentric activation, and upon landing, these muscles act eccentrically to prevent excessive ankle dorsiflexion. Similarly, during running activities, the gastrocnemius and soleus appear to have their greatest activity during the midstance phase (Reber et al. 1993). Strengthening programs can begin with Theraband exercises and can be advanced to toe raises with weight partially unloaded. The strengthening program should increase in difficulty through full weightbearing toe raises and jumping activities. For individuals with mild weakness, a solid ankle cushion heel (SACH) may be added to force the foot into smooth plantarflexion at initial contact, and a rocker bar shoe modification can help provide a smooth push-off (Ragnarsson 1993).

The other muscles likely to become weak with an S1 injury are very important for ankle-foot mechanics. The intrinsic muscles of the foot are vital to the control of the foot throughout the early to late stance phases.

The quadratus plantae, in particular, maintains the arch of the foot during midfoot pronation and assists the plantar fascia in producing the *windlass mechanism* of the foot. Weakness of the posterior tibialis may lead to hyperpronation, and thereby to loss of arch and calcaneal varus control. Foot intrinsic strengthening with toe raises, towel scrunches, and picking up weights with the toes may help. Orthoses that support the medial arch may assist with medial arch control. Taping for the medial arch may be another alternative for decreased eccentric control but often needs to be reapplied frequently during activity, due to loss of tape strength.

> **windlass mechanism**—The action of the arch and plantar fascia on the bony structures of the foot as the foot moves from early into midstance phase. The bones of the tarsal and metatarsal region tighten in response to the arch's stresses, leading to a more stable midfoot and forefoot during these phases.

As with L5 injuries, when an S1 nerve injury is detected, the care provider should assume proprioceptive losses and initiate exercises for the entire lower extremity as soon as possible.

FEMORAL NEUROPATHY

Femoral neuropathy appears to be uncommon in sport activity (Feinberg et al. 1997) and occurs mostly in association with trauma or obstetrical complications (An et al. 1987, Susens et al. 1968, Winternitz et al. 1992). For more information on anatomy, signs, and symptoms of femoral neuropathy, and for specific case reports, see chapter 6 (pages 107-110). Femoral neuropathies high within the pelvis cause neurologic deficits of hip, knee, and thigh. They mostly affect hip flexion (due to the loss of the iliacus and rectus femoris muscles) and knee extension (due to the loss of the quadriceps muscles). Exercises that target the iliopsoas, rectus femoris, and the accessory hip flexors (such as the tensor fascia lata and adductors) should strengthen hip flexion weakness when it is mild. The athlete initially can perform hip flexion against Theraband resistance, advancing as appropriate to ankle weights and machine-based exercises. Adduction and abduction against resistance will help strengthen the adductors and tensor fascia lata, respectively. The loss of hip flexion supplied by the iliacus and rectus femoris can be only partially compensated for by the flexion capacity of the adductors and tensor fascia lata. Proprioception may be affected at the hip, knee, or ankle, through either the femoral nerve proper or the saphenous nerve, but losses typically are minimized by the multiple nerve supply to each of the lower-extremity joints.

If the femoral nerve supply to the iliacus is spared, the primary muscle loss will only be to knee extension; if any proprioceptive losses occur, they will affect only the knee and ankle joints, sparing the hip. When loss is minor, quadriceps strengthening can be done with the techniques described on pages 211-212. Other local muscle groups cannot adequately compensate for more severe extension deficits. Attempts can be made to strengthen the adductor group (supplied by the obturator and tibial nerves), which may have a muscular bundle investing into the vastus medialis (O'Rahilly 1986b). When the knee is already in extension, the tensor fascia lata (via the lateral retinaculum) may have some minor knee extension capacity, and attempts should be made to strengthen this muscle. Additionally, the gastrocnemius, by primarily acting as a flexor at the knee, may be able to act by a *reverse origin-insertion* mechanism to reduce excessive knee extension/recurvatum through eccentric activation. Similarly, the hamstrings (biceps femoris, semitendinosus, and semimembranosus) may be able to activate eccentrically in a reverse origin-insertion capacity to reduce excessive knee extension and recurvatum. As with injuries to the femoral nerve at higher levels, these injuries usually require a knee orthosis capable of preventing genu recurvatum. As with femoral nerve injuries above the hip, proprioceptive losses that occur with injuries below the hip are probably well tolerated due to compensation by other local peripheral nerves that supply the knee and ankle joints. Therefore, proprioceptive exercises targeting the affected lower extremity will probably allow for rapid return to baseline proprioceptive capacity.

> **reverse origin-insertion**—Muscular activation that occurs when the axis of rotation reverses to cause the muscular origin to move toward the point of muscular insertion.

OBTURATOR NEUROPATHY

The obturator nerve supplies the hip joint both directly and possibly through the accessory obturator nerve (when present), and to a variable degree, it supplies the knee joint (Bradshaw et al. 1997, Kennedy et al. 1982, O'Rahilly 1986b). The obturator nerve also provides cutaneous sensation to the medial thigh. Deficits resulting from obturator nerve damage will vary depending upon the degree of injury. The adductor group of muscles has four activities during gait:

1. Eccentric control of hip extension at terminal stance phase
2. Concentric initiation of swing phase

3. Concentric activation at initial contact, to advance the pelvis in relation to the limb in stance phase

4. Minor eccentric activation throughout stance phase, to prevent excessive hip abduction produced by the gluteus medius and minimus muscles

The adductor muscles significantly decrease energy expenditure of gait by limiting the motion of the body's center of gravity (Saunders et al. 1953). Weak or absent adductor activity leads to abnormal gait patterns characterized by a slinging forward of the limb and trunk to initiate swing phase, shortening of stance phase on the affected side, and/or a vaulting of the pelvis to initiate swing phase on the unaffected side. Compensation for loss of adductor activity is critical for lower-extremity function and for reducing energy expenditures.

Initiation of swing phase via combined adduction and flexion, however, is difficult to compensate for with obturator nerve injuries. The extensor/adductor portion of the adductor magnus supplied by the tibial nerve may provide some compensation and should be strengthened as described for hip adduction. The rectus femoris can advance the limb through concentric activation but adds a small moment of abduction to this action. Due to its insertion into the lesser trochanter, the iliopsoas can act as a weak adductor of the limb. The semitendinosus and semimembranosus have very weak adduction capacity in addition to their ability to flex the knee and extend the hip. The adduction component of the semitendinosus and semimembranosus muscles should also be strengthened as much as possible to try to compensate for the adduction loss. Proprioceptive losses are likely to be mild due to the significant overlap of innervation to the hip and knee joint from other local peripheral nerves, but they should be evaluated and treated with appropriate exercise protocols if losses are identified. Appropriate exercises are provided earlier in the chapter for addressing these proprioceptive losses, and chapter 7 includes an entire section on closed- and open-chain exercises; see also discussions of the use of minitrampolines, Pro-Fitters, and BAPS boards in this chapter (pages 212-214).

SUPERIOR GLUTEAL NEUROPATHY

The superior gluteal nerve, which has no cutaneous sensory innervation (O'Rahilly 1986a), supplies the gluteus medius, gluteus minimus, and the tensor fascia lata. It also supplies the hip joint. The primary function of the gluteus medius, gluteus minimus, and tensor fascia lata is to be active during the stance phase to prevent tipping of the pelvis and to allow for a fluid gait cycle. As with L5, and to a lesser extent, S1 radiculopathies, hip abductor weakness from a superior gluteal neuropathy may lead to a

Trendelenburg gait (compensated or uncompensated). Superior gluteal neuropathies are more likely than lumbosacral radiculopathies to lead to this gait deviation, due to the loss of nerve function to the only major hip abductors. In contrast to lumbosacral radiculopathies, the surrounding hip musculature should be unaffected with superior gluteal neuropathy—but strengthening programs will typically be of less benefit due to the lack of compensatory musculature. Attempts should still be made to strengthen the hip flexors (see page 211) and extensors (see page 212), since these muscles have minor hip abduction capacity (particularly when the hip is already in partial abduction). Proprioception should be addressed, tapping the capacity of other nerves that innervate the hip joint.

INFERIOR GLUTEAL NEUROPATHY

The inferior gluteal nerve supplies the gluteus maximus muscle, which is the major hip extensor. During initial contact in the gait cycle, the gluteus maximus prevents excessive hip flexion via an eccentric activation. The hip extensors are also responsible for eccentrically controlling hip flexion during swing phase. Injury to this muscle can lead to a type of gait known as a gluteal "lurch," characterized by excessive hip extension and lumbar lordosis at initial contact. Strengthening the hamstrings via Theraband exercises (see figure 9.8 on page 217), stool walking (see figure 9.10 on page 218), free weights, or a hip machine may compensate for mild gluteal weakness by helping the hamstrings to act as secondary hip extensors.

TIBIAL NEUROPATHY

The tibial component of the sciatic nerve supplies muscles responsible for hip extension and knee flexion, while the actual tibial nerve innervates the ankle plantarflexors, invertors, and all intrinsic foot musculature. A variable degree of proprioceptive information from the knee, ankle, and foot joints travels within the tibial nerve. Sensory fibers from the medial sural cutaneous branch combine with the peroneal communicating branch of the common peroneal nerve to form the sural nerve (Williams 1954).

Injury Above the Knee

The tibial component of the sciatic nerve can be injured by direct trauma to the posterior thigh or by compression due to tumor or *myositis ossificans*. Injury to the tibial nerve within the popliteal fossa has been documented with knee dislocations (Santi and Botte 1996). When the tibial nerve innervation to the hamstrings is spared, hip extension remains at full strength and knee flexion should be at normal or near-normal strength. Knee flexion strength may be diminished owing to the loss of the gastrocnemius muscle. As with injury at the hip, proprioception may be affected from the knee, ankle, or foot joints and should be addressed if present, taking advantage of multiple other innervating nerves to the joints of the leg (see pages 212-214).

Injury Below the Knee

Tibial nerve compression under the soleal arch, as well as other local traumatic events, can lead to impaired tibial nerve function to the distal lower leg and foot, sparing only the gastrocnemius and soleus muscles. Ankle dislocations or fractures can cause tibial disruption, sparing the plantarflexors and long toe flexors/inverters (Santi and Botte 1996). Proprioception in ankle and intertarsal joints may also be affected with tibial injury at this level and should be treated. Compression of the medial plantar nerve, lateral plantar nerve, or both can occur at the tarsal tunnel, resulting in various deficits of foot musculature strength and sensation (Mann 1994, Mondelli et al. 1998). Flexor tenosynovitis within the flexor retinaculum or local ankle degenerative changes can result in posterior tibial nerve compression (Schneck CD, personal communication 1997). Weakness of the foot intrinsic musculature may diminish stability and strength during the push-off phase of late stance. Medial arch control may also be affected during all phases of stance and can possibly lead to other clinical lower-extremity syndromes due to overload in this area.

Clinically significant tarsal tunnel syndrome probably occurs infrequently. Stretch techniques and ultrasound may be attempted to improve flexor retinaculum flexibility and reduce tibial nerve compression. Stretching for the long flexors is important when overuse is suspected as the cause for tenosynovitis. Strengthening should target the long toe flexors and the intrinsic foot musculature as much as possible (see pages 220-221). Correction of excessive pronation through use of orthoses (Jackson and Haglund 1991) may help people with this abnormality. Orthoses should maintain the medial arch, maintain the subtalar joint in neutral alignment, and control the forefoot as well. A rocker bar added to the sole of the shoe can assist weakened push-off. Radin (1983) noted that heel varus and forefoot pronation are often present in cases of tarsal tunnel and reported that use of a lateral heel wedge ameliorated symptoms. Steroid injection, ice application, or NSAID use may be considered (Jackson and Haglund 1991) prior to surgical intervention. Most athletes will tolerate mild tarsal tunnel syndrome without significant modifications or need for orthoses, but more severe cases may limit athletic competition if the intrinsic muscles are atrophied and proprioception or cutaneous sensation is diminished.

PERONEAL NEUROPATHIES

The common peroneal nerve supplies ankle dorsiflexion and eversion, toe extension, and a minimal degree of knee flexion (short head of the biceps femoris). Peroneal nerve injury can obstruct proprioceptive information from the knee (common peroneal), ankle (deep peroneal and sural nerves), and intertarsal joints (deep peroneal and accessory deep peroneal nerves) .

Injury to the Common Peroneal

The sciatic nerve comprises the common peroneal and tibial nerves. The peroneal nerve fibers lie more lateral to those of the tibial, the funiculi are larger than those of the tibial, and the nerve is anchored at the fibular head (Feinberg et al. 1997). These factors make the common peroneal nerve more susceptible to injury than the tibial division. Injury to the common peroneal component of the sciatic nerve at the hip can occur during hip surgery or from local trauma. Injury to the common peroneal division at the hip differs little with respect to functional significance from an injury at the popliteal fossa above the separation of the deep and superficial peroneal nerves. The only muscle to be affected by hip injury that is not affected by an injury at the popliteal fossa is the short head of the biceps femoris. Loss of function to the short head of the biceps femoris is not functionally significant. Functional impairment arises primarily from a loss of dorsiflexion and loss of foot and ankle eversion capacity. A spring action device can be used to assist dorsiflexion and make gait and running more functional, but athletic capacity will still be significantly impaired. Advice similar to that in figure 9.7 on page 216 may be used for mild cases of dorsiflexor weakness. More severe cases of weakness may require a double upright AFO or a dorsiflexion assist AFO. Even mild common peroneal injuries can affect athletic function. Strengthening should attempt to restore function through Theraband dorsiflexion (see figure 9.6 on page 215) and eversion (see figure 9.15 on page 222) exercises. Proprioception may be diminished from the knee, ankle, or intertarsal joints. Proprioceptive information may still be transmitted via the other nerves supplying these joints and should be utilized when possible. Cutaneous sensory losses will encompass the anterior lower leg, dorsum of the foot, and possibly a portion of the sural cutaneous distribution, due to its partial supply from the peroneal communicating branch of the common peroneal nerve.

Tables A.3, A.4, A.7, A.8, and A.9 in the appendix (see page 239) provide reference information to the reader concerning innnervation of the lower extremities.

Injury at the popliteal fossa occurs most commonly with trauma, either direct or via stretch to the nerve (Feinberg et al. 1997, Kim and Kline 1996, Meals 1977, Moeller et al. 1997, Williams et al. 1996). Exercise-induced peroneal nerve entrapment at the fibular head also appears to occur with some frequency (Leach et al. 1989, Mitra et al. 1995).

Injury to the Deep Peroneal

Tibia or fibula fractures, compartment syndromes, or surgical traction injuries can result in superficial or deep peroneal nerve dysfunction. The deep peroneal nerve supplies the ankle dorsiflexors and toe extensors. These muscles are primarily responsible for dorsiflexion. Sensory supply to the ankle and foot joints may come from the deep peroneal nerve or its branches. Strengthening should target the dorsiflexors as previously described (see figure 9.6 on page 215). Proprioception exercise should target these areas to take advantage of the remaining supply from the tibial and saphenous nerves. Sensory loss is of little functional significance.

Injury to the Superficial Peroneal

Superficial peroneal nerve injury occurs more commonly than injury to the deep peroneal branch (Santi and Botte 1996). Injury to the superficial peroneal nerve can occur with inversion ankle sprains (Kleinrensink et al. 1994) and has been seen by the author on several occasions after blunt trauma to the mid lower leg. The major functional loss with impairment of this division is decreased or absent eversion capacity (peroneus longus and brevis). This loss alters gait and predisposes the athlete to risk of recurrent ankle sprains and of damage to the lateral ligament complex of the ankle. Bracing and strength training for eversion weakness has been discussed previously in this section. It is important to note that the peroneus tertius has deep peroneal nerve supply and can act as a minor evertor and should be strengthened when possible. Additionally, the long toe extensors can perform minor eversion and can be strengthened in a fashion very similar to ankle dorsiflexor strengthening. Here, the Theraband is placed over the toes, and they are dorsiflexed against resistance. Severe weakness can lead to significant functional deficit even with bracing and may preclude able-bodied participation. The superficial peroneal nerve probably does not supply the ankle or foot joints, and cutaneous sensory loss is of little or no clinical importance.

SCIATIC NEUROPATHY

The sciatic nerve is usually injured by direct trauma or via stretch mechanisms. Injury generally occurs in the hip or buttock region but can happen

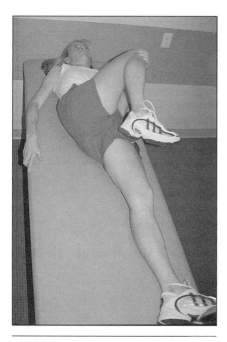

Figure 9.17 Stretching the hip and buttock, with specific attention to the piriformis muscle. The athlete brings the knee toward the opposite shoulder to obtain a posterior buttock stretch.

at any level where the tibial and peroneal components travel together. Piriformis syndrome—compression of the sciatic nerve between the small external rotators of the hip—has been touted by many as a frequent cause of sciatic neuropathy. Spindler and Pappas (1995) and the author believe that most cases of buttock pain with or without sciatica are usually secondary to a radiculopathy until proven otherwise. If, in fact, the piriformis is found to cause sciatic compression, then an aggressive hip and buttock stretching program should be instituted, with special attention to the piriformis muscle. This can be accomplished by having the athlete lie supine and bring the knee to the opposite shoulder (figure 9.17). Adding internal rotation may further stretch the piriformis. It is important to have the athlete maintain the ipsilateral pelvis and buttock close to the plinth or ground while performing this stretch; otherwise the lumbosacral spine will rotate and the appropriate muscular area will not be stretched. Stretching exercises for the gluteal muscles (figure 9.18) and

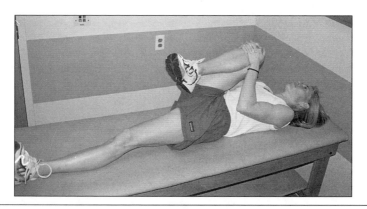

Figure 9.18 Gluteal stretch. The athlete brings the knee toward the chest to obtain a proximal buttock stretch.

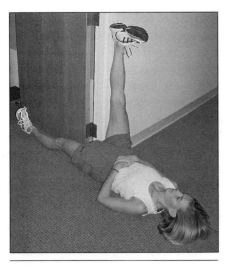

Figure 9.19 Hamstring stretch. The athlete lies supine in a doorway. The left leg in this figure is extended through the doorway and the right hamstring is stretched by placing it onto the door casing. The right leg should be relaxed throughout this stretch routine.

hamstrings (figure 9.19) can also improve local hip extensor flexibility, which will make piriformis stretching easier to perform. Post-traumatic sequelae, such as myositis ossificans after hamstring injury, have been documented by others (Carmody and Prietto 1995) and by the author as a cause of sciatic neuropathy. When the sciatic nerve is injured, the resulting deficits depend upon the degree of injury to the peroneal and tibial divisions. Rehabilitation is much more complicated, as muscles normally used to compensate for lost function may also be affected. The clinician must evaluate the athlete carefully, performing serial examinations to determine how much recovery has occurred and what muscles are available to compensate. Injuries to the tibial and peroneal branches have been discussed separately at length above (see pages 227-230). Clinicians should use their judgment to determine which muscles should be rehabilitated first, applying the strengthening and proprioception protocols described in the preceding sections.

LATERAL FEMORAL CUTANEOUS NEUROPATHY

The lateral femoral cutaneous nerve is a small sensory branch that supplies the skin of the anterior and lateral upper leg. This nerve has no muscular branches and does not innervate any joints. It is infrequently injured in athletes, and when it is affected by compression, traction, or direct trauma it causes insignificant clinical deficits. This nerve injury is best prevented as opposed to being treated. As most lesions to this nerve are caused by repetitive trauma, treatment is to minimize further trauma once identified. In those cases where compression is thought to be the cause, local corticosteroid injection may be of benefit. Surgical decompression in this author's experience has not provided good results and should be discouraged.

SAPHENOUS NEUROPATHY

The saphenous nerve is the termination of the femoral nerve. It provides cutaneous sensation to the skin of the medial lower leg from approximately the knee to the medial malleolus and provides sensory branches to the knee and possibly to the ankle joint. Loss of saphenous nerve function causes sensory deficits in the distribution described but usually lead to very little joint proprioceptive loss, since multiple other larger nerves are present to compensate for any saphenous losses.

SURAL NEUROPATHY

The sural nerve provides cutaneous sensation to the posterior lower leg and lateral foot and innervation to the ankle joint. Injury to the sural nerve will only produce sensory deficit in the area of distribution and clinically insignificant proprioceptive losses at the ankle, due to overlapping local innervation.

MEDIAL AND LATERAL PLANTAR NEUROPATHIES

The medial plantar nerve supplies the medial muscles of the foot (abductor hallucis, flexor digitorum brevis, flexor hallucis brevis, and first lumbrical), provides cutaneous sensory information to the plantar medial foot, and innervates the medial intertarsal and tarsometatarsal/intermetatarsal joints. The medial plantar nerve forms just prior to, within, or just distal to the flexor retinaculum. Injury to the medial plantar branch has been described in the section on tibial nerve entrapment within the flexor retinaculum and may result in weakness of the muscles described above as well as sensory deficits of the medial plantar foot. Muscular weakness from medial plantar neuropathy may reduce midfoot and forefoot pronation control during mid- and late-stance phase. Athletes often can compensate for such weakness by strengthening the lateral plantar-innervated muscles (if spared) and the long toe flexors (flexor hallucis longus and flexor digitorum longus) and by using medial arch support orthoses. The sensory deficit can impair athletic function in the early stages but can usually be overlooked by the athlete as time from the injury increases. If the medial plantar nerve is entrapped within the abductor hallucis, this muscle is usually spared, with variable involvement to the more distal muscles. Athletes who suffer from this problem will probably notice only a sensory disturbance in the form of either paresthesia or dysesthesia and will likely not be aware of any gait abnormality. Strengthening should be directed toward the long toe extensors and other intrinsic muscles. Arch-supporting orthoses are probably not necessary, but in some cases they are helpful in reducing pronation and allowing for more effective push-off.

The lateral plantar nerve supplies the remaining intrinsic foot muscles not supplied by the medial plantar nerve and provides cutaneous sensory information to the lateral plantar foot; it also innervates the lateral intertarsal and tarsometatarsal/intermetatarsal joints. The lateral plantar nerve also forms proximal to, within, or just distal to the flexor retinaculum and may be compressed secondary to tarsal tunnel syndrome. The major weakness identified is to the quadratus plantae—an arch-supporting muscle that helps reduce midfoot pronation during early and midstance phase and allows for controlled push-off. A full-length arch orthosis may be all that is necessary with most lateral plantar branch entrapments. Paresthesia or dysesthesia may also be present, but they are less problematic than those affecting the medial plantar branch, due to its smaller sensory supply of the foot. Other aspects of treatment of tarsal tunnel syndrome have been described above (see "Tibial Neuropathy," pages 227-228), and apply to medial and lateral plantar nerve entrapments at the flexor retinaculum. Entrapment of the abductor digiti minimi muscular branch of the lateral plantar has been described. This may occur with excessive supination and trauma or may occur due to an anomalous fibrous band that compresses the nerve. There is no gait deviation with this neuropathy. The athlete typically describes an ache along the lateral foot, without other sensory disturbance. If excessive supination leads to the neuropathy, talar-neutral orthoses should be used to correct the gait deviation. Stretching to the tarsal and metatarsal joints may help if an anomalous fibrous arch is present. Entrapments that don't respond to stretching, strengthening, or orthoses may be injected with a steroid-based preparation or may need surgical decompression if the steroid is unsuccessful.

DIGITAL NEUROPATHIES

The most common digital neuropathies are due to neuromas. Cutaneous sensory loss may be present to a varying degree, but the primary disability to athletes is typically from the dysesthesia that results with forefoot progression from the fifth metatarsophalangeal joint to the first and second metatarsophalangeal joints. It is during this mid- to late-stance phase that the digital nerve is compressed and irritated, sometimes causing significant pain and decreased capacity. Treatment is geared toward "opening up" the midfoot and forefoot to reduce the compression onto the neuroma that has formed. This can be performed by stretching the plantar arch and intermetatarsophalangeal joints. The athlete places one hand on each side of the foot and stretches with either a plantar- or dorsal-directed force in the midline. Arch-supporting orthoses and metatarsal pads similarly will reduce neuroma compression and should be considered. Because this condition occurs commonly in women who wear shoes with a tight, narrow toe box, changing to shoes with a wider toe box should reduce symptoms. Local icing may also reduce symptoms. If local treatments do not improve symptoms, corticosteroid injection or surgical intervention may be considered.

PUDENDAL NEUROPATHY

As described in chapter 6, pudendal neuropathies in athletics occur most often in cyclists. The pudendal nerve provides penile sensation and assists with the parasympathetic component of erection. Because loss of pudendal function leads only to sexual dysfunction without affecting athletic capacity, no sports rehabilitation is required. This nerve injury is best prevented as opposed to being treated.

CONCLUSION

Rehabilitation of lower-extremity nerve injuries requires that the clinician be an expert in neuroanatomy, biomechanics, and the use of orthoses. The clinician must evaluate the epidemiology of the injury, determine the extent of damage, and apply this knowledge to obtain the best functional outcome for the athlete. Since the same nerve injury can produce very different deficits and patterns of recovery in different people, it is crucial that athletes not be placed into a "cookbook" rehabilitation program. Frequent serial examinations of strength and proprioception should be performed by medical staff to update the rehabilitation program as needed. With proper institution of these principles, one can expect to maximize athletic return and can determine as early as possible whether an individual can return to able-bodied competition or will need to compete at an adapted level.

REFERENCES

An HS, Simpson JM, and Gale S. Acute anterior compartment syndrome in the thigh: a case report and review of the literature. J Orthop Trauma 1987; 1:180-182.

Baba H, Uchida K, Furusawa N, Maezawa Y, Azuchi M, Kamitani K, Annen S, Imura S, and Tomita K. Posterior limbus vertebral lesions causing lumbosacral radiculopathy and the cauda equina syndrome. Spinal Cord 1996; 34:427-432.

Barrett JR, Tanji JL, Drake C, Fuller D, Kawasaki RI, and Fenton RM. High- versus low-top shoes for the prevention of ankle sprains in basketball players: a prospective randomized study. Am J Sports Med 1993; 21(4):582-585.

Berger AR and Schaumburg HH. Rehabilitation of focal nerve injuries. J Neuro Rehab 1988; 2(2):65-91.

Borenstein DG, Wiesel SW, and Boden SD. Mechanical disorders of the lumbosacral spine: acute herniated nucleus pulposus. In: Borenstein DG, Wiesel SW, and Boden SD (eds.), *Low back pain: medical diagnosis and comprehensive management,* 2nd edition. Philadelphia: Saunders, 1995:191-197.

Bradshaw C, McCrory P, Bell S, and Brukner P. Obturator nerve entrapment: a cause of groin pain in athletes. Am J Sports Med 1997; 25(3):402-408.

Brozin IH, Martfel J, Goldberg I, and Kurtizky A. Traumatic closed femoral nerve neuropathy. J Trauma 1982; 22(2):158-160.

Carmody C and Prietto C. Entrapment of the sciatic nerve as a late sequela of injury to the hamstring muscles. J Bone Joint Surg [Am] 1995; 77(7):1100-1107.

Champetier J. Innervation de l'articulation tibio-tarsienne (articulatio talocruralis). Acta Anat 1970; 77:398-421.

Crafts RC. The hip area. In: Crafts RC (ed.), *A textbook of human anatomy*. New York: Wiley Medical, 1985:416-449.

Deyo RA, Diehl AK, and Rosenthal M. How many days of bed rest for acute low back pain? A randomized clinical trial. N Engl J Med 1986; 315(17):1064-1070.

Donelson R, Aprill C, Medcalf R, and Grant W. A prospective study of centralization of lumbar and referred pain. A predictor of symptomatic discs and anular competence. Spine 1997; 22(10):1115-1122.

Donelson R, Grant W, Kamps C, and Metcalf R. Pain response to sagittal end-range spinal motion. Spine 1991; 16(6 Suppl):S206-212.

Einarsson G and Grimby G. Strengthening exercise program in post-polio subjects. In: Halstead LS and Weichers DO (eds.), *Research and clinical aspects of the late effects of poliomyelitis*. White Plains, New York: March of Dimes Birth Defects Foundation, 1987:275-283.

Feinberg JH, Nadler SF, and Krivickas LS. Peripheral nerve injuries in the athlete. Sports Med 1997; 24(6):385-408.

Feldman RM and Soskolne CL. The use of non-fatiguing strengthening exercises in post-polio syndrome. In: Halstead LS and Weichers DO (eds.), *Research and clinical aspects of the late effects of poliomyelitis*. White Plains, New York: March of Dimes Birth Defects Foundation, 1987:335-341.

Feuerbach JW, Grabiner MD, Koh TJ, and Weiker GG. Effect of an ankle orthosis and ankle ligament anesthesia on ankle joint proprioception. Am J Sports Med 1994; 22(2):223-229.

Fritz JM, Delitto A, Vignovic M, and Busse RG. Interrater reliability of judgments of the centralization phenomenon and status change during movement testing in patients with low back pain. Arch Phys Med Rehabil 2000; 81(1):57-61.

Fuentes RJ and Rosenberg JM. Questions and answers. In: Fuentes RJ and Rosenberg JM (eds.), *Athletic drug reference '99*. Durham, NC: Clean Data, Inc./Glaxo-Wellcome, 1999:44.

Gardner E. The innervation of the knee joint. Anat Rec 1948; 101:109-130.

Gardner E and Gray DJ. The innervation of the foot joints. Anat Rec 1968; 161(2):141-148.

Greene TA and Hillman SK. Comparison of support provided by a semirigid orthosis and adhesive ankle taping before, during and after exercise. Am J Sports Med 1990; 18:498-506.

Huittinen VM. Lumbosacral nerve injury in fracture of the pelvis: a postmortem radiographic and patho-anatomical study. Acta Chir Scand [Suppl] 1972; 429:3-43.

Huittinen VM and Slätis P. Nerve injury in double vertical pelvic fractures. Acta Chir Scand 1972; 138:571-575.

Infante E and Kennedy WR. Anomalous branch of the peroneal nerve detected by electromyography. Arch Neurol 1970; 22(2):162-165.

Jackson DL and Haglund B. Tarsal tunnel syndrome in athletes: case reports and literature review. Am J Sports Med 1991; 19(1):61-65.

Karas R, McIntosh G, Hall H, Wilson L, and Melles T. The relationship between nonorganic signs and centralization of symptoms in the prediction of return to work for patients with low back pain. Phys Ther 1997; 77(4):354-360.

Kennedy JC, Alexander IJ, and Hayes KC. Nerve supply of the human knee and its functional importance. Am J Sports Med 1982; 10(6):329-335.

Kim DH and Kline DG. Management and results of peroneal nerve lesions. Neurosurgery 1996; 39(2):312-319.

Kleinrensink GJ, Stoeckart R, Meulstee J, Kanselar Sukul DM, Vleeming A, Snijders CJ, and van Noort A. Lowered motor conduction velocity of the peroneal nerve after inversion trauma. Med Sci Sports Exerc 1994; 26(7):877-883.

Lambert EH. The accessory deep peroneal nerve: a common variation in innervation of extensor digitorum brevis. Neurology 1969; 19(12):1169-1176.

Leach RE, Purnell MB, and Akiyoshi S. Peroneal nerve entrapment in runners. Am J Sports Med 1989; 17(2):287-291.

Ljunggren AE. Natural history and clinical role of the herniated disc. In: Wiesel SW, Weinstein JN, Herkowitz H, Dvorák J, and Bell G (eds.), *The lumbar spine,* 2nd edition. Philadelphia: Saunders, 1996:473-491.

Manfroy PP, Ashton-Miller JA, and Wojtys EM. The effect of exercise, prewrap, and athletic tape on the maximal active and passive ankle resistance to ankle inversion. Am J Sports Med 1997; 25(2):156-163.

Mann RA. Entrapment neuropathies of the foot. In: DeLee JC and Drez D (eds.), *Orthopaedic sports medicine: principles and practice.* Philadelphia: Saunders, 1994:1831-1833.

McKenzie RA. The lumbar spine: mechanical diagnosis and therapy. In: McKenzie RA (ed.), *The lumbar spine: mechanical diagnosis and therapy.* Waikane, New Zealand: Spinal Publications, 1981.

Meals RA. Peroneal nerve palsy complicating ankle sprain. J Bone Joint Surg [Am] 1977; 59(7):966-968.

Miller EH and Benedict FE. Stretch of the femoral nerve in a dancer: a case report. J Bone Joint Surg [Am] 1985; 67(2):315-317.

Mitra A, Stern JD, Perrotta VJ, and Moyer RA. Peroneal nerve entrapment in athletes. Ann Plast Surg 1995; 35:366-368.

Moeller JL, Monroe J, and McKeag DB. Cryotherapy-induced common peroneal nerve palsy. Clin J Sport Med 1997; 7(3):212-216.

Mondelli M, Giannini F, and Reale F. Clinical and electrophysiological findings and follow-up in tarsal tunnel syndrome. Electroencephalogr Clin Neurophysiol 1998; 109(5):418-425.

Montgomery WH, Pink M, and Perry J. Electromyographic analysis of hip and knee musculature during running. Am J Sports Med 1994; 22(2):272-278.

Nachemson AL. Disc pressure measurements. Spine 1981; 6(1):93-97.

Norris CM. *Back stability.* Champaign, IL: Human Kinetics, 2000.

O'Rahilly RO. The gluteal region. In: O'Rahilly RO (ed.), *Gardner, Gray and O'Rahilly's anatomy: a regional study of human structure,* 5th edition. Philadelphia: Saunders, 1986a:197-201.

O'Rahilly RO. The thigh, hip joint, and knee. In: O'Rahilly RO (ed.), *Gardner, Gray and O'Rahilly's anatomy: a regional study of human structure,* 5th edition. Philadelphia: Saunders, 1986b:202-223.

Radin EL. The tarsal tunnel syndrome. Clin Orthop 1983; 181(Dec):167-170.

Ragnarsson KT. Lower extremity orthotics, shoes and gait aids. In: DeLisa JA and Gans BM (eds.), *Rehabilitation medicine: principles and practice,* 2nd edition. Philadelphia: Lippincott, 1993:492-506.

Reber L, Perry J, and Pink M. Muscular control of the ankle in running. Am J Sports Med 1993; 21(6):805-810.

Saal JA and Saal JS. Nonoperative treatment of herniated lumbar intervertebral disc with radiculopathy: an outcome study. Spine 1989; 14(4):431-437.

Saal JA, Saal JS, and Herzog RJ. The natural history of lumbar intervertebral disc extrusion treated nonoperatively. Spine 1990; 15(7):683-686.

Sammarco GJ and Stephens MM. Neurapraxia of the femoral nerve in a modern dancer. Am J Sports Med 1991; 19(4):413-414.

Santi MS and Botte MJ. Nerve injury and repair in the foot and ankle. Foot & Ankle International 1996; 17(7):425-439.

Saunders JBM, Inman VT, and Eberhart HD. The major determinants in normal and pathological gait. J Bone Joint Surg [Am] 1953; 35(3):543-558.

Spangfort EV. The lumbar disk herniation: a computer-aided analysis of 2,504 operations. Acta Orthop Scand [Suppl] 1972; 142:1-95.

Spindler KP and Pappas J. Neurovascular problems. In: Nicholas JA and Hershman EB (eds.), *The lower extremity & spine in sports medicine*, 2nd edition. St. Louis: Mosby, 1995:1345-1358.

Sufka A, Hauger B, Trenary M, Bishop B, Hagen A, Lozon R, and Martens B. Centralization of low back pain and perceived functional outcome. J Orthop Sports Phys Ther 1998; 27(3):205-212.

Susens GP, Hendrikson CG, Mulder J, and Sams B. Femoral nerve entrapment secondary to a heparin hematoma. Ann Intern Med 1968; 69(3):575-579.

Weber H. Lumbar disc herniation: a controlled, prospective study with ten years of observation. Spine 1983; 8(2):131-140.

Wertheimer LG. The sensory nerves of the hip joint. J Bone Joint Surg [Am] 1952; 34(2):477-487.

White AH, McKenzie R, Paris SV, Stein D, Floman Y, and Mayer TG. Rehabilitation. In: Weinstein JN and Wiesel SW (eds.), *The lumbar spine*. Philadelphia: Saunders, 1990:772-779.

Williams DD. A study of the human fibular communicating nerve. Anat Rec 1954; 120(3):533-543.

Williams P, Shenolikar A, Roberts RC, and Davies RM. Acute non-traumatic compartment syndrome related to soft tissue injury. Injury 1996; 27(7):507-508.

Winternitz WA, Metheny JA, and Wear LC. Acute compartment syndrome of the thigh in sports related injuries not associated with femoral fractures. Am J Sports Med 1992; 20(4):476-478.

Appendix

Table A.1   Upper-Extremity Nerves With Muscle Groups Innervated and Major Root Supply

Nerve	Muscle group innervated	Major root supply
Musculocutaneous	Shoulder flexion	C5, C6, C7
	Elbow flexion	C5, C6, C7
	Elbow supination	C5, C6
Median	Elbow flexion	C6, C7
	Forearm pronation	C6, C7
	Wrist flexion	C6, C7
	Finger flexion	C7, C8, T1
	Thumb abduction	C8, T1
Axillary	Shoulder flexion	C5, C6
	Shoulder extension	C5, C6
	Shoulder abduction	C5, C6
	Shoulder external rotation	C5, C6
Ulnar	Elbow flexion	C7, C8
	Finger flexion	C8, T1
	Finger abduction	C8, T1
	Finger adduction	C8, T1
Radial	Shoulder extension	C5, C6, C7, C8, T1
	Elbow flexion	C5, C6, C7
	Elbow extension	C6, C7, C8, T1
	Forearm supination	C5, C6
	Wrist extension	C6, C7, C8
	Finger extension	C7, C8

Data from Magee, D.J.: Orthopedic Physical Assessment. Second Edition. Philadelphia, W.B. Saunders Co., 1992, pp. 104, 149, 185.

Table created by Robert Savarese.

Table A.2 Primary Innervation of Upper-Extremity Joints

Joint	Primary innervation (nerve and roots)
Shoulder	Dorsal scapular Axillary Lateral pectoral Medial pectoral Musculocutaneous Subscapular Thoracodorsal Radial Suprascapular Accessory Cranial nerve XI C5 C6 C7 C8 T1
Elbow	Musculocutaneous Radial Median Ulnar C5 C6 C7 C8 T1
Wrist	Median Ulnar Radial C6 C7 C8
Hand	Median Ulnar Radial C7 C8 T1

Table created by Robert Savarese.

Table A.3 Primary Innervation of Lower-Extremity Joints

Joint	Primary innervation (nerve and roots)
Hip	Obturator Accessory obturator (when present) Femoral Nerve to the quadratus femoris Superior gluteal L2 L3 L4 L5 S1
Knee	Femoral Saphenous Common peroneal Tibial ? Obturator ? L2 L3 L4 ? L5
Ankle	Tibial Deep peroneal Sural Accessory deep peroneal (when present) ? Saphenous L4 ? L5 S1
Foot	Medial plantar (tibial) Lateral plantar (tibial) Deep peroneal Accessory deep peroneal (when present) L5 S1 S2

A question mark indicates disagreement among anatomists.

Table created by Brian A. Davis.

Table A.4 Lower-Extremity Peripheral Nerves With Muscle Groups Innervated and Major Root Supply

Nerve	Muscle groups innervated	Major root supply
Femoral	Spine flexors	L2, L3
	Hip flexors	L2, L3
	Knee extensors	L2, L3, L4
Obturator	Hip adductors	L2, L3, L4
	? Knee extensors (adductor magnus-vastus medialis)	L2, L3, L4
Sciatic	Through peroneal and tibial nerves—no direct innervation	L4, L5, S1, S2
Peroneal	Ankle dorsiflexors	L4, L5
	Ankle evertors	L5, S1
	Toe extensors	L5, S1
Tibial	Hip extensors	L5, S1, S2
	Knee flexors	L5, S1, S2
	Ankle plantarflexors	L5, S1, S2
	Ankle invertors	L5, S1, S2
	Toe flexors	L5, S1, S2
	Foot intrinsics	S1, S2

A question mark indicates disagreement among anatomists.

Table created by Brian A. Davis.

Table A.5 Innervation of Shoulder and Arm Muscles

Muscle	Nerve	Root supply
Trapezius	Spinal accessory C3 and 4 (?sensory)	**CN XI** **Cervical roots 3 and 4 (?sensory)**
Levator scapulae	Dorsal scapular C3 and 4 (?sensory)	**C5** **Cervical roots 3 and 4 (?sensory)**
Sternocleidomastoid	Spinal accessory C2, C3 (?sensory)	**CN XI** **Cervical roots 2 and 3 (?sensory)**
Scalenes	?Branches of the ventral rami of cervical plexus	**?Cervical roots 1-4**
Rhomboids	Dorsal scapular	**C5**
Serratus anterior	Long thoracic	**C5, C6, C7**
Pectoralis muscles	Lateral pectoral Medial pectoral	**C5-7** **C8, T1**
Subclavius	Nerve to subclavius	**C5**, C6
Deltoid	Axillary	**C5, C6**
Coracobrachialis	Musculocutaneous	**C5, C6**
Biceps brachii	Musculocutaneous	**C5, C6**
Latissimus dorsi	Thoracodorsal	C6, **C7, C8**
Teres major	Lower subscapular	**C5, C6**
Teres minor	Axillary	**C5, C6**
Supraspinatus	Suprascapular	**C5, C6**
Infraspinatus	Suprascapular	**C5, C6**
Subscapularis	Upper subscapular Lower subscapular	**C5** **C5, C6**
Triceps	Radial	C6, **C7, C8**
Anconeus	Radial	**C7, C8**
Brachioradialis	Radial	**C5, C6**
Brachialis	Musculocutaneous Radial	**C5, C6** **C7**
Supinator	Posterior interosseous/ deep branch of radial	**C5, 6,** C7
Pronator teres	Median	**C6,** C7
Pronator quadratus	Anterior interosseous	C6, C7, **C8, T1** (Kimura - **C7, C8**)
Palmaris longus	Median	**C7, C8,** T1

(continued)

Table A.5 *(continued)*

Muscle	Nerve	Root supply
Flexor carpi radialis	Median	**C6, C7**
Flexor digitorum superficialis	Median	**C7, C8, T1**
Flexor pollicis longus	Anterior interosseous	**C7, C8, T1**
Flexor digitorum profundus	Anterior interosseous (digits 2 and 3)	C7, **C8, T1**
	Ulnar (digits 4 and 5)	C7, **C8, T1**
Abductor pollicis longus	Posterior interosseous	**?C7-T1** (Kimura **C7, C8**)
Extensor pollicis brevis	Posterior interosseous	**?C7-T1** (Kimura **C7, C8**)
Extensor pollicis longus	Posterior interosseous	**?C7-T1** (Kimura **C7, C8**)
Extensor indicis	Posterior interosseous	**?C7-T1** (Kimura **C7, C8**)
Extensor carpi ulnaris	Posterior interosseous	**?C7, C8**
Extensor carpi radialis longus	Radial	**C6, C7,** C8 (Kimura **C5, C6**)
Extensor carpi radialis brevis	Radial	**C6, C7,** C8 (Kimura **C5, C6**)
Extensor digiti minimi	Posterior interosseous	**C7, C8**
Extensor digitorum communis	Posterior interosseous	C6, **C7, C8** (Kimura **C7, C8**)
Flexor carpi ulnaris	Ulnar	C7 (Kimura), **C8, T1**

Bold = major root; regular print = less consistent or questionable

Kimura J. Anatomic basis for localization. In: Kimura J. (ed.), Electrodiagnosis in diseases of nerve and muscle: principles and practice, 3rd edition. Oxford: Oxford Press, 2001:16-17.

A question mark indicates disagreement among anatomists.

Table created by Brian H. Davis.

Table A.6 Innervation of Hand Muscles

Muscle	Nerve	Root supply
Palmaris brevis	Superficial branch of ulnar	**C8, T1**
Opponens digiti minimi	Deep branch of ulnar	**C8, T1**
Abductor digiti minimi	Deep branch of ulnar	**C8, T1**
Flexor digiti minimi brevis	Deep branch of ulnar	**C8, T1**
Flexor pollicis brevis	Median (superficial head)	**C8, T1**
	Deep branch of ulnar (deep head)	**C8, T1**
Abductor pollicis brevis	Median	**C8, T1**
Opponens pollicis	Median	**C8, T1**
Adductor pollicis	Deep branch of ulnar	**C8, T1**
Lumbricals	Median (digits 2 and 3)	**C8, T1**
	Ulnar (digits 4 and 5)	**C8, T1**
Interossei	Deep branch of ulnar	**C8, T1**

Bold = major root; regular print = less consistent or questionable

Table created by Brian H. Davis.

Table A.7 Innervation of Abdomen/Hip/Pelvis Muscles

Muscle	Nerve	Root supply
Rectus abdominis	Thoracoabdominal + subcostal	T5, T6, **T7-12**, L1
External oblique	Thoracoabdominal + subcostal	**T7-12**
Internal oblique	Ilioinguinal + hypogastric	T7, T8, **T9-12, L1**
Quadratus lumborum	Subcostal and lumbar plexus	**T12, L1, L2**, L3
Serratus posterior inferior	Ventral rami or spinal nerve branches	**T9-11**, T12
Transversus abdominis	Thoracoabdominals + subcostal	**T7-12, L1**
Pyramidalis	Subcostal	**T12**
Psoas muscles	Lumbar plexus Ventral rami	L1, **L2, L3**, L4, L5
Iliacus	Femoral	**L2, L3, L4**
Gluteus maximus	Inferior gluteal	**L5, S1, S2**
Gluteus medius	Superior gluteal	**L4, L5, S1**, S2
Gluteus minimus	Superior gluteal	**L4, L5, S1**
Tensor fascia lata	Superior gluteal	**L4, L5, S1**
Pectineus	Femoral + obturator + accessory obturator	**L2**, L4, L5
Adductor brevis	Obturator	**L2-4**
Adductor longus	Obturator	**L2, L3**, L4, L5
Adductor magnus	Obturator (anterior/adductor/flexor head)	**L3-5**
	Tibial (posterior/extensor/adductor head)	L2, S1
Piriformis	Ventral rami + nerve to piriformis	L5, **S1, S2**
Obturator externus	Obturator	L2, **L3, L4**
Obturator internus	Nerve to obturator internus	**L5, S1, L2**
Superior gemellus	Nerve to obturator internus	**L5, S1, L2**
Inferior gemellus	Nerve to quadratus femoris	**L4, L5, S1**, S2
Quadratus femoris	Nerve to quadratus femoris	**L4, L5, S1**, S2

Bold = major root; regular print = less consistent or questionable

Table created by Brian H. Davis.

Table A.8 Innervation of Leg Muscles

Muscle	Nerve	Root supply
Sartorius	Femoral	**L2, L3,** L4
Gracilis	Obturator	**L2-4**
Biceps femoris	Tibial (long head)	**L5, S1, S2**
	Common peroneal (short head)	**L5, S1, S2**
Semitendinosus	Tibial	L4, **L5, S1,** S2
Semimembranosus	Tibial	L4, **L5, S1,** S2
Quadriceps	Femoral	**L2-4**
Popliteus	Tibial	**L4, L5, S1**
Tibialis anterior	Deep peroneal	**L4, L5,** S1
Extensor digitorum longus	Deep peroneal	**L4, L5, S1**
Extensor hallucis longus	Deep peroneal	**L4, L5, S1**
Peroneus longus	Superficial peroneal	L4, **L5, S1,** S2
Peroneus brevis	Superficial peroneal	L4, **L5, S1,** S2
Peroneus tertius	Deep peroneal	L4, **L5, S1**
Gastrocnemius	Tibial	L5, **S1, S2**
Soleus	Tibial	L5, **S1, S2**
Plantaris	Tibial	**L4, L5, S1,** S2
Flexor digitorum longus	Tibial	**L5, S1, S2,** S3
Flexor hallucis longus	Tibial	**L5, S1, S2,** S3
Tibialis posterior	Tibial	L4, **L5, S1,** S2

Bold = major root; regular print = less consistent or questionable

Table created by Brian H. Davis.

Table A.9 Innervation of Foot Muscles

Muscle	Nerve	Root supply
Abductor hallucis	Medial plantar	**L5, S1,** S2, S3
Flexor digitorum brevis	Medial plantar	**L5, S1,** S2, S3
Abductor digiti minimi	Lateral plantar	L5, **S1, S2,** S3
Quadratus plantae	Lateral plantar	L5, **S1, S2,** S3
Lumbricals	Medial plantar (digit 2) Lateral plantar (digits 3, 4, and 5)	**L5, S1, S2,** S3 **L5, S1, S2,** S3
Flexor hallucis brevis	Medial plantar	**L5, S1,** S2, S3
Adductor hallucis	Lateral plantar	**L5, S1, S2,** S3
Flexor digiti minimi brevis	Lateral plantar	**L5, S1, S2,** S3
Dorsal interossei	Lateral plantar	**L5, S1, S2,** S3
Palmar interossei	Lateral plantar	**L5, S1, S2,** S3
Extensor digitorum brevis	Deep peroneal	**L4, L5, S1,** S2
Extensor hallucis brevis	Deep peroneal	**L4, L5, S1,** S2

Bold = major root; regular print = less consistent or questionable

Table created by Brian H. Davis.

Glossary

adventitia—The outer layer that makes up a tubular organ or structure, is composed of collagenous and elastic fibers, and is not covered with peritoneum.

allodynia—Pain produced by nonnoxious stimulation of the skin in the territory of a damaged nerve.

annulus fibrosus—A concentric ring of fibers that forms the outer portion of an intervertebral disc.

anterior tarsal tunnel syndrome—Deep peroneal nerve compression beneath the inferior extensor retinaculum of the ankle.

antidromic—Relating to propagation of an impulse along an axon in a direction the reverse of the normal.

Baker's cyst—Synovial cyst in the popliteal fossa formed by accumulation of fluid in a noncommunicating bursa, or by distension of a bursa by fluid from the knee joint.

burner—A syndrome commonly seen in football where an athlete usually experiences a burning or stinging sensation down one upper limb after a block or tackle. Symptoms usually last less than one or two minutes and are believed to be caused by a stretched or compressed cervical root or brachial plexus.

cancellous bone—Bone that has a lattice- or spongy-like structure.

cauda equina syndrome—Paresthesias in the bladder, sacrum, or perineum secondary to compression of the spinal nerve roots that can lead to areflexic paralysis.

Cedell fracture—Fracture of the medial tubercle of the posterior process of the talus.

centralization—A treatment technique that the examiner uses to determine what lumbar positions reduce leg pain (i.e., "centralize" the pain to the lumbar or gluteal regions). Activities are initiated in this position of centralization to reduce disc pressures and nerve irritability.

closed-chain exercise—One in which the limb is fixed to either the wall or the ground.

coaptor—A muscle or other structure that assists with joint stability by bringing joint surfaces together.

compartment syndrome—Elevated pressure in a fascial compartment, caused by swelling or hemorrhage of the contents; it can produce nerve injury and/or muscle necrosis.

concentric contraction—Muscle contraction that results in the approximation of the muscle's origin and insertion.

conduction block—Failure of action potential propagation along a nerve, caused by demyelination or damage to the myelin sheath. Conduction block occurs in neurapraxic injuries. Conduction is possible, however, below the point of block.

conduction velocity—Speed of propagation of an action potential along a nerve or muscle fiber.

deafferentation—The removal of afferent (incoming) nerve supply.

demyelination—Destruction or loss of myelin from a peripheral nerve.

dentate ligaments—A band of fibrous pia mater extending along the spinal cord on each side between the dorsal and ventral roots; these tissues suspend the spinal cord from the dura mater and help maintain the central position of the cord.

depolarization—Decrease and ultimate reversal of the transmembrane potential of a muscle (or nerve) fiber. An initial step leading to muscle contraction.

dermatome—The area of skin supplied by a single posterior nerve root.

disc herniation—The nucleus pulposis (inner portion) of the intervertebral disc has ruptured through the annulus (outer portion) and posterior longitudinal ligament.

disc protrusion—Bulging of the nucleus pulposis through a weakened annulus fibrosis.

dorsal ramus—A branch of a spinal nerve that supplies the posterior area of the body.

dorsal root—Sensory branch of a spinal nerve that enters the dorsal part of the spinal cord.

dorsal root ganglion—Collection of nerve cell bodies in the dorsal root.

dysesthesia—A condition whereby disagreeable sensation is produced by ordinary stimulation.

eccentric contraction—Muscle contraction that results in a lengthening of the muscle's origin and insertion.

electrodiagnostic study (EDX)—The clinical electromyographic (EMG) study performed to diagnose a peripheral nerve injury. This study should include both a set of nerve conduction studies and a needle electrode examination of selected muscles in order to be considered complete.

electromyography (electomyographic)—Of or pertaining to the use of examining the electrical signals from within the muscle/nerve units.

engram—Patterns of movement, including velocity, vector, position, and multiple other variables, that are stored in central and peripheral centers for subsequent use.

extruded disc—A type of disc herniation in which the nucleus pulposus protrudes through the annulus fibrosus and the nuclear material remains attached to the disc.

fabella syndrome—Entrapment of the common peroneal nerve by an accessory ossicle (the fabella) in the lateral gastrocnemius muscle.

facet joint—Term used to describe the zygapophyseal joint. It is comprised of the superior articular process of one vertebra and the inferior articular process of the vertebra above. It is a synovial joint.

fasciotomy—Surgical incision of the fascia overlying muscle, generally performed to release excessive pressure build up.

fibrillation potential—Biphasic spikes of short duration and an initial positive phase associated with a spontaneously contracting muscle fiber; indicative of denervation.

fluoroscopy (fluoroscopic)—The use of or pertaining to the use of cineradiographic imaging.

genu recurvatum—Hyperextension of the knee to form a convex posterior curve of the lower extremity. Also known as "back knee."

hip pointer—Contusion to the anterior superior iliac spine (ASIS), commonly occurring in football, basketball, soccer, and hockey.

heterotopic ossification—Abnormal bone formation in soft-tissue structures. Myositis ossificans is a form of heterotopic ossification.

hypesthesia—Diminished sensitivity to stimulation.

hypothenar—Related to the fleshy mass on the medial side of the palm.

intervertebral foramen—The opening formed by the inferior and superior notches on the pedicles of adjacent vertebrae that transmits the spinal nerve.

iontophoresis—A physical modality in which soluble salts (most commonly steroids) are introduced into the body through the skin via an electrical current.

ipsilateral rotation—Rotation to the same side as that on which the patient experiences symptoms.

isokinetic exercise—One in which the muscle moves at a constant angular velocity during activation.

isometric contraction—Muscle contraction that increases tension without a shortening or lengthening of the muscle.

isometric exercise—One in which the muscle is activated without change in the joint angle (i.e., the muscle does not shorten with activation).

isotonic contraction— Muscle contraction that results in a shortening of the muscle without a change in its tension.

isotonic exercise—One in which a muscle shortens and moves a load (maintains constant tension).

kinesiology—The science or the study of movement and the active and passive structures involved.

lymphedema—Swelling in subcutaneous tissues as a result of obstruction of lymphatic vessels or lymph nodes.

meralgia paresthetica syndrome—Neuropathy of the lateral femoral cutaneous nerve.

Morton's neuroma—Mechanically induced degenerative neuropathy of the interdigital nerves of the foot, most commonly in the second or third web space.

myositis ossificans—Calcification that develops in a muscle after an injury such as a severe contusion or strain.

myotome—A group of muscles innervated from a single spinal segment.

nerve glide—Normal physiologic movement of a nerve within connective tissue as a response to bodily movements.

nerve gliding—A nerve has flexibility within its connective tissue that allows it to glide.

neurapraxia—Mild nerve injury in which only the myelin sheath, and not the axon, is damaged.

neurapraxic—An injury to the myelin that results in a temporary conduction block to the axons involved. There is no axonal degeneration. Only the myelin sheath, and not the axon, is damaged.

neuritis—Nerve inflammation or irritation.

neuropathic pain—Refers to pain that is proposed to be generated secondary to nerve dysfunction.

neuropathy—A functional disturbance or pathologic change in the peripheral nervous system.

nociceptor—A receptor that responds to tissue damage, or the chemical mediators associated with tissue damage. They signal the sensation the brain interprets as pain.

nucleus pulposus—A semifluid mass that forms the central portion of an intervertebral disc.

opiate—Naturally occurring compound from the opium plant.

opioid—Synthetically produced compound mimicking the actions of opiates.

open-chain exercise—One in which the limb is not fixed to either the wall or the ground.

orthodromic—Denoting the propagation of an impulse along an axon in the normal direction.

orthosis (orthoses)—Any device used to assist function. Can include devices made of plastic, metal, canvas, tape, or any other material as needed to improve function.

paresthesia—An abnormal touch sensation, such as burning or prickling, in the absence of an external stimulus.

pars interarticularis—The segment of bone between the superior and inferior articular processes of a lumbar vertebra.

piriformis syndrome—Buttock and posterior thigh pain purported to be caused by compression of the sciatic nerve by the piriformis muscle.

plyometric exercise—One in which the muscle is stretched and then activated to achieve a very forceful muscular response.

polyphasic potential—An action potential having five or more phases associated with the process of reinnervation.

positive sharp wave—A biphasic, positive-negative action potential recorded from a muscle fiber when damage has occurred to its innervating axon or to the muscle fiber itself.

posting—Part of wind-up phase of pitching motion where the pitcher is stabilized on one limb.

proprioceptive neuromuscular facilitation (PNF)—Exercise programs designed to facilitate recovery using neuromuscular patterns and sensory receptors to either enhance or inhibit movement.

radiculopathy—A clinical condition caused by compression of a nerve root by a prolapsed disk or other anatomic factors that lead to compression of a nerve root; more generally, any disease of spinal nerve roots or spinal nerves; "radiculitis" is a synonym.

recruitment—The successive activation of the same and additional motor units with increasing strength of voluntary muscle contraction.

reinnervation—The restoration of nerve control of a paralyzed muscle or organ by means of regrowth of nerve fibers.

relative stenosis—A spinal canal that is narrow relative to an arbitrary ratio that has been defined by Pavlov (1987), as opposed to absolute stenosis that is defined by anatomic guidelines.

reverse origin-insertion—Muscular activation that occurs when the axis of rotation reverses to cause the muscular origin to move toward the point of muscular insertion.

sequestered disc—A type of disc herniation in which a free fragment is in the spinal canal outside of the annulus fibrosus and the nuclear material is no longer attached to the disc.

shoulder abduction relief sign—Physical exam technique designed to help diagnose a cervical radiculopathy at the C5 or C6 level by reducing neural tension. The maneuver is performed by passively abducting the shoulder of the symptomatic side overhead and thus reducing the radicular symptoms.

spondylolisthesis—Forward displacement of the body of one vertebra on the vertebra below it, most commonly due to a defect in the pars interarticularis.

Spurling maneuver—Physical exam provocative maneuver to help diagnose a cervical radiculopathy by reproducing radicular symptoms. The patient's head and neck are obliquely extended to the side of symptoms and then axially loaded.

stabilization exercise—One that places the injured spine area into the most balanced position (usually neutral) while maintaining that position through the use of muscular contraction. These exercises are advanced from basic to advanced activities while maintaining the spine in a balanced, anatomic pain-free state.

straight-leg raising test—Physical examination maneuver in which the examiner passively lifts the supine patient's leg by flexing the hip with the knee extended. If this maneuver produces back pain radiating into the leg, it is suggestive of a lumbosacral radiculopathy.

supraclavicular—Above the clavicle.

tai chi quan—An exercise program that involves changes in posture in linked movements. It focuses on balance, coordination, concentration, and stress relief.

tarsal tunnel syndrome—Entrapment of the tibial nerve or one of its terminal branches in the fibro-osseous canal formed by the flexor retinaculum and the bones of the foot posterior to the medial malleolus.

temporal dispersion—Relative desynchronization of portions of an action potential due to different rates of conduction of the evoked components.

tendinitis—Inflammation of a tendon.

tenosynovitis—Inflammation of the tendon sheath.

thenar—Related to the fleshy mass on the lateral side of the palm.

thoracic outlet syndrome—Compression of the neurovascular bundle (subclavian artery, subclavian vein, brachial plexus) from either a cervical rib, hypertrophic scalenes, constriction from the pectoralis minor, a narrowed costoclavicular space, or prominent first thoracic rib. Symptoms include numbness, tingling, and weakness corresponding usually to the lower trunk of the brachial plexus. Patients may also complain of pain in the neck or the shoulder girdle region.

Tinel's sign—Electric shock sensation produced in the territory of a nerve when the nerve is tapped or palpated.

trap-door experiment—Research design where ankle is suddenly forced into new position by dropping out a trapdoor. The most commonly used design is forced inversion (ankle varus).

Trendelenburg gait—Abnormal gait pattern that occurs when hip abduction weakness is present. The individual will either lean or vault to the side opposite hip weakness (uncompensated Trendelenburg gait) or to the side of hip weakness (compensated Trendelenburg gait).

ultrasound—Sound waveform produced by energy bombardment of a quartz crystal. Used for its heating and purported healing properties.

Valleix sign—Tenderness to palpation proximal or distal to the tarsal tunnel, a physical examination finding suggestive of tarsal tunnel syndrome.

ventral ramus—A branch of a spinal nerve that supplies the anterior area of the body and the extremities.

ventral root—Motor branch of a spinal nerve that enters the ventral part of the spinal cord.

vertebral foramen—Also known as the neuroforamen. A bony canal through which the nerve roots exit the spinal canal, and a common site for nerve root compression. There are several anatomic causes for nerve root compression, including uncovertebral bone spurs, disc protrusions, and facet joint hypertrophy.

vertebral transverse process—A process that projects on the dorsilateral aspect of each side of the vertebra's neural arch.

windlass mechanism—The action of the arch and plantar fascia on the bony structures of the foot as the foot moves from early into midstance phase. The bones of the tarsal and metatarsal region tighten in response to the arch's stresses, leading to a more stable midfoot and forefoot during these phases.

Index

Note: The italicized *f* and *t* following page numbers refer to figures and tables, respectively.

About the Editors

Joseph H. Feinberg, MD, MS, graduated from Albany Medical College in 1983. He completed his residency training in physical medicine and rehabilitation at the Rusk Institute at NYU in 1990 and has completed fellowships in orthopedic pathology at the Hospital for Special Surgery and in biomechanics at the University of Iowa. He was the director of sports medicine at the Kessler Institute for Rehabilitation from 1993 to 1998 and is currently the director of electrodiagnostics in the department of physiatry at the Hospital for Special Surgery, where he is also the fellowship director. He has been the team physician for Seton Hall University, Jersey City State College, and the Jersey Dragons soccer team; and he is currently the team physician for St. Peter's College. He was recognized by *New York* magazine as one of New York City's best doctors in 2001 and 2002.

Dr. Feinberg's research efforts include the study of nerve regeneration, muscle fatigue, and muscle kinesiology. He has authored multiple publications on peripheral nerve injuries, nerve regeneration, burner syndrome, muscle kinesiology, and muscle fatigue. He has given presentations on these topics at the American College of Sports Medicine (ACSM); the American Academy of Physical Medicine and Rehabilitation; the Physiatric Association of Spine, Sports, and Occupational Rehabilitation (PASSOR); and the Orthopedic Research Society. He is a fellow of the ACSM, a fellow of the American Academy of Electrodiagnostic Medicine (AAEM), and a member of the AAEM training exam committee.

Dr. Feinberg is director of AFICIA (Aid for Children in Africa with Disabilities), an organization that provides medical volunteer care to disabled children in Africa. He has been a triathlete since 1990 and currently lives in Montville, New Jersey.

Neil I. Spielholz, PT, PhD, FAPTA, was trained at Columbia University in New York in 1955 and licensed in New York and Florida as a physical therapist. He also earned a PhD from the department of physiology and biophysics at New York University School of Medicine in New York City. He then spent almost 30 years on the faculty of the department of rehabilitation medicine at New York University Medical Center in the electrodiagnostic laboratory. After retiring from NYU, he continued teaching and doing research at the University of Miami School of Medicine's department of orthopaedics and rehabilitation, division of physical therapy, for the next 10 years. In 2001 he retired from the University of Miami as research professor, and was made professor emeritus. Today, his retirement remains only partial, as he continues to lecture and write.

Dr. Spielholz has coauthored two books on clinical neurophysiology and has written 15 book chapters and 40 papers on the topics of electromyography, nerve conduction studies, intraoperative use of somatosensory-evoked potentials, electrotherapy, and the basic neurophysiology related to all of the preceding. He serves as an editorial board member and as a peer reviewer for various journals.